Emergency Neuroradiology

Guest Editors

ALEXANDER J. NEMETH, MD
MATTHEW T. WALKER, MD

RADIOLOGIC CLINICS
OF NORTH AMERICA

www.radiologic.theclinics.com

Consulting Editor
FRANK H. MILLER, MD

January 2011 • Volume 49 • Number 1

SAUNDERS an imprint of ELSEVIER, Inc.

W.B. SAUNDERS COMPANY
A Division of Elsevier Inc.

1600 John F. Kennedy Boulevard • Suite 1800 • Philadelphia, Pennsylvania 19103-2899

http://www.theclinics.com

RADIOLOGIC CLINICS OF NORTH AMERICA Volume 49, Number 1
January 2011 ISSN 0033-8389, ISBN 13: 978-1-4557-0500-9

Editor: Barton Dudlick
Developmental Editor: Natalie Whitted

Radiologic Clinics of North America (ISSN 0033-8389) is published bimonthly by Elsevier Inc., 360 Park Avenue South, New York, NY 10010-1710. Months of issue are January, March, May, July, September, and November. Periodicals postage paid at New York, NY and additional mailing offices. Subscription prices are USD 386 per year for US individuals, USD 610 per year for US institutions, USD 185 per year for US students and residents, USD 450 per year for Canadian individuals, USD 766 per year for Canadian institutions, USD 556 per year for international individuals, USD 766 per year for international institutions, and USD 266 per year for Canadian and foreign students/residents. To receive student and resident rate, orders must be accompanied by name of affiliated institution, date of term and the signature of program/residency coordinatior on institution letterhead. Orders will be billed at individual rate until proof of status is received. Foreign air speed delivery is included in all *Clinics* subscription prices. All prices are subject to change without notice. **POSTMASTER:** Send address changes to *Radiologic Clinics of North America*, Elsevier Health Sciences Division, Subscription Customer Service, 3251 Riverport Lane, Maryland Heights, MO63043. **Customer Service: Telephone: 1-800-654-2452** (U.S. and Canada); **1-314-447-8871** (outside U.S. and Canada). **Fax: 1-314-447-8029. E-mail: journalscustomerservice-usa@ elsevier.com** (for print support); **journalsonlinesupport-usa@elsevier.com** (for online support).

Reprints. For copies of 100 or more of articles in this publication, please contact the Commercial Reprints Department, Elsevier Inc., 360 Park Avenue South, New York, New York 10010-1710. Tel.: (+1) 212-633-3812; Fax: (+1) 212-462-1935; E-mail: reprints@elsevier.com.

Radiologic Clinics of North America also published in Greek Paschalidis Medical Publications, Athens, Greece.

Radiologic Clinics of North America is covered in *MEDLINE/PubMed (Index Medicus), EMBASE/Excerpta Medica, Current Contents/Life Sciences, Current Contents/Clinical Medicine, RSNA Index to Imaging Literature, BIOSIS, Science Citation Index,* and *ISI/BIOMED.*

Printed in the United States of America.

Contributors

CONSULTING EDITOR

FRANK H. MILLER, MD
Professor of Radiology; Chief, Body Imaging
Section and Fellowship Program and GI
Radiology, Medical Director MRI, Department
of Radiology, Northwestern University Feinberg
School of Medicine, Chicago, Illinois

GUEST EDITORS

ALEXANDER J. NEMETH, MD
Assistant Professor of Radiology, Director,
Neuroradiology Magnetic Resonance Imaging,
Neuroradiology Section, Radiology Department,
Northwestern Memorial Hospital, Feinberg
School of Medicine, Northwestern University,
Chicago, Illinois

MATTHEW T. WALKER, MD
Associate Professor of Radiology, Section Chief,
Neuroradiology Section, Radiology Department,
Northwestern Memorial Hospital, Feinberg
School of Medicine, Northwestern University,
Chicago, Illinois

AUTHORS

LAURA L. AVERY, MD
Assistant Radiologist, Department of Radiology,
Division of Emergency Radiology, Massachusetts
General Hospital; Instructor in Radiology,
Harvard Medical School, Boston,
Massachusetts

PATRICK D. BARNES, MD
Chief, Pediatric Neuroradiology;
Co-Director, Pediatric MRI and CT Center ,
Lucile Packard Children's Hospital; Professor,
Department of Radiology, Stanford University
Medical Center, Stanford, California

ENZO A. CENTO, MD
Clinical Assistant in Emergency Radiology
and Clinical Fellow, Department of Radiology,
Harvard Medical School, Boston,
Massachusetts

JEFFREY DESANTO, MD
Fellow, Neuroradiology Department, Barrow
Neurological Institute, St. Joseph's Hospital
and Medical Center, Phoenix, Arizona

CLIFFORD J. ESKEY, MD, PhD
Associate Professor of Radiology and Surgery,
Director of Interventional Neuroradiology,
Director, Division of Neuroradiology,
Department of Radiology, Dartmouth-Hitchcock
Medical Center, Lebanon, New Hampshire

ADAM FLANDERS, MD
Professor of Radiology and Rehabilitation
Medicine, Division of Neuroradiology,
Department of Radiology, Thomas Jefferson
University Hospital, Philadelphia, Pennsylvania

TAREK A. HIJAZ, MD
Assistant Professor of Radiology, Section
of Neuroradiology, Department of Radiology,
Feinberg School of Medicine, Northwestern
University, Chicago, Illinois.

MARA M. KUNST, MD
Clinical Fellow, Section of Neuroradiology,
Instructor of Radiology, Department of Radiology,
Harvard Medical School, Massachusetts
General Hospital, Boston, Massachusetts

iv Contributors

SEAMUS LOOBY, MD
Fellow in Neuroradiology, Division of
Neuroradiology, Department of Radiology,
Thomas Jefferson University Hospital,
Philadelphia, Pennsylvania

ERIN N. MCCOMB, MD
Assistant Professor of Radiology, Director,
Molecular Imaging; Neuroradiology Section,
Radiology Department, Northwestern Memorial
Hospital, Feinberg School of Medicine,
Northwestern University, Chicago, Illinois

GUL MOONIS, MD
Staff Radiologist, Department of Radiology,
Massachusetts Eye and Ear Infirmary;
Department of Radiology, Beth Israel
Deaconess Medical Center, Harvard Medical
School, Boston, Massachusetts

MARK E. MULLINS, MD, PhD
Department of Radiology, Emory University
School of Medicine, Atlanta, Georgia

ALEXANDER J. NEMETH, MD
Assistant Professor of Radiology, Director,
Neuroradiology Magnetic Resonance Imaging,
Neuroradiology Section; Radiology Department,
Northwestern Memorial Hospital, Feinberg
School of Medicine, Northwestern University,
Chicago, Illinois

ROBERT A. NOVELLINE, MD
Director of Emergency Radiology, Department
of Radiology, Division of Emergency Radiology,
Massachusetts General Hospital; Professor
of Radiology, Harvard Medical School, Boston,
Massachusetts

BOJAN D. PETROVIC, MD
Neuroradiology Attending, Neuroradiology
Section, Department of Radiology, NorthShore
University HealthSystem, Evanston, Illinois

RICH S. RANA, MD
Radiology Resident, Senior Teaching Faculty,
Harvard Radiology Core Clerkship, Department of
Radiology, Beth Israel Deaconess Medical Center,
Harvard Medical School, Boston, Massachusetts

JEFFREY S. ROSS, MD
Staff Neuroradiologist, Neuroradiology
Department, Barrow Neurological Institute,
St. Joseph's Hospital and Medical Center,
Phoenix, Arizona

PAMELA W. SCHAEFER, MD
Associate Director of Neuroradiology,
Neuroradiology Fellowship Director, Clinical
Director of MRI, Section of Neuroradiology,
Associate Professor of Radiology, Department
of Radiology, Harvard Medical School,
Massachusetts General Hospital, Boston,
Massachusetts

SCOTT D. SMITH, MD
Neuroradiology Fellow, Department of Radiology,
Dartmouth-Hitchcock Medical Center, Lebanon,
New Hampshire

SRINIVAS M. SUSARLA, MD, DMD, MPH
Resident, Department of Oral and Maxillofacial
Surgery, Massachusetts General Hospital,
Boston, Massachusetts

MATTHEW T. WALKER, MD
Associate Professor of Radiology; Section Chief,
Neuroradiology Section, Radiology Department,
Northwestern Memorial Hospital, Feinberg
School of Medicine, Northwestern University,
Chicago, Illinois

Contents

Mara M. Kunst and Pamela W. Schaefer

The goal of stroke imaging is to appropriately select patients for different types of therapeutic management in order to optimize outcome and minimize potential complications. To accomplish this, the radiologist has to evaluate each case and tailor an imaging protocol to fit the patient's needs and best answer the clinical question. This review outlines the routinely used, current neuroimaging techniques and their role in the evaluation of the acute stroke patient. The ability of computed tomography and magnetic resonance imaging to adequately evaluate the infarcted brain parenchyma, the cerebral vasculature, and the ischemic, but potentially viable tissue, often referred to as the "ischemic penumbra," is compared The authors outline an imaging algorithm that has been employed at their institution, and briefly review endovascular therapies that can be used in specific patients for stroke treatment.

Scott D. Smith and Clifford J. Eskey

When patients present to the emergency room with sudden onset of focal neurologic symptoms or altered consciousness, hemorrhagic stroke is a major focus of emergency diagnostic evaluation. The entities that compose hemorrhagic stroke, intracerebral and subarachnoid hemorrhage, are readily diagnosed with advanced imaging. This article reviews current imaging options for the detection of acute hemorrhage, along with the expected imaging findings for each modality. Common and unusual causes and their distinguishing imaging features are discussed. Imaging strategies and recent work in specific imaging findings that may guide patient management in the future are also addressed.

Mark E. Mullins

Infectious and inflammatory processes of the intracranial compartment often result in acute clinical presentations. The possible causes are legion. Clues to the diagnosis involve clinical presentation, laboratory analysis, and neuroimaging. This article reviews some of the salient factors in understanding intracranial infection/ inflammation, including pathophysiology and neuroimaging protocols/findings, and provides some examples and a few "pearls and pitfalls."

Bojan D. Petrovic, Alexander J. Nemeth, Erin N. McComb, and Matthew T. Walker

Posterior reversible encephalopathy syndrome (PRES) and venous thrombosis are frequently encountered first in the emergency setting and share some common characteristics. The clinical presentation in both entities is vague, and the brain parenchymal findings of PRES syndrome may resemble those of venous thrombosis in some ways. Both entities often occur in a bilateral posterior distribution and may be associated with reversible parenchymal findings if the inciting factor is treated. These diagnoses should be at the forefront of the differential diagnosis when confronted with otherwise unexplained brain edema, among other findings described in this article.

symptoms and the complications of these conditions are often determined by the precise anatomic site involved, anatomic considerations are stressed. Familiarity with the fascial layers, spaces of the neck, and the contents of each space is helpful for this discussion. The fascial layers of the neck are important barriers to infection, and once infection is established, the fascial layers play a part in directing its spread.

Interpretation of images associated with the traumatically injured face is challenging. The complexity of facial anatomy, coupled with the superimposition of numerous bony structures on plain radiographs, poses specific obstacles to accurate interpretation of facial injury. Although plain radiographs can be helpful in cases of isolated injuries, CT is the most useful modality for evaluating facial injury. This article reviews facial anatomy as it pertains to traumatic injury, emphasizes the clinical findings associated with various types of facial injury, and simplifies the diagnosis of facial injury on CT.

Because of the controversy involving the determination of child abuse, or nonaccidental injury (NAI), radiologists must be familiar with the issues, literature, and principles of evidence-based medicine to understand the role of imaging. Children with suspected NAI must receive protective evaluation along with a timely and complete clinical and imaging work-up. Imaging findings cannot stand alone and must be correlated with clinical findings, laboratory testing, and pathologic and forensic examinations. Only the child protection investigation may provide the basis for inflicted injury in the context of supportive clinical, imaging, biomechanical, or pathology findings.

GOAL STATEMENT

The goal of the *Radiologic Clinics of North America* is to keep practicing radiologists and radiology residents up to date with current clinical practice in radiology by providing timely articles reviewing the state of the art in patient care.

ACCREDITATION

The *Radiologic Clinics of North America* is planned and implemented in accordance with the Essential Areas and Policies of the Accreditation Council for Continuing Medical Education (ACCME) through the joint sponsorship of the University of Virginia School of Medicine and Elsevier. The University of Virginia School of Medicine is accredited by the ACCME to provide continuing medical education for physicians.

The University of Virginia School of Medicine designates this educational activity for a maximum of 15 *AMA PRA Category 1 Credits*™ for each issue, 90 credits per year. Physicians should only claim credit commensurate with the extent of their participation in the activity.

The American Medical Association has determined that physicians not licensed in the US who participate in this CME activity are eligible for a maximum of *15 AMA PRA Category 1 Credits*™ for each issue, 90 credits per year.

Credit can be earned by reading the text material, taking the CME examination online at http://www.theclinics.com/home/cme, and completing the evaluation. After taking the test, you will be required to review any and all incorrect answers. Following completion of the test and evaluation, your credit will be awarded and you may print your certificate.

FACULTY DISCLOSURE/CONFLICT OF INTEREST

The University of Virginia School of Medicine, as an ACCME accredited provider, endorses and strives to comply with the Accreditation Council for Continuing Medical Education (ACCME) Standards of Commercial Support, Commonwealth of Virginia statutes, University of Virginia policies and procedures, and associated federal and private regulations and guidelines on the need for disclosure and monitoring of proprietary and financial interests that may affect the scientific integrity and balance of content delivered in continuing medical education activities under our auspices.

The University of Virginia School of Medicine requires that all CME activities accredited through this institution be developed independently and be scientifically rigorous, balanced and objective in the presentation/discussion of its content, theories and practices.

All authors/editors participating in an accredited CME activity are expected to disclose to the readers relevant financial relationships with commercial entities occurring within the past 12 months (such as grants or research support, employee, consultant, stock holder, member of speakers bureau, etc.). The University of Virginia School of Medicine will employ appropriate mechanisms to resolve potential conflicts of interest to maintain the standards of fair and balanced education to the reader. Questions about specific strategies can be directed to the Office of Continuing Medical Education, University of Virginia School of Medicine, Charlottesville, Virginia.

The faculty and staff of the University of Virginia Office of Continuing Medical Education have no financial affiliations to disclose.

The authors/editors listed below have identified no financial or professional relationships for themselves or their spouse/partner:
Laura L. Avery, MD; Patrick D. Barnes, MD; Enzo A. Cento, MD; Jeffrey DeSanto, MD; Barton Dudlick, (Acquisitions Editor); Tarek A. Hijaz, MD; Theodore E. Keats, MD, (Test Author); Mara M. Kunst, MD; Seamus Looby, MD; Erin N. McComb, MD; Frank H. Miller, MD (Consulting Editor); Gul Moonis, MD; Robert A. Novelline, MD; Bojan D. Petrovic, MD; Rich S. Rana, MD; Pamela W. Schaefer, MD; Scott D. Smith, MD; Srinivas M. Susarla, MD, DMD, MPH; and Matthew T. Walker, MD (Guest Editor).

The authors/editors listed below have identified the following financial or professional relationships for themselves or their spouse/partner:
Clifford J. Eskey, MD, PhD is a consultant, is on the Advisory Committee/Board, and is a stockholder for Relievant Medsystems, Inc.
Adam Flanders, MD is a consultant for Geron.
Mark E. Mullins, MD, PhD is a visiting professor for the University of Kentucky and Bluegreass Society, is an invited lecturer for the Grand Rapids Medical Education and Research Center for Health Professions/Spectrum Health, and is employed by Emory.
Alexander J. Nemeth, MD (Guest Editor) is employed by and is on the Speakers' Bureau for Northwestern Medical Faculty Foundation and Schwab Rehabilitation Hospital.
Jeffrey S. Ross, MD receives royalties from Amirsys, Inc.

Disclosure of Discussion of Non-FDA Approved Uses for Pharmaceutical Products and/or Medical Devices.
The University of Virginia School of Medicine, as an ACCME provider, requires that all faculty presenters identify and disclose any off-label uses for pharmaceutical and medical device products. The University of Virginia School of Medicine recommends that each physician fully review all the available data on new products or procedures prior to clinical use.

TO ENROLL

To enroll in the Radiologic Clinics of North America Continuing Medical Education program, call customer service at 1-800-654-2452 or sign up online at http://www.theclinics.com/home/cme. The CME program is available to subscribers for an additional annual fee USD 245.

Radiologic Clinics of North America

THE CLINICS ARE NOW AVAILABLE ONLINE!

Access your subscription at:
www.theclinics.com

Preface
Emergency Neuroradiology

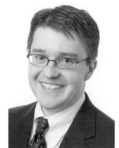
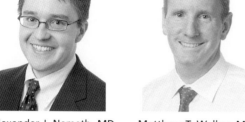

Alexander J. Nemeth, MD   Matthew T. Walker, MD
Guest Editors

Our primary goal was to make this issue of the *Radiologic Clinics* an outstanding edition of high quality and exceptional educational value. To this end, we attempted to include every subject relevant to neuroradiology that one may expect to encounter in a general emergency radiology practice. This includes the most important concepts in emergent brain, spine, head and neck imaging, as well as pediatric nonaccidental trauma. While this text is not all inclusive, we believe that it provides an excellent starting point for learning the fundamentals of emergency neuroradiology and can serve as a reference for those wishing to reinforce their current knowledge base. We hope that even experienced radiologists may learn something new.

After establishing the scope of this issue, we set out to find authors who we thought would make outstanding contributions to our goals. The contributors represent major centers from widespread regions across the United States and have provided a sampling of different techniques and styles that should result in a strong educational experience in the aggregate. We feel very fortunate to have received their input and support, as we believe their combined expertise has made this issue a truly vital volume of the current concepts in emergency neuroradiology. We would like to acknowledge the kind assistance of Hugh D. Curtin, MD, from the Massachusetts Eye and Ear Infirmary in Boston, and of V. Michelle Silvera, MD, from Children's Hospital Boston, in the planning of this issue.

We would like to thank our Chairman, Eric J. Russell, MD, for his support and encouragement, and Frank Miller, MD, for his invitation to participate in this edition. We could not have completed this project without the support of the neuroradiology attendings in our section to whom we are grateful, including Michelle Naidich, Steve Futterer, Achilles Karagianis, Tarek Hijaz, Benjamin P. Liu, Erin McComb, Sandra Horowitz, and Guilherme Dabus. We would also like to acknowledge the support and contributions of the radiology residents and neuroradiology fellows at the Feinberg School of Medicine of Northwestern University.

Finally, thank you to our families (Theresa and Alexander Nicolas; Karen, Grace, and Owen) for their patience during the preparation of this *Clinics* issue.

Alexander J. Nemeth, MD
Department of Radiology
Northwestern Memorial Hospital
Northwestern University Feinberg
School of Medicine
676 North Saint Clair Street
Suite 1400
Chicago, IL 60611-2927, USA

Matthew T. Walker, MD
Department of Radiology
Northwestern Memorial Hospital
Northwestern University Feinberg
School of Medicine
676 North Saint Clair Street
Suite 1400
Chicago, IL 60611-2927, USA

E-mail addresses:
a-nemeth@northwestern.edu (A.J. Nemeth)
mwalker@nmff.org (M.T. Walker)

Radiol Clin N Am 49 (2011) xi
doi:10.1016/j.rcl.2010.11.003

Ischemic Stroke

Mara M. Kunst, MD*, Pamela W. Schaefer, MD

KEYWORDS

- Ischemia • Infarction • Stroke imaging • Penumbra
- Perfusion

Acute ischemic stroke affects more than 659,000 Americans each year. If detected and treated early, accepted and emerging therapies have the ability to dramatically improve patient outcome. The goal of stroke imaging is to appropriately select patients for different types of therapeutic management in order to optimize outcome and minimize potential complications. To accomplish this, the radiologist has to evaluate each case and tailor an imaging protocol to fit the patient's needs and best answer the clinical question. This review outlines the routinely used, current neuroimaging techniques and their role in the evaluation of the acute stroke patient. In doing so, the ability of computed tomography (CT) and magnetic resonance (MR) imaging to adequately evaluate the infarcted brain parenchyma, the cerebral vasculature, and the ischemic, but potentially viable tissue, often referred to as the "ischemic penumbra," is compared. The authors outline an imaging algorithm that has been employed at their institution, and briefly review endovascular therapies that can be used in specific patients for stroke treatment.

IMAGING OF THE BRAIN PARENCHYMA

In the setting of acute ischemic stroke, both CT and MR imaging can be used to evaluate the cerebral parenchyma. The goals of both modalities are similar: (1) to exclude the presence of hemorrhage and mimics of stroke such as infection, inflammation, and neoplasm (among other entities), and (2) to detect and quantify infarcted tissue.

Imaging the Brain Parenchyma with CT

CT offers several practical advantages to MR imaging in the emergency setting. CT scanners are more widely available and patients can be brought to and from the scanner with minimal delay. Compared with MR imaging, CT requires much less prescreening; only contrast allergies and renal function need to be assessed. Furthermore, metallic equipment can safely accompany the patient in the CT scanner, allowing for easier monitoring of potentially unstable acute stroke patients.

Exclusion of hemorrhage

The presence of intracranial hemorrhage is an absolute contraindication to the administration of intravenous recombinant tissue plasminogen activator (rtPA), the only therapy with proven clinical benefit for the treatment of acute infarction. Non-contrast CT (NCCT) has long been the gold standard for detecting the presence of intracranial hemorrhage based on data from early CT scanners and practical experience.[1,2] A negative NCCT is required before the administration of rtPA according to guidelines established in 1995 by the National Institute for Neurologic Diseases and Stroke (NINDS) trial.[3,4]

Detection of infarcted tissue

Tissue that appears hypodense on NCCT is usually irreversibly infarcted, and likely represents all or part of the infarct core (discussed in subsequent sections). More subtle signs of cerebral ischemia may be detected on NCCT within a few hours of symptom onset. These signs have been well described in the literature and include the hyperdense vessel sign, the insular ribbon sign, obscuration of the lentiform nucleus, blurring of gray-white matter differentiation, and sulcal effacement (**Fig. 1**). Although well described, accurate detection and quantification of these signs remain highly reader dependent.

Section of Neuroradiology, Department of Radiology, Harvard Medical School, Massachusetts General Hospital, 55 Fruit Street, Boston, MA, USA
* Corresponding author.
E-mail address: marakunst@gmail.com

Radiol Clin N Am 49 (2011) 1–26
doi:10.1016/j.rcl.2010.07.010
0033-8389/11/$ – see front matter © 2011 Elsevier Inc. All rights reserved.

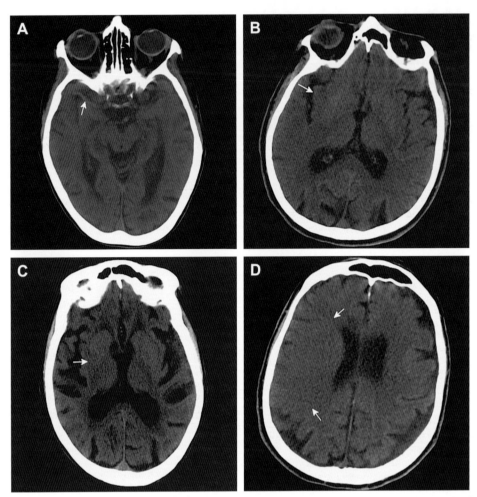

Fig. 1. Early signs (<6 hours) of cerebral infarction on noncontrast head CT. High density in the proximal middle cerebral artery (MCA) is thought to represent an acute thrombus lodged in the middle cerebral artery, and is referred to as the "hyperdense MCA sign" (*arrow* in *A*). The presence of edema in the distribution of the lenticulostriate arteries produces loss of the normal striated appearance of the insular cortex or "insular ribbon sign" (*arrow* in *B*) and local hypoattenuation in the basal ganglia, or "obscuration of the lentiform nuclei" (*arrow* in *C*). Loss of gray white matter differentiation and sulcal effacement (region between the 2 *arrows* in *D*) indicate diffuse cerebral swelling and, of the above signs, carry the poorest clinical prognosis.

Detecting signs of early ischemia on NCCT is influenced by several factors including the severity of the infarct, as measured by clinical examination and National Institutes of Health Stroke Scale (NIHSS) (**Table 1**), and the time between symptom onset and imaging.[5] The detection rate for signs of early ischemia within the 3-hour time window is 67% or less in most trials,[6–8] and may be as low as 31%.[5] Sensitivity is improved, up to 71%, by using narrow window width and center level settings (8 HU and 32 HU, respectively) to accentuate the contrast between normal and edematous tissue (**Fig. 2**).[9] The rate of detection increases to approximately 82% at 6 hours, which is outside the therapeutic window for intravenous rtPA.[10]

Quantifying the extent of infarction is also subject to great interreader variability. Specifically, when asked to determine if ischemic changes on NCCT involve greater than one-third of the middle cerebral artery (MCA) territory, even experienced clinicians show only 39% agreement.[7] In response, the Alberta Stroke Program Early CT Score (ASPECTS) was developed in 2001 to quantify acute ischemia on NCCT images by using a 10-point topographic scoring system (**Fig. 3**).[11] ASPECTS increased interreader reliability by up to 71% to 89%, and correlated well with functional outcome and risk of symptomatic intracranial hemorrhage (sensitivity/specificity 78%/96% and 90%/62%).[12] Despite this significant improvement,

Table 1
The National Institutes of Health (NIH) Stroke Scale

1a. Level of Consciousness	0 = Alert 1 = Not alert 2 = Not alert 3 = Responds only with reflex motor or autonomic effects or totally unresponsive, flaccid, and areflexic
1b. LOC Questions: The patient is asked the month and his/her age	0 = Answers both questions correctly 1 = Answers one question correctly 2 = Answers neither question correctly
1c. LOC Commands: The patient is asked to open and close the eyes and then to grip and release the nonparetic hand	0 = Performs both tasks correctly 1 = Performs one task correctly 2 = Performs neither task correctly
2. Best Gaze: Only horizontal eye movements will be tested	0 = Normal 1 = Partial gaze palsy 2 = Forced deviation
3. Visual: Visual fields (upper and lower quadrants) are tested by confrontation, using finger counting or visual threat	0 = No visual loss 1 = Partial hemianopia 2 = Complete hemianopia 3 = Bilateral hemianopia
4. Facial Palsy:	0 = Normal 1 = Minor paralysis 2 = Partial paralysis 3 = Complete paralysis
5. Motor Arm: 5a. Left Arm 5b. Right Arm	0 = No drift 1 = Drift 2 = Some effort against gravity 3 = No effort against gravity; limb falls 4 = No movement UN = Amputation or joint fusion, explain:_____
6. Motor Leg: 6a. Left Leg 6b. Right Leg	0 = No drift 1 = Drift 2 = Some effort against gravity 3 = No effort against gravity 4 = No movement UN = Amputation or joint fusion, explain:_____
7. Limb Ataxia:	0 = Absent 1 = Present in one limb 2 = Present in two limbs UN = Amputation or joint fusion, explain:_____
8. Sensory:	0 = Normal 1 = Mild to moderate sensory loss 2 = Severe to total sensory loss
9. Best Language:	0 = No aphasia; normal 1 = Mild to moderate aphasia 2 = Severe aphasia 3 = Mute, global aphasia
10. Dysarthria:	0 = Normal 1 = Mild to moderate dysarthria 2 = Severe dysarthria UN = Intubated or other physical barrier, explain:_____
11. Extinction and Inattention (formerly Neglect):	0 = No abnormality 1 = Visual, tactile, auditory, spatial, or personal inattention 2 = Profound hemi-inattention

The NIH Stroke Scale is a standardized method used by physicians and other health care professionals to measure the level of impairment caused by a stroke. The level of stroke severity as measured by this scoring system is: 0 = no stroke; 1–4 = minor stroke; 5–15 = moderate stroke; 15–20 = moderate/severe stroke; 21–42 = severe stroke.

ASPECTS is based on evaluating specific structures on 2 axial CT slices, making the system highly dependent on the imaging plane. More recently, the "ABC/2" method has been used to rapidly and accurately calculate the volume of infarcted tissue (**Fig. 4**).[13] Although originally described in MR, the technique, which measures lesions in 3 perpendicular axes, can by applied to both CT and MR, is independent of the imaging plane, and has shown high intrarater and interrater reliability (71%–99%).[13]

The importance of detecting and quantifying these early signs of infarction was demonstrated in the European Cooperative Acute Stroke Studies (ECASS I and II), where patients with large infarcts and early swelling were shown to have an increased incidence of hemorrhage and poor outcome following rtPA therapy.[3,14] Despite

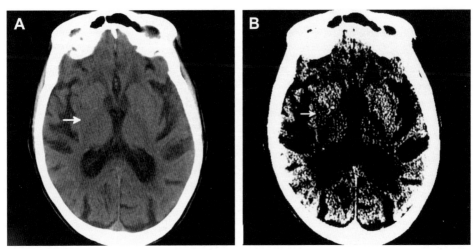

Fig. 2. Window level setting in stroke. Asymmetric low attenuation within the right posterior putamen (*arrows* in *A* and *B*) is subtle using standard brain window width and center level settings (*A*) (level 35, window 100), but becomes much more conspicuous with lower center level and narrower window width (*B*) (level 8, window 32).

some controversy,[5,15] these findings have resulted in the current consensus among stroke experts that the criteria for withholding rtPA in the first 3 hours after symptom onset include hemorrhage or definite signs of ischemia that exceed one-third of the MCA territory (correlating roughly to an ASPECTS score <7 and an ABC/2 volume >100 cm³).[13,16] The recently published ECASS III trial indicates that this time window may now safely be increased to 4.5 hours.[17]

Imaging the Brain Parenchyma with MR Imaging

MR imaging with its multiple sequences provides excellent evaluation of the brain parenchyma for

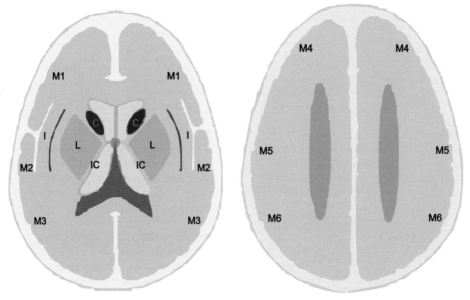

Fig. 3. ASPECTS Schematic. The ASPECTS scoring system is based on assessing 10 distinct regions of the MCA distribution on 2 axial slices. Once slice is centered at the level of the basal ganglia and thalami (*left*). Another slice is centered at the level of the centrum semiovale (*right*). Each demarcated region accounts for 1 point in the ASPECTS system: M1, M2, M3, M4, M5, M6, the insula (I), the caudate (C), the lentiform nucleus (L), and the internal capsule (IC). For each area involved by ischemia, 1 point is subtracted from a total score of 10 on each side. A sharp increase in dependent or fatal outcomes occurs with ASPECTS of 7 or less, corresponding roughly with an infarct involving greater than one-third of the MCA territory.

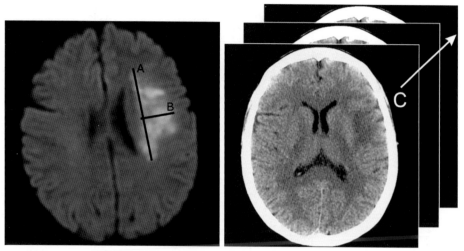

Fig. 4. ABC/2. The ABC/2 formula produces rapid and easy clinical assessment by correlating the region of infarction to the volume of an ellipsoid. The region of abnormal signal intensity (DWI, *left*) or reduced attenuation (CT, *right*) can be measured via 3 multiplanar, perpendicular axes. A and B are measured on the axial slice with the largest region of involvement (DWI, *left*). C is calculated from the number of axial slices the abnormality appears on, multiplied by the slice thickness (CT, *right*). A, B, and C are then multiplied, and the product is divided by 2 for the volume of infarcted tissue. A lesion between 70 and 100 cm^3 roughly correlates with one-third of the MCA territory and implies a poor prognosis.

stroke and its many mimics. MR imaging is also becoming widely available and can be found in the emergency rooms of some hospitals. Despite this, the previously mentioned practical considerations, including need for more extensive patient screening and incompatibility with routine patient monitoring equipment, remain the largest limitation for the use of MR imaging as the first-line imaging modality in acute stroke.

Exclusion of hemorrhage

The sensitivity of MR imaging for the detection of hemorrhage is primarily dependent on the age of the hemorrhage and the sequences used (**Table 2**). In the first 6 hours (the time frame that is critical for the treatment of acute ischemia), hemorrhage is mostly composed of oxyhemoglobin, with deoxyhemoglobin occurring in increasing amounts along the periphery (**Fig. 5**). Because oxyhemoglobin is isointense to the brain parenchyma on T1, hyperintense on T2, and diamagnetic, it may be overlooked on T1, T2, and gradient echo (GRE) sequences, particularly near cerebrospinal fluid (CSF) spaces. Deoxyhemoglobin may also be subtle on conventional sequences, as it is isointense on T1- and hypointense on T2-weighted sequences; however, its paramagnetism and resultant T2* effect make it conspicuous on GRE sequences. Although the high protein content of oxyhemoglobin makes it detectable in the subarachnoid space on

fluid-attenuated inversion recovery (FLAIR) sequences, the appearance is nonspecific and can be mimicked by several pathologic and nonpathologic conditions, including flow artifact, meningitis, leptomeningeal metastases, oxygen therapy, and propofol administration.[18,19] These potential pitfalls continue to limit definitive exclusion of hemorrhage on MR imaging alone.

As any known prior intracranial hemorrhage is an absolute contraindication to intravenous rtPA therapy, the relatively common presence of chronic microhemorrhages has raised appropriate concern about intravenous rtPA administration in patients in whom they are seen. Chronic microhemorrhages can be defined as homogeneous rounded areas of signal loss that measure less than 5 mm in diameter without surrounding edema on GRE sequences. Recent studies have found no increased risk of hemorrhagic conversion of acute ischemic stroke treated with thrombolytic therapy in patients with up to 10 microhemorrhages detected on routine GRE sequences.[20,21] The risk in patients with more than 10 microhemorrhages remains undetermined.

Detection of infarcted or ischemic tissues

MR diffusion-weighted imaging (DWI) is the single most accurate method for detecting acute ischemia. DWI is based on the principle that the random (brownian) motion of water molecules in

Table 2
Stages of hemorrhage on MR and CT

Stage	Time Course	CT	T1	T2	Gradient Echo	Mass Effect	Components
Hyperacute	<6 h	High density	Low intensity	High intensity with peripheral low intensity	Centrally isointense, peripherally hypointense	+++	High protein, central oxyhemoglobin, peripheral deoxyhemoglobin
Acute	≈ 8–72 h	High density	Isointense to low intensity	Low intensity	Hypointense centrally and peripherally	+++	High protein, deoxyhemoglobin
Early subacute	≈ 3 d to 1 wk	High density	High intensity	Low intensity	Hypointense centrally and peripherally	+++/++	High protein, intracellular methemoglobin
Late subacute	≈ 1 wk to months	Isodense	High Intensity	High intensity with rim of low intensity	Isointense	±	Diluted protein, extracellular methemoglobin
Chronic	≈ months to years	Low density	Low intensity	Low intensity	Hypointense	-	Protein absorbed, hemosiderin

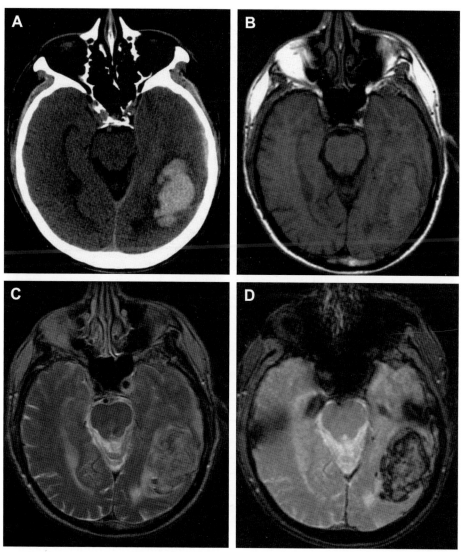

Fig. 5. Hyperacute (<6 hours) hemorrhage on CT and MR imaging. Hyperacute hemorrhage is hyperdense on non-contrast CT (*A*), isointense to the surrounding brain parenchyma on T1-weighted image (*B*), hyperintense to surrounding brain parenchyma on T2 (*C*), and demonstrates susceptibility artifact in increasing amounts along the periphery of the hemorrhage on gradient echo sequences (*D*), as oxyhemoglobin changes to deoxyhemoglobin.

living tissues can be quantitatively measured. Following application of equal and opposite strong gradient pulses combined with a spin-echo, echo-planar pulse sequence, loss of tissue signal is proportional to the rate of water diffusion. In the setting of acute ischemia, failure of the energy-dependent Na^+/K^+ transporter in neuronal and glial cells results in increased intracellular Na^+ and net translocation of water to the intracellular space. Intracellular water motion is relatively restricted by the presence of cell membranes

and by the breakdown of organelles. Resultant cell swelling compresses the extracellular space, leading to more restricted movement of protons in that space as well. This decreased diffusion results in hyperintense signal on DW images that can be reliably detected within the first 30 minutes of stroke symptom onset, at a time when other MR imaging sequences and CT remain negative.

Contrast on DW images is exponentially related to differences in diffusion and linearly related to underlying T2 signal. To remove the T2 contrast, a map of apparent diffusion coefficient (ADC) values is created by obtaining 2 image sets, one with a very low b value and one with b = 1,000 s/mm^2. By plotting the natural logarithm of the signal intensity versus b for these 2 b values, the ADC can be determined from the slope of this line. Alternatively, the DWI can be divided by the echoplanar spin-echo (SE) T2 image (or low b value image), to give an "exponential image" (EXP), the signal intensity of which is exponentially related to the apparent diffusion coefficient.[19] A DWI hyperintense lesion with truly restricted diffusion will be dark on ADC maps and bright on EXP images, whereas a lesion that is hyperintense on DWI due to the T2 component ("T2 shine-through") but has elevated diffusion will appear bright on ADC and dark on EXP images.

The high sensitivity and specificity of DWI is invaluable in reliably detecting the presence of and evaluating the extent of infarcted tissue.

Reported sensitivities range from 88% to 100%, and reported specificities range from 86% to 100%.[3,22,23] Infarctions not identified on DWI (false negatives) are usually very small and located in the brainstem, deep gray nuclei, or cortex.[24] False-positive hyperintense DWI signal may result from T2 shine-through of subacute or early chronic infarctions, an error that is easily avoided by interpreting the DWI images in combination with ADC maps or exponential images. It is also well known that several nonischemic conditions can produce restricted diffusion, mimicking acute infarction on DW, ADC, and EXP imaging (**Table 3**). When reviewed in conjunction with conventional MR images and clinical history, these lesions can usually be distinguished from acute infarctions.[20] Reversible restricted diffusion (abnormal on initial DW, ADC, and EXP images, but normal on follow-up images) is very rare, but can occur more often with very early reperfusion, usually

---

Table 3
Nonischemic conditions that may cause restricted diffusion on MR imaging (hyperintense on DWI, hypointense on ADC)

Condition	Cause
Mass Lesions	
Epidermoid mass	Hypercellular tumor
Lymphoma	Hypercellular tumor
Glioblastoma	Hypercellular tumor
Medulloblastoma	Hypercellular tumor
Traumatic	
Diffuse axonal injury (most cases)	Cytotoxic edema
Hemorrhage (oxyhemoglobin)	Intracellular, high protein content
Hemorrhage (extracellular methemoglobin)	High protein content
Infectious	
Abscess or pyogenic infection	Increased viscosity
Herpes encephalitis	Cytotoxic edema
Creutzfeldt-Jakob syndrome	Spongiform change
Inflammatory	
Multiple sclerosis (a few acute lesions)	Myelin vacuolization
Other	
Hemiplegic migraine	Na$^+$/K$^+$ adenosine triphosphatase (ATPase) activity decrease, spreading depression
Seizure activity	Na$^+$/K$^+$ ATPase activity decrease
Transient global amnesia	Unknown,? ischemia
Heroin leukoencaphalopathy	Myelin vacuolization
Flagyl	? Axonal swelling limiting extracellular space
Hypoglycemia	Na$^+$/K$^+$ ATPase activity decrease

following intravenous and/or intra-arterial thrombolysis. Despite these potential pitfalls, DWI has emerged as the most sensitive and specific imaging technique for detecting acute infarction and as the gold standard for delineating infarction core.[16] The size of the DWI lesion may also have a role in predicting patient outcome. In particular, at least 2 studies have demonstrated that large initial DWI volumes predict poor outcome and increased risk of intracranial hemorrhage.[25,26] As a result, those patients with an initial DWI lesion volume of greater than one-third of the MCA territory or greater than 100 cm^3 are typically excluded from acute stroke trials.

Other MR imaging sequences can support the diagnosis of and help estimate the age of infarction. The MR correlates of the CT "hyperdense vessel sign" are focal vessel hyperintensity on FLAIR, vascular susceptibility artifact on GRE, and loss of a normal flow void on T2 sequences. Of these, vessel hyperintensity on FLAIR images is the most sensitive, with one study showing detection rates comparable to MR angiography (MRA) in both middle and posterior cerebral arteries.[27] Effacement of sulci, cisterns, and ventricles due to mild swelling can be seen within the first few hours after stroke symptom onset, prior to any parenchymal signal abnormality.[28] Edema associated with infarction presents earliest on FLAIR sequences, but still only achieves a sensitivity of 29% in the first 6 hours after stroke onset.[29] By 8 hours, hyperintense signal develops on T2-weighted images and by 16 hours, low signal intensity is noted on T1-weighted images (**Table 4**).[28] With this approximate guideline in mind, for patients in whom the time of stroke onset is not known (eg, a "wake-up-stroke") and in whom MR imaging confirms an infarct on DWI and ADC, but shows no or minimal FLAIR hyperintense signal, the time of onset is likely less than 6 hours (**Fig. 6**). Although these patients cannot receive rtPA by NINDS criteria, ongoing research is investigating whether they may benefit from interventional therapies.

IMAGING OF THE CEREBRAL VASCULATURE

Vascular imaging in the acute ischemic stroke patient most commonly extends from the aortic arch to the cranial vertex. Evaluation of the intracranial circulation is performed to identify and characterize the vascular lesion, and to quantify the extent of collateral flow. In general, vascular lesions in the proximal, large vessels result in the largest infarcts with the greatest likelihood of hemorrhagic transformation, and the greatest

potential benefit from neuroendovascular intervention. In these cases, the presence and extent of collateral vessels helps to determine the territory at risk. In the absence of a visible occlusion, infarcts may be caused by lesions in small arteries that cannot be imaged, or by an embolus in a large proximal artery that has broken up spontaneously. In general, such patients have relatively favorable outcomes.[22]

Evaluation of the extracranial circulation is mainly performed to identify and characterize a potentially thrombotic or embolic source and to help determine whether treatment should be medical or surgical. Correctly characterizing a diseased vessel segment is critical for patient care, as occlusions are typically treated pharmacologically, whereas endarterectomy or stent placement is indicated for symptomatic patients with greater than 70% stenosis. Diagnosis of potentially treatable diseases, such as vasculitis, may benefit from cross-sectional imaging that adequately evaluates the vessel lumen, wall, and adjacent soft tissues. Patients with a history of atrial fibrillation may benefit from extended vascular imaging to exclude the presence of a left atrial or ventricular thrombus.

Although digital subtraction angiography (DSA) remains the reference standard for vascular imaging, it is an invasive procedure that carries risks, is costly, and is time-consuming. For these reasons, noninvasive techniques have replaced DSA in the initial, emergent evaluation of the acute stroke patient. The techniques, advantages, and disadvantages of the 2 most common noninvasive vascular imaging modalities, CT and MRA, are now discussed.

CT Angiography

Technique

CTA techniques vary largely by institution. At the authors' institution, CTA is typically performed by injecting 80 mL of intravenous contrast at 3.5 to 5 mL/s through a power injector with a saline chaser. Image acquisition is synchronized to the peak arterial enhancement by a bolus-triggering method. Images are acquired with a maximally overlapping pitch and a thin overlapping slice reconstruction (1.25 mm thick by 0.625 interval), and are reconstructed with a soft tissue algorithm for improved 3-dimensional (3D) reformatting. Postprocessing is essential for complete vessel analysis and includes thick section maximum intensity projections (MIPs) created at the scanner, and 3D volume rendered reformatted images, which are performed in time for final review.

Table 4
Time course of infarction on MR imaging

Stage	DWI	ADC	EXP	T1	T2/FLAIR
Hyperacute (0–6 h)	Hyperintense	Hypointense	Hyperintense	Isointense—perhaps some loss of sulci	Isointense
Acute (6 h to 4 d)	Hyperintense	Hypointense	Hyperintense	Iso- to hypointense—mass effect	Hyperintense (FLAIR becomes reliably hyperintense slightly before T2)
Subacute (4–14 d)	Hyperintense due to T2 shine-through	Iso- to hyperintense (pseudonormalization)	Iso- to hypointense	Hypointense	Hyperintense
Chronic	Hyperintense due to T2 shine-through	Hyperintense (encephalomalacia)	Hypointense	Smaller area of hypointense signal	Hyperintense

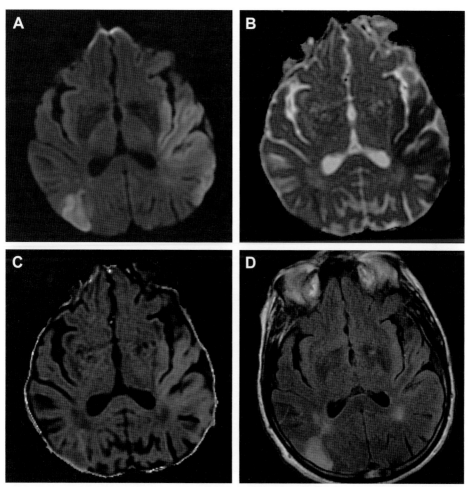

Fig. 6. Estimating the age of infarction. A 73-year-old man presented 3 hours after sudden onset of aphasia. Hyperintense DWI signal within the left posterior insula and temporal lobe (*A*) with corresponding low signal intensity on ADC maps (*B*), hyperintense signal on EXP (*C*), and only subtle hyperintense signal and edema on FLAIR (*D*) is consistent with a hyperacute (<6 hours) infarction, and is likely the cause of the patient's new onset deficit. A second, smaller infarction in the right parieto-occipital region is mostly hyperintense on DWI (*A*), isointense on ADC maps (*B*), isointense on EXP maps (*C*), and hyperintense on FLAIR (*D*), findings that are more consistent with a subacute timeframe (5–10 days), and was clinically silent.

Advantages

In addition to more widespread availability, CTA offers several practical benefits for vascular imaging in the acute stroke setting. Most CT scanners are capable of performing CTA immediately following NCCT. Once hemorrhage has been excluded, rtPA therapy can be initiated immediately without requiring personnel and equipment to be screened for safety. Modern multidetector CT scanners afford a short acquisition time, which decreases the incidence of motion-related artifacts and venous contamination. CTA uses a true intravascular contrast agent, and is therefore less susceptible to artifactual vessel narrowing caused by turbulent or slow flow on time-of-flight MRA images. In addition, CTA is not susceptible to the phase and susceptibility artifacts that may affect Gadolinium contrast-enhanced MRA (CE MRA). The spatial resolution of CTA is also approximately twice that of MRA.

Several studies evaluating the accuracy of CTA in the intracranial circulation have focused on the proximal large intracranial vessels, including the internal carotid arteries, and first and second segments of the anterior, middle and posterior cerebral arteries. In one study using DSA as the gold standard, CTA demonstrated 98.4% sensitivity and 98.1% specificity for detecting proximal vessel acute occlusive thrombus.[23] In another study, DSA was significantly more sensitive than time-of-flight (TOF) MRA for both intracranial stenosis (98% vs 70%, P<.001) and occlusion (100% vs 87%, P = .02).[24] CTA MIPs increase conspicuity of vascular stenosis/occlusion in both proximal and distal vessels (**Fig. 7**); they are also the most accurate method for quantifying the degree of collateral circulation, which has shown an inverse correlation with the final infarct volume.[30]

For evaluation of the extracranial circulation, CTA is also generally preferred to MRA. Although controversial, several studies have demonstrated CTA to have the strongest correlation with DSA, citing better spatial resolution, less flow dependence, and the ability to demonstrate both luminal and extraluminal abnormalities that augment evaluation of vascular narrowing.[31–38] A 2004 meta-analysis pooled data from 28 studies comparing CTA with DSA, and found CTA to have 85% sensitivity and 93% specificity for detection of a 70% to 99% stenosis, and 97% sensitivity and 99% specificity for detecting an occlusion.[39] Studies comparing CTA and MRA for carotid and vertebral artery dissection vary widely by technique. A recently published meta-analysis found both modalities to have similar correlation with DSA (sensitivities and specificities ranging from 51% to 100% and 67% to 100% for CTA, and 50% to

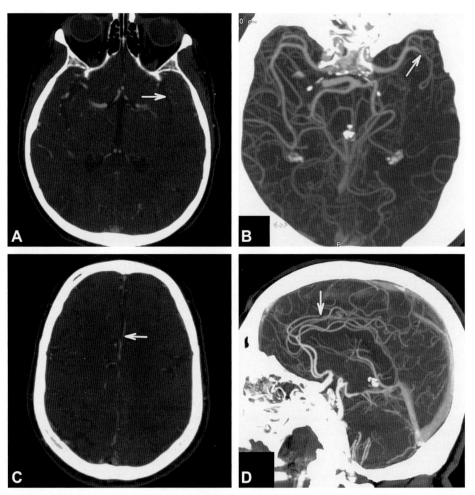

Fig. 7. Benefits of MIPs in vessel evaluation. Vessel occlusion or thrombus in the distal intracranial circulation is complicated by small vessel caliber and tortuosity. MIPs are created by "stacking" axial CT slices on top of one another and "windowing" to highlight areas of high radiodensity. The 3D volume can be used to evaluate a single, distal tortuous vessel along its length. A vessel occlusion in the left MCA superior division was oriented perpendicular to the axial CTA source images (*arrow* in *A*), making visualization difficult. The occlusion was clearly identified on the axial MIP as a vessel cutoff (*arrow* in *B*). In the same patient, a subtle left distal anterior cerebral artery occlusion was not prospectively visualized on the axial CTA source images (*arrow* in *C*), but was identified on the sagittal MIPs (*arrow* in *D*).

100% and 29% to 100% for MRA, respectively).[40] Despite this, certain limitations of MR imaging and MRA, including obscuration of mural hematoma by hyperintense signal from an adjacent occlusive thrombus, as well as lack of hyperintense signal within mural hematoma on T1-weighted images in early dissection, are overcome by CTA.[40,41]

CTA may also have a role in evaluation of the brain parenchyma in acute stroke patients. If imaging is appropriately timed to the contrast bolus, both the large vessels and the microvasculature become opacified and hypoperfused brain becomes visibly hypodense on CTA source images (CTA-SI). CTA-SIs increase the detection of acute ischemia,[42] and increase the utility of ASPECTS as compared with NCCT. On 4- and 16-detector row CT scanners, lesion volumes on CTA-SI correlate closely with those on DWI, and with the final infarct volume in patients who reperfuse, suggesting that they identify the infarct core.[43,44] However, although 4- and 16-detector row scanners allow the contrast bolus to achieve a "steady state" during which the microvasculature becomes opacified, newer 64 and higher detector row CT scanners can outpace the flow of contrast-opacified blood; consequently, CTA-SIs on these scanners show areas of hypodensity that are larger than the DWI abnormality and overestimate the final infarct size (Hu R. and colleagues, unpublished data, 2010).

Disadvantages

The main disadvantage of CTA is radiation exposure, which requires an additional dose of approximately 2.5 mSv for a CTA of the head, and 9.5 mSv for a CTA of the head and neck.[45] In the acute stroke setting, additional delayed-phase CTA may also be necessary for accurate image interpretation. For example, apparent vascular occlusions require delayed images to differentiate between true occlusion and delayed opacification due to slow flow. Furthermore, if the major venous sinuses are not adequately opacified and there is suspicion of venous infarction, delayed images of the head should be obtained to exclude venous sinus thrombosis. The most critical aspect of limiting radiation exposure in the acute stroke setting is active monitoring of image acquisition, and tailoring additional sequences to those that are necessary for accurate interpretation with the constant, conscious goal of minimizing the patient's overall radiation dose.

CTA also requires injection of iodine-based contrast material, which has the potential to exacerbate already impaired renal function and may trigger adverse allergic reactions. A recent review evaluated the incidence of contrast-induced nephropathy in patients receiving both CTA and CT perfusion (CTP) imaging for the evaluation of acute stroke. Of the 198 patients studied, none developed chronic kidney disease or required dialysis, and 2.9% experienced a significant increase in baseline creatinine values.[46] The risk of allergic reaction has decreased significantly with the now widespread use of low-osmolar nonionic contrast media, with a reported overall incidence of 0.15%, less than 0.03% of which require medical treatment.[47] Decisions about whether to proceed with intravenous contrast administration should be made with these data in mind, and in close consultation with the clinical team.

Interpretation of CTA can be limited by several artifacts that may result in partial or significant obscuration of adjacent arteries. Streak artifact commonly results from metallic hardware in the upper chest (pacemaker) or neck (dental hardware), from photon starvation between the shoulders, or from slow-flowing contrast material in the adjacent veins. Heavy atherosclerotic calcification may also produce streak artifact that can overestimate vessel stenosis and/or mimic an occlusion. In addition, CTA performed on 64-detector scanners[48] is susceptible to flow artifacts and misrepresentation of flow dynamics (eg, pseudodissection or pseudo-occlusion). Most of these artifacts can be accurately identified by an experienced reader. Targeted delayed imaging or correlation with another vascular imaging modality may also be helpful.

MR Angiography

Technique
MRA describes any of several MR imaging techniques used to depict arteries. In the setting of acute stroke, a typical protocol is a 3D TOF sequence through the circle of Willis, and a CE MRA or a 2-dimensional (2D) TOF sequence through the neck. TOF is a GRE technique that images vascular flow by repeatedly (with a short repetition time [TR]) applying a radiofrequency pulse to a given volume of tissue, perpendicular to the direction of blood flow. The short TR interval allows saturation of stationary tissue, while protons within flowing blood remain bright. Maximum flow signal is achieved when a totally new column of blood enters the slice every TR period. A saturation pulse placed superior to the volume of tissues eliminates venous contamination. TOF MRA is most commonly acquired from sequential axial slices (2D), or a single large volume (3D) depending on the coverage required and the range of flow velocities under examination. 2D TOF MRA is more sensitive to slow flow,

making it ideal for longer vessel segments with limited tortuosity (eg, neck vessels). 3D TOF MRA takes longer to perform and is less sensitive to slow flow, but has a relatively higher signal to noise ratio and higher spatial resolution, making it the better choice for small, tortuous vessels (eg, the intracranial vessels).

CE MRA of the neck is most commonly performed using a technique that is conceptually similar to that used for CTA. An intravenous injection of a short dense bolus of gadolinium is imaged on its first pass through the arterial system. In high concentrations, the gadolinium markedly shortens the T1 of the intermixed blood. The extremely short TR values ensure saturation of almost all stationary tissues and produce a high sensitivity to the gadolinium-enhanced blood. Images are typically acquired in the coronal plane and the peak of the contrast bolus is mapped to the center of k space.

Of note, phase-contrast MRA is another non-contrast technique that generates both magnitude and phase images, displaying blood vessel anatomy and direction of flow, respectively. The technique has some advantages over TOF MRA, including decreased sensitivity to some flow-related artifacts and superior background suppression; however, increased acquisition time and technical variability make it less useful in the acute stroke population, and it is not discussed further here.

Advantages

In the setting of acute stroke, TOF MRA techniques provide an invaluable imaging alternative for patients with renal insufficiency or intravenous contrast allergy. Although the sensitivity and specificity for detecting intracranial stenoses and occlusions is inferior to CTA (discussed in the section on CTA advantages), 3D TOF MRA still provides excellent evaluation of the proximal, large intracranial vessels, particularly when combined with additional sequences (DWI, vascular susceptibility signal on GRE, and FLAIR hyperintense vessel signal).

For evaluation of the extracranial vasculature, both CE MRA and 2D TOF techniques are comparable to CTA. A recent study compared both MRA techniques with CTA in the evaluation of greater than 70% carotid stenosis, and demonstrated an accuracy of 92.9% for 2D TOF MRA and 93.8% for CE MRA.[49] CE MRA is usually preferred because it performs better than 2D TOF MRA in evaluation of the proximal arch vessels, and the visualization of such findings as hairline occlusion, dissection, or tandem lesions, detection of which can have important implications for patient management.[50–52] TOF MRA is typically used for patients with renal failure and contrast allergies, and when direction of flow needs to be evaluated, such as suspected subclavian steal.

Disadvantages

Aside from the practical considerations inherent to the MR imaging technique, both TOF and CE MRA have technical limitations that reduce their specificity. In 2D TOF MRA, turbulent flow from stenotic vessel segments results in intravoxel dephasing, which appears as signal-intensity drop-out (or flow void).[53,54] Although this flow void correlates well with a stenosis of greater than 70%, on both CTA[49] and DSA[55] the exact percentage of narrowing cannot be measured. 3D TOF is less sensitive to slow flow and is vulnerable to saturation effects, which refer to a gradual loss of T1 signal caused by repeated excitation with radiofrequency pulses. Both of these factors contribute to poor visualization of the distal intracranial vessels on MRA, and therefore inability to assess the collateral circulation. CE MRA is highly technique dependent, and overestimation of carotid artery narrowing can result from several sources, including dephasing artifacts along the margin of the lumen (which become exaggerated in areas of tight narrowing) (**Fig. 8**), susceptibility artifacts from a dense bolus contrast injection, the signal-intensity threshold used to create the MIPs, and the section thickness causing partial volume averaging effect.[56–58]

CE MRA requires the administration of gadolinium, which has been associated with nephrogenic systemic fibrosis (NSF), a progressive fibrosing dermopathy. Although the exact pathophysiology of NSF is unclear, it is likely caused by a combination of decreased kidney function, presence of inflammation, and exposure to gadolinium-based contrast agents.[59,60] The highest reported incidence of NSF was 8.8% in patients whose glomerular filtration rate (GFR) was less than 15 mL/min, were not undergoing hemodialysis, and received high, nonstandard doses of gadolinium.[61] The incidence of NSF has disappeared with the now routine screening of renal function in at-risk patients prior to gadolinium administration.

EVALUATING TISSUE VIABILITY/PERFUSION IMAGING

Perfusion imaging techniques evaluate capillary, tissue-level circulation, which is beyond the resolution of traditional anatomic imaging. In general, both CT and MR perfusion techniques use rapid serial imaging to dynamically trace the wash-in and wash-out of a contrast bolus power injected into a peripheral vein through an intravenous catheter. In the setting of CT, the iodine-based contrast

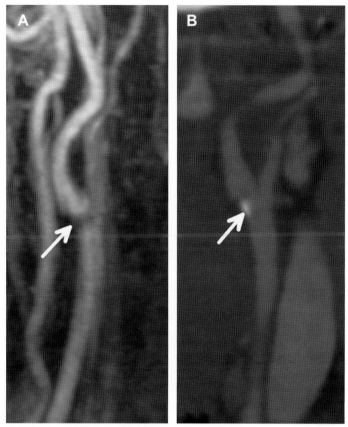

Fig. 8. MRA versus CTA. A 57-year-old woman with transient ischemic attack. Coronal gadolinium-enhanced MRA MIP (*A*) was slightly motion degraded, and loss of signal in the left distal common carotid artery (*arrow*) was thought to be compatible with a moderate to severe stenosis. CTA was recommended and CTA MIP (*B*) showed a corresponding focal calcification (*arrow*) with mild to moderate stenosis.

bolus causes a transient increase, then decrease in the density of the brain parenchyma over time. In the setting of MR imaging, the signal intensity of the brain parenchyma decreases, then increases over time because of susceptibility artifact on the T2* GRE echo planar images. These images are then analyzed by a computer and converted into contrast versus time curves, which can be used to estimate particular perfusion measurements in each part of the brain: mean transit time (MTT), cerebral blood volume (CBV), and cerebral blood flow (CBF).

MTT is measured in seconds and represents the average time required by a red blood cell to cross the capillary network. CBV is measured in milliliters per 100 g of brain tissue and reflects the blood pool content of each pixel. Knowledge of these 2 values can be used to calculate CBF according to the *central volume theorem*: CBF = CBV/MTT. CBF is measured in milliliters per 100 g of brain tissue per minute and reflects the amount of blood flowing through each pixel in 1 minute. Additional transit time measures used for MR imaging are time to peak (TTP) (which reflects the time it takes

to reach maximal susceptibility effect) and Tmax (which is the time to peak of the deconvolved residue function).

Conceptually, CBF, CBV, and MTT reflect the following. Distal to an occlusion, cerebral perfusion pressure decreases, resulting in a heterogeneous reduction in CBF that is largely dependent on the local cerebral perfusion pressure and collateral flow. With mild reduction in CBF, compensatory vasodilation and capillary recruitment results in an increase in the amount of blood in each pixel (CBV) and a prolongation in the amount of time it takes for a red blood cell to cross the capillary network (MTT). In this tissue oxygen delivery is maintained, thereby preserving oxidative metabolism and neuronal function. In areas where CBF has decreased beyond the support of local autoregulatory mechanisms, microvascular collapse occurs, resulting in decreased CBV. In these areas oxygen delivery is impaired, leading within seconds to cessation of neuronal electrical activity, and within minutes to deterioration of the energy state and ion homeostasis.[62]

In practice, perfusion maps are most frequently interpreted by inspecting them for "lesions" representing abnormal CBV, CBF, or MTT. In this interpretation, the terms "infarct core" and "ischemic penumbra" are often used. The core, which often lies near the center of the ischemic region, is defined as the tissue that has been irreversibly damaged and is unlikely to survive regardless of therapeutic intervention. This tissue is represented by decreased CBV, severely decreased CBF, and increased MTT. The term "ischemic penumbra" is often used to describe a region of tissue that is threatened by ischemia, but may be saved by rapid reperfusion. This only moderately ischemic tissue often surrounds the ischemic core, where collateral vessels provide some degree of residual perfusion; this region typically has preserved or increased CBV, mildly decreased CBF, and increased MTT (**Fig. 9**). Discrimination between the infarct core and its surrounding potentially salvageable penumbra has been the focus of functional imaging over the past decade, spurred by

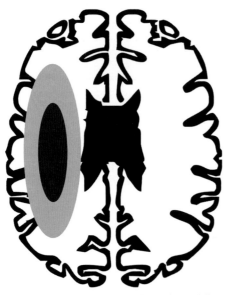

Fig. 9. Acute infarction. Within the right middle cerebral artery vascular territory infarction, the central, darker gray oval represents the infarct "core," or tissue that is irreversibly damaged. In practice, this region is best delineated by restricted diffusion. Hypodense regions on NCCT and CTA-SI (on 4- and 16-detector scanners) also depict infarct core. On perfusion imaging, this region is represented by severely decreased CBF, increased MTT, and decreased CBV. The peripheral lighter gray oval represents the "ischemic penumbra," tissue that is threatened by ischemia but may be saved by rapid reperfusion. In practice, this region is represented by mildly decreased CBF, increased MTT, and preserved or increased CBV.

the hope that patients with a large penumbra and small infarct core may benefit from thrombolysis well beyond the initial hours of stroke symptom onset. Since that time, there has been near-continuous debate over which imaging modality (MR or CT) is best suited to clinically make this distinction. A summary of CT and MR techniques for defining the infarct core and penumbra is provided in **Table 5**.

CT Perfusion

Technique
CTP techniques vary largely by institution. At the authors' institution, CTP studies are performed on a 64-slice scanner. Two sequential 4-cm thick sections are selected, starting at the level of the basal ganglia on unenhanced CT. Following a 37-mL bolus contrast injection at 7 mL/s, cine CT scanning is initiated at 1 image/s for a duration of 45 seconds. After this, 5 sets of axial images are obtained every 15 seconds for an additional 75 seconds. The process is then repeated for the next section.

CTP data are analyzed at an imaging workstation equipped with commercially available software. Postprocessing involves placement of freehand-drawn regions of interest in an input artery (eg, the A1 segment of the anterior cerebral artery) and an input vein (eg, the torcula Herophili), for which contrast-enhancement curves are generated. CBV is calculated from the area under the curve in a parenchymal pixel divided by the area under the curve in an arterial pixel. Deconvolution analysis of arterial and tissue time attenuation curves is used to obtain the MTT. CBF is then calculated according to the central volume theorem (see equation given earlier). The software then generates color-coded CBF, CBV, and MTT maps.

Interpretation
On CTP, CBV maps are usually used to define the infarct core. Tissue that appears normal on CBV maps but abnormal in CBF or MTT maps is thought to represent the ischemic penumbra (**Fig. 10**). Several studies have validated the ability of CTP to distinguish between core and penumbra within and beyond the 3-hour time window, some by comparing perfusion parameters to the contralateral brain parenchyma,[63] to MR imaging (both MR perfusion [MRP][64] and DWI/FLAIR[65]), and to a combination of DWI and NIHSS.[66] At present, however, no large clinical trials have been successfully completed using only CTP to select patients for reperfusion therapy during the 3- to 9-hour time window. Smaller trials beyond the 3-hour time window have suggested that the most effective method to distinguish between

Table 5
Summary of CT and MR techniques for defining infarct core and penumbra

Modality	Infarct Core	Penumbra
CT	• Hypodensity reveals all or part of the infarct core • Specific, but not sensitive	• Subtle CT ischemic signs are not sensitive or specific

MR imaging	• DWI is the most sensitive and specific imaging marker
	• Core >100 cm^3 ≈ one-third of the MCA territory
	   • Poor patient prognosis
	   • Contraindication to thrombolysis
		• Cannot define

CTA	• CTA source images have been used to define the infarct core • Results are highly dependent on technique	• Cannot define
MRA	• Cannot define	• Cannot define

CTP	• Best estimated by low CBV
	• Threshold values have not been established
	• Less sensitive & specific than DWI
		• Tissue that is:
		   • Normal on CBV maps
		   • Abnormal in CBF or MTT maps
		• Threshold values have not been established

MRP	• DWI is most sensitive and specific marker • CBV reduction is a generally accepted marker—should correlate with restricted diffusion	• Definite perfusion parameter has not been clearly defined • CBF reduction and MTT prolongation are sensitive indicators • MRP/DWI mismatch has been shown useful in small clinical trials

infarct core and penumbra applies thresholds to the MTT, CBF, and CBV values.[65–68] In one study, PCT was compared with DWI (infarct core) and follow-up FLAIR image abnormalities in patients with persistent occlusion (infarct penumbra). An absolute CBV of less than 2 ml per 100 g best defined infarct core and a relative MTT of greater than 145% best defined infarct penumbra.[64] In another study, comparing hypoperfused tissue on CT-CBV and CT-CBF to follow-up infarction, a relative CBV of 0.60 and a relative CBF of 0.48 best discriminated between infarcted and noninfarcted tissue.[66] In a third study, ischemic regions with greater than 66% reduction in CT-CBF ratio had a 95% positive predictive value for infarction regardless of recanalization status.[67] To date, however, there is no high-level evidence or consensus for these core and penumbra thresholds.[16,69]

Advantages

Compared with MRP, CTP has advantages of speed, lower cost, and widespread availability. CTP can be performed immediately following unenhanced CT (to exclude hemorrhage, large hypodense infarct, or mass lesion) and CTA (to evaluate for the presence of a vascular lesion). CTP parameters of CBV, CBF, and MTT may be more easily quantified than their MRP counterparts, owing in part to the linear relationship between iodinated CT contrast concentrations and CT image density. The major clinical advantage of CTP is that it can safely be used in patients who cannot undergo MR imaging. CTP, particularly when combined with CTA, provides an invaluable alternative for the estimation of both the infarct and the ischemic penumbra, and a significant improvement in the detection of infarction over NCCT alone.[70,71]

Disadvantages

One major disadvantage of CTP is that it is not as sensitive as DWI for the detection of acute ischemia. There is no universally accepted correlate for DWI, leaving the infarct core to be estimated by either one or a combination of perfusion parameters. Different postprocessing software from different manufacturers tested on the same data sets give a wide range of absolute and relative CBV, CBF, and MTT thresholds for

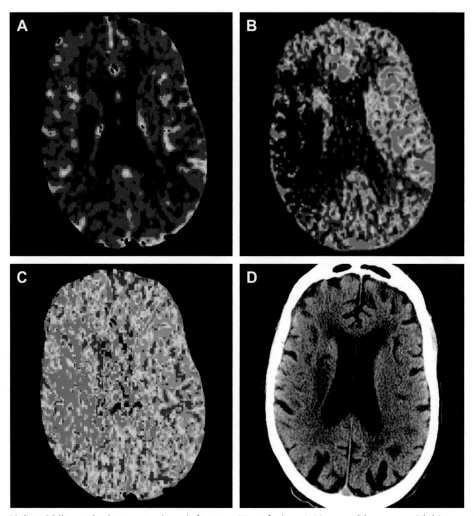

Fig. 10. Right middle cerebral artery territory infarct on CT perfusion. A 78-year-old woman with history of atrial fibrillation presenting 3 hours following left face, arm, and leg weakness, and dysarthria. CBV maps (*A*) demonstrate focal decreased cerebral blood volume in the right corona radiata. CBF maps (*B*) demonstrate a much broader region of decreased cerebral blood flow conforming to the right middle cerebral artery vascular territory. There is corresponding prolonged mean transit time on MTT maps (*C*). Intravenous rtPA was administered. Follow-up NCCT (*D*) at 1 month demonstrates the completed infarct involving mainly the corona radiata and closely approximating the original cerebral blood volume map lesion. In this case, the entire ischemic penumbra recovered.

infarct core and penumbra. This variability needs to be addressed in definitive trials, with validation of optimal postprocessing and image interpretation procedures, followed by standardization of methodology.[69] Once standardized, the technique must be confirmed by large clinical trials before the additional radiation exposure (approximately 3.35–6.7 mSv)[45] and contrast boluses are justified for routine clinical use.

The other major disadvantage of CTP is limited coverage. Although coverage varies depending on manufacturer and generation of multidetector scanner, a 16-detector scanner is able to image a 2-cm thick section per contrast bolus and a 64-detector scanner can image up to 4 cm. By way of reference, evaluation of the anterior circulation requires 8 cm of craniocaudal coverage. Several techniques have attempted to increase coverage, but have their own trade-offs. With the "shuttle-mode perfusion technique," the scanner table moves back and forth switching between 2 different cine views, albeit at a reduced temporal resolution of data acquisition.[72] Alternatively, 2 boluses can be used to acquire 2 slabs of CTP data at different levels, doubling the overall coverage.[66] Unlike the shuttle mode, this technique requires twice the amount of contrast and twice the radiation dose. Coverage volume will continue to increase with enlarging detector arrays and improved technology. Cutting-edge scanners with 320 detector rows offer the possibility of 16-cm coverage without the decreased temporal resolution required with the shuttle-mode technique.

MR Perfusion

Technique

MRP imaging is generally performed with a bolus tracking technique, dynamic susceptibility contrast (DSC) imaging. DSC relies on the decrease in signal caused by magnetic susceptibility effects of gadolinium as it passes through the intracranial vasculature. Because blood passes through the brain parenchyma rapidly, the most commonly used sequence is a single-shot, GRE echo planar sequence capable of multiple slice acquisitions from a single TR. Typically, gadolinium is injected rapidly (5–7 mL/s) into a peripheral intravenous catheter, and then images are obtained repeatedly as the contrast agent passes through the brain. The technique takes approximately 1 to 2 minutes, and is performed so as to track the first pass of the contrast bolus through the intracranial vasculature, without recirculation effects. Approximately 60 images are obtained for each 5-mm brain slice, covering the entire brain.[22] The images obtained in the examination are converted by a computer to contrast agent concentration-versus-time curves. The CBV is proportional to the area under the curve. The CBF and MTT are typically computed with an arterial input function and deconvolution methodology. As with CTP, the echo planar imaging data are transferred to a separate workstation on which the perfusion maps are produced.

Interpretation

With MRP, the ischemic penumbra is usually defined as the region of brain tissue that is abnormal on perfusion but normal on DWI images, that is, the region of so-called diffusion-perfusion mismatch (DPM) (Fig. 11). The perfusion parameter that is used to calculate this mismatch, however, has not been clearly defined. Physiologic evidence indicates that CBF reduction and MTT prolongation are more sensitive indicators of ischemic, but potentially viable tissue. CBV reduction is a generally accepted marker of infarct core, and should correlate with the region of restricted diffusion. This definition is also consistent with empiric observations that the volume of a lesion seen in early CBF or MTT maps tends to overestimate the ultimate infarct volume, and is less well correlated with final infarct volume than is initial

DWI or CBV lesion volume.[73–75] Usually the MTT is used for visual interpretation, because contrast-to-noise ratios are higher on these maps than in others.

The DPM concept and its ability to successfully select patients for treatment guidance beyond 3 hours has been successfully demonstrated in several clinical trials. The Desmoteplase in Acute Ischemic Stroke trial (DIAS)[74] and the Dose Escalation of Desmoteplase for Acute Ischemic Stroke trial (DEDAS)[75] used a 20% mismatch between the MTT and DWI lesions in addition to a DWI lesion volume less than one-third of the MCA territory as trial entry criteria. Patients were given intravenous desmoteplase (a thrombolytic agent derived from bat venom) or placebo between 3 and 9 hours after symptom onset. These trials demonstrated that administration of desmoteplase was associated with dose-dependent rates of higher reperfusion and better clinical outcomes compared with placebo. In the DEFUSE (Diffusion Weighted Imaging Evaluation for Understanding Stroke) study, 74 patients recruited on the basis of a negative NCCT received intravenous rtPA within 3 to 6 hours after stroke onset. Early reperfusion was associated with a significantly increased chance of a favorable clinical response in patients with at least a 20% DWI–perfusion-weighted imaging (PWI) mismatch, whereas patients without a mismatch did not benefit from early reperfusion.[76] In the Echoplanar Imaging Thrombolytic Evaluation Trial (EPITHET), 101 patients were recruited on the basis of a negative NCCT and received intravenous tPA or placebo within 3 to 6 hours after stroke onset; of these, 86% had a DWI-PWI mismatch. Although there was no significant difference in infarct growth between patients who received placebo and those who received intravenous tPA, there was increased reperfusion in those with a mismatch, and reperfusion was associated with less infarct growth and improved clinical outcomes.[77]

When mismatch as a target for therapy was first introduced, it was arbitrarily defined as PWI lesion 20% larger than the baseline DWI lesion volume. However, some investigators have suggested using a larger mismatch. For example, the DEFUSE investigators retrospectively determined an optimum DPM ratio of 2.6 (ie, MRP lesion 2.6 times larger than the DWI lesion) for the best chance of favorable outcome after early reperfusion.[54] More recently, Copen and colleagues[76] demonstrated that if vascular imaging demonstrates a proximal arterial occlusion, the majority of patients (80%) have a greater than 20% mismatch for up to 24 hours after stroke onset.

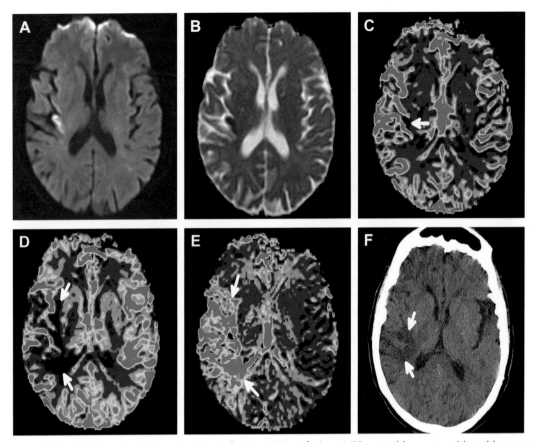

Fig. 11. Right middle cerebral artery territory infarct on MR perfusion: A 76-year-old woman with sudden-onset left-sided facial droop and weakness presented 6 hours following onset. DWI (*A*) and ADC (*B*) images revealed restricted diffusion in the right posterior insula and external capsule. There was corresponding low signal on CBV maps (*arrow* in *C*). A much larger region corresponding with the right middle cerebral artery superior division demonstrated decreased cerebral blood flow (black region indicated by *arrows* in *D*) and increased mean transit time (red and green area indicated by *arrows* in *E*). Intravenous rtPA could not be administered because the patient was outside of the therapeutic window. A follow-up CT obtained 2 days later (*F*) showed that the infarct extended into part, but not all, of the ischemic penumbra.

These studies raise the possibility that imaging-based treatment protocols may appropriately select patients who may benefit from thrombolysis well beyond the initial hours of stroke symptom onset.

Advantages

The major clinical advantage of MRP is the fact that it can be easily combined with DWI, the single best imaging method for identifying infarct core, and unlike CT, it provides whole brain coverage. In addition, as already described, the use of the DPM to select patients for therapy and potentially improve patient outcomes has been validated in small clinical trials. The major technical advantages of MRP over CTP include whole brain coverage and lack of radiation. MRP also produces images with a higher contrast-to-noise ratio.

Disadvantages

The major technical disadvantage of MRP is the lack of linearity between signal intensity and contrast concentration, which makes quantification of perfusion parameters very difficult and unreliable. The major clinical disadvantage is that although widely accepted and used in practice, the diagnostic and clinical utility of MRP has not been proven in controlled, adequately powered studies. Individual centers have demonstrated that different MRP parameters are generally predictive of tissue fate and clinical outcome; however, there has been no determination of which technique is most accurate. Contributing to the lack of consensus is the variability in definitions of what represents ischemic core, penumbra, and final infarct size, and how they relate to clinical outcome on which the measures of accuracy are based.

IMAGING AND TREATMENT ALGORITHM

Based on the practical considerations and clinical trial data mentioned here, the authors have developed the following algorithm for imaging management of acute stroke patients in their Emergency Department (ED) (**Fig. 12**). On arrival and initial clinical assessment, including the NIHSS, patients are quickly transported to the ED CT scanner. Noncontrast head CT is obtained and evaluated at the scanner by the on-call radiologist to exclude hemorrhage and infarction in greater than one-third of the MCA territory or 100 cm³ (measured by ABC/2). If neither is present and the patient has no other contraindications, intravenous rtPA can be administered by the clinical team. CTA of the head and neck vessels is then obtained, with an additional immediate delay scan from the aortic arch to the circle of Willis if there is incomplete arterial opacification. The decision of whether to give intravenous contrast is a clinical one, based in part on the patient's estimated risk of renal impairment and NIHSS score. The CTA source images and immediate postprocessed triplane MIP images are then reviewed by the radiologist at the scanner. Whether to perform CTP imaging, which requires an additional contrast bolus, is decided by the stroke neurologist, largely based

on the patient's MR compatibility, clinical stability, and renal function. If the patient can undergo MR scanning, he or she is transferred from CT to a mobile MR table and brought to the MR imaging scanner. If MR imaging is not deemed appropriate and there is concern for a potentially large ischemic penumbra, CTP can be obtained.

For MR imaging, DWI is always obtained because it is the best method for determining infarct core. FLAIR is obtained if the time of stroke onset is unknown because a DWI abnormality without a FLAIR abnormality likely represents an infarction that is less than 6 hours old. If the region of restricted diffusion is large (>100 cm³), no intervention is indicated and additional imaging is not needed. If the region of completed infarction is small (<100 cm³), indicating that there is a potentially large territory at risk, MRP imaging should be considered. Lastly, MRA can be performed if the vessels have not already been adequately evaluated with CTA.

BEYOND IMAGING: METHODS OF TREATMENT

Neuroendovascular interventions, which include procedures such as local intra-arterial thrombolysis and the mechanical removal of thrombus, are

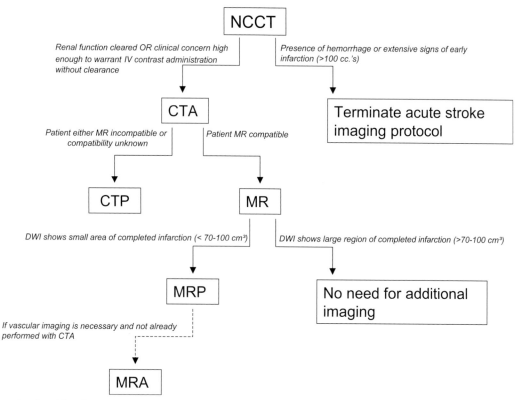

Fig. 12. Algorithm for imaging management of acute stroke patients in the authors' Emergency Department.

largely reserved for acute ischemic stroke patients who cannot safely receive (ie, present outside of the 3–4.5 hour time window), or who have failed intravenous rtPA therapy, and in whom imaging has shown a large region of potentially salvageable tissue. A complete review of these interventions is beyond the scope of this article, however, interested readers are referred to recent reviews by Janjua and Brisman[78] and Nogueira and colleagues.[79,80]

Although guidelines for the endovascular treatment of acute ischemic stroke vary largely by institution, general inclusion and exclusion criteria have been established by large clinical trials. First and foremost, the level of clinical concern prior to intervention must be high. This level is usually assessed using the NIHSS score, and several studies have used a score of at least 10 to triage patients for adjunctive endovascular treatment.[81,82] Convincing data support the safety of local intra-arterial thrombolysis if performed within 6 hours of symptom onset.[83–85] Mechanical thrombectomy is safe and effective for revascularizing occluded vessels in patients up to 8 hours after symptom onset.[81,86,87] For strokes involving the posterior circulation, the therapeutic window can be increased to 24 hours.[88–90] This unconventional time window is allowed because untreated basilar occlusion has a nearly uniform fatal outcome, and the regions served by the posterior circulation may be more resistant to reperfusion injury and hemorrhage owing to their collateral blood supply patterns.[91]

At their institution, the authors honor additional specific guidelines based on clinical data mentioned above. If a patient has a proximal vessel occlusion and an infarct core (DWI, NCCT, CT-CBV) less than 100 cm^3, then intra-arterial recanalization should be considered. If a patient is not a candidate for recanalization and has a proximal or distal occlusion with a core penumbra (usually MTT or other transit time measures) mismatch, then the patient should be closely monitored in the intensive care unit with special attention to keeping his or her blood pressure relatively high to preserve cerebral perfusion pressure to the ischemic tissue at risk of infarction. If the core and penumbra volumes are matched, the infarction is not at risk of extending and aggressive therapy is not required.

SUMMARY

Nearly 1.5 decades after the introduction of systemic thrombolysis for the treatment of acute ischemic stroke, we are now entering an era of newer imaging and image-guided interventions that can both extend the time window for potential treatment and provide a targeted, patient-specific therapeutic approach. Both CT and MR imaging provide promising tools for evaluating the brain parenchyma, with distinct advantages that can be maximized for the individual patient's needs. Although further work and investigation are required to standardize practice guidelines and improve patient access, advanced imaging techniques and endovascular treatments will hopefully offer alternatives to patients who are otherwise without therapeutic options.

REFERENCES

1. Paxton R, Ambrose J. The EMI scanner. A brief review of the first 650 patients. Br J Radiol 1974;47 (561):530–65.
2. Jacobs L, Kinkel WR, Heffner RR Jr. Autopsy correlations of computerized tomography: experience with 6,000 CT scans. Neurology 1976;26(12): 1111–8.
3. Hacke W, Kaste M, Fieschi C, et al. Intravenous thrombolysis with recombinant tissue plasminogen activator for acute hemispheric stroke. The European Cooperative Acute Stroke Study (ECASS). JAMA 1995;274(13):1017–25.
4. Tissue plasminogen activator for acute ischemic stroke. The national institute of neurological disorders and stroke rt-PA Stroke Study Group. N Engl J Med 1995;333(24):1581–7.
5. Patel SC, Levine SR, Tilley BC, et al. Lack of clinical significance of early ischemic changes on computed tomography in acute stroke. JAMA 2001;286(22):2830–8.
6. von Kummer R, Meyding-Lamadé U, Forsting X, et al. Sensitivity and prognostic value of early CT in occlusion of the middle cerebral artery trunk. AJNR Am J Neuroradiol 1994;15(1):9–15 [discussion: 16–8].
7. Grotta JC, Chiu D, Lu M, et al. Agreement and variability in the interpretation of early CT changes in stroke patients qualifying for intravenous rtPA therapy. Stroke 1999;30(8):1528–33.
8. Roberts HC, Dillon WP, Furlan AJ, et al. Computed tomographic findings in patients undergoing intra-arterial thrombolysis for acute ischemic stroke due to middle cerebral artery occlusion: results from the PROACT II trial. Stroke 2002;33(6):1557–65.
9. Lev MH, Farkas J, Gemmete JJ, et al. Acute stroke: improved nonenhanced CT detection—benefits of soft-copy interpretation by using variable window width and center level settings. Radiology 1999; 213(1):150–5.
10. von Kummer R, Nolte PN, Schnittger H, et al. Detectability of cerebral hemisphere ischaemic infarcts by

CT within 6 h of stroke. Neuroradiology 1996;38(1): 31–3.

11. Pexman JH, Barber PA, Hill MD, et al. Use of the Alberta Stroke Program Early CT Score (ASPECTS) for assessing CT scans in patients with acute stroke. AJNR Am J Neuroradiol 2001;22(8):1534–42.

12. Barber PA, Demchuk AM, Zhang J, et al. Validity and reliability of a quantitative computed tomography score in predicting outcome of hyperacute stroke before thrombolytic therapy. ASPECTS study group. Alberta Stroke Programme Early CT Score. Lancet 2000;355(9216):1670–4.

13. Sims JR, Gharai LR, Schaefer PW, et al. ABC/2 for rapid clinical estimate of infarct, perfusion, and mismatch volumes. Neurology 2009;72(24): 2104–10.

14. Hacke W, Kaste M, Fieschi C, et al. Randomised double-blind placebo-controlled trial of thrombolytic therapy with intravenous alteplase in acute ischaemic stroke (ECASS II). Second European-Australasian Acute Stroke Study Investigators. Lancet 1998;352(9136):1245–51.

15. Schellinger PD, Fiebach JB, Hacke W. Imaging-based decision making in thrombolytic therapy for ischemic stroke: present status. Stroke 2003;34(2): 575–83.

16. Latchaw RE, Alberts MJ, Lev MH, et al. Recommendations for imaging of acute ischemic stroke. A scientific statement from the American Heart Association. Stroke 2009;40(11):3646–78.

17. Hacke W, Kaste M, Bluhmki E, et al. Thrombolysis with alteplase 3 to 4.5 hours after acute ischemic stroke. N Engl J Med 2008;359(13):1317–29.

18. Tha KK, Terae S, Kudo K, et al. Differential diagnosis of hyperintense cerebrospinal fluid on fluid-attenuated inversion recovery images of the brain. Part II: non-pathological conditions. Br J Radiol 2009;82(979):610–4.

19. Tha KK, Terae S, Kudo K, et al. Differential diagnosis of hyperintense cerebrospinal fluid on fluid-attenuated inversion recovery images of the brain. Part I: pathological conditions. Br J Radiol 2009;82 (977):426–34.

20. Kim HS, Lee DH, Ryu CW, et al. Multiple cerebral microbleeds in hyperacute ischemic stroke: impact on prevalence and severity of early hemorrhagic transformation after thrombolytic treatment. AJR Am J Roentgenol 2006;186(5):1443–9.

21. Boulanger JM, Coutts SB, Eliasziw M, et al. Cerebral microhemorrhages predict new disabling or fatal strokes in patients with acute ischemic stroke or transient ischemic attack. Stroke 2006;37(3): 911–4.

22. Arnold M, Nedeltchev K, Brekenfeld C, et al. Outcome of acute stroke patients without visible occlusion on early arteriography. Stroke 2004;35 (5):1135–8.

23. Lev MH, Farkas J, Rodriguez VR, et al. CT angiography in the rapid triage of patients with hyperacute stroke to intraarterial thrombolysis: accuracy in the detection of large vessel thrombus. J Comput Assist Tomogr 2001;25(4):520–8.

24. Bash S, Villablanca JP, Jahan R, et al. Intracranial vascular stenosis and occlusive disease: evaluation with CT angiography, MR angiography, and digital subtraction angiography. AJNR Am J Neuroradiol 2005;26(5):1012–21.

25. Arenillas JF, Rovira A, Molina CA, et al. Prediction of early neurological deterioration using diffusion- and perfusion-weighted imaging in hyperacute middle cerebral artery ischemic stroke. Stroke 2002;33(9): 2197–203.

26. Yoo AJ, Verduzco LA, Schaefer PW, et al. MRI-based selection for intra-arterial stroke therapy: value of pretreatment diffusion-weighted imaging lesion volume in selecting patients with acute stroke who will benefit from early recanalization. Stroke 2009;40(6):2046–54.

27. Assouline E, Benziane K, Reizine D, et al. Intra-arterial thrombus visualized on T2* gradient echo imaging in acute ischemic stroke. Cerebrovasc Dis 2005;20(1):6–11.

28. Yuh WT, Crain MR, Loes DJ, et al. MR imaging of cerebral ischemia: findings in the first 24 hours. AJNR Am J Neuroradiol 1991;12(4):621–9.

29. Perkins CJ, Kahya E, Roque CT, et al. Fluid-attenuated inversion recovery and diffusion- and perfusion-weighted MRI abnormalities in 117 consecutive patients with stroke symptoms. Stroke 2001;32(12):2774–81.

30. Tan JC, Dillon WP, Liu S, et al. Systematic comparison of perfusion-CT and CT-angiography in acute stroke patients. Ann Neurol 2007;61(6):533–43.

31. Wintermark M, Jawadi SS, Rapp JH, et al. High-resolution CT imaging of carotid artery atherosclerotic plaques. AJNR Am J Neuroradiol 2008;29(5): 875–82.

32. Napoli A, Fleischmann D, Chan FP, et al. Computed tomography angiography: state-of-the-art imaging using multidetector-row technology. J Comput Assist Tomogr 2004;28(Suppl 1):S32–45.

33. Saba L, Mallarini G. MDCTA of carotid plaque degree of stenosis: evaluation of interobserver agreement. AJR Am J Roentgenol 2008;190(1):W41–6.

34. Bartlett ES, Walters TD, Symons SP, et al. Carotid stenosis index revisited with direct CT angiography measurement of carotid arteries to quantify carotid stenosis. Stroke 2007;38(2):286–91.

35. Bartlett ES, Walters TD, Symons SP, et al. Diagnosing carotid stenosis near-occlusion by using CT angiography. AJNR Am J Neuroradiol 2006;27(3): 632–7.

36. Randoux B, Marro B, Koskas F, et al. Carotid artery stenosis: prospective comparison of CT,

three-dimensional gadolinium-enhanced MR, and conventional angiography. Radiology 2001;220(1): 179–85.

37. Bartlett ES, Walters TD, Symons SP, et al. Quantification of carotid stenosis on CT angiography. AJNR Am J Neuroradiol 2006;27(1):13–9.

38. Saba L, Sanfilippo R, Pirisi R, et al. Multidetector-row CT angiography in the study of atherosclerotic carotid arteries. Neuroradiology 2007;49(8):623–37.

39. Koelemay MJ, Nederkoorn PJ, Reitsma JB, et al. Systematic review of computed tomographic angiography for assessment of carotid artery disease. Stroke 2004;35(10):2306–12.

40. Provenzale JM, Sarikaya B. Comparison of test performance characteristics of MRI, MR angiography, and CT angiography in the diagnosis of carotid and vertebral artery dissection: a review of the medical literature. AJR Am J Roentgenol 2009; 193(4):1167–74.

41. Elijovich L, Kazmi K, Gauvrit JY, et al. The emerging role of multidetector row CT angiography in the diagnosis of cervical arterial dissection: preliminary study. Neuroradiology 2006;48(9):606–12.

42. Hunter GJ, Hamberg LM, Ponzo JA, et al. Assessment of cerebral perfusion and arterial anatomy in hyperacute stroke with three-dimensional functional CT: early clinical results. AJNR Am J Neuroradiol 1998;19(1):29–37.

43. Coutts SB, Lev MH, Eliasziw M, et al. ASPECTS on CTA source images versus unenhanced CT: added value in predicting final infarct extent and clinical outcome. Stroke 2004;35(11):2472–6.

44. Lev MH, Segal AZ, Farkas J, et al. Utility of perfusion-weighted CT imaging in acute middle cerebral artery stroke treated with intra-arterial thrombolysis: prediction of final infarct volume and clinical outcome. Stroke 2001;32(9):2021–8.

45. Almandoz JD, et al. CT Angiography of the carotid and cerebral circulation. Radiol Clin North Am 2010; 48(2):265–81.

46. Hopyan JJ, Gladstone DJ, Mallia G, et al. Renal safety of CT angiography and perfusion imaging in the emergency evaluation of acute stroke. AJNR Am J Neuroradiol 2008;29(10):1826–30.

47. Hunt CH, Hartman RP, Hesley GK. Frequency and severity of adverse effects of iodinated and gadolinium contrast materials: retrospective review of 456,930 doses. AJR Am J Roentgenol 2009;193(4):1124–7.

48. Kim JJ, Dillon WP, Glastonbury CM, et al. Sixty-four-section multidetector CT angiography of carotid arteries: a systematic analysis of image quality and artifacts. AJNR Am J Neuroradiol 2010;31(1):91–9.

49. Babiarz LS, Romero JM, Murphy EK, et al. Contrast-enhanced MR angiography is not more accurate than unenhanced 2D time-of-flight MR angiography for determining > or = 70% internal carotid artery stenosis. AJNR Am J Neuroradiol 2009;30(4):761–8.

50. Carr JC, Shaibani A, Russell E, et al. Contrast-enhanced magnetic resonance angiography of the carotid circulation. Top Magn Reson Imaging 2001; 12(5):349–57.

51. Timaran CH, Rosero EB, Valentine RJ, et al. Accuracy and utility of three-dimensional contrast-enhanced magnetic resonance angiography in planning carotid stenting. J Vasc Surg 2007;46(2): 257–63 [discussion 263–4].

52. Romero JM, Ackerman RH, Dault NA, et al. Noninvasive evaluation of carotid artery stenosis: indications, strategies, and accuracy. Neuroimaging Clin N Am 2005;15(2):351–65, xi.

53. Mustert BR, Williams DM, Prince MR. In vitro model of arterial stenosis: correlation of MR signal dephasing and trans-stenotic pressure gradients. Magn Reson Imaging 1998;16(3):301–10.

54. Yang CW, Carr JC, Futterer SF, et al. Contrast-enhanced MR angiography of the carotid and vertebrobasilar circulations. AJNR Am J Neuroradiol 2005;26(8):2095–101.

55. Nederkoorn PJ, van der Graaf Y, Eikelboom BC, et al. Time-of-flight MR angiography of carotid artery stenosis: does a flow void represent severe stenosis? AJNR Am J Neuroradiol 2002;23(10):1779–84.

56. Babiarz LS, Astor B, Mohamed MA, et al. Comparison of gadolinium-enhanced cardiovascular magnetic resonance angiography with high-resolution black blood cardiovascular magnetic resonance for assessing carotid artery stenosis. J Cardiovasc Magn Reson 2007;9(1):63–70.

57. Yamagiwa H. [Clinicopathological study of 65 cases of aberrant pancreas in the stomach]. Rinsho Byori 1990;38(12):1387–91 [in Japanese].

58. Cosottini M, Pingitore A, Puglioli M, et al. Contrast-enhanced three-dimensional magnetic resonance angiography of atherosclerotic internal carotid stenosis as the noninvasive imaging modality in revascularization decision making. Stroke 2003;34 (3):660–4.

59. Gibson SE, Farver CF, Prayson RA. Multiorgan involvement in nephrogenic fibrosing dermopathy: an autopsy case and review of the literature. Arch Pathol Lab Med 2006;130(2):209–12.

60. Sadowski EA, Bennett LK, Chan MR, et al. Nephrogenic systemic fibrosis: risk factors and incidence estimation. Radiology 2007;243(1):148–57.

61. Prince MR, Zhang H, Morris M, et al. Incidence of nephrogenic systemic fibrosis at two large medical centers. Radiology 2008;248(3):807–16.

62. Astrup J, Siesjo BK, Symon L. Thresholds in cerebral ischemia—the ischemic penumbra. Stroke 1981;12(6):723–5.

63. Eastwood JD, Lev MH, Azhari T, et al. CT perfusion scanning with deconvolution analysis: pilot study in patients with acute middle cerebral artery stroke. Radiology 2002;222(1):227–36.

64. Eastwood JD, Lev MH, Wintermark M, et al. Correlation of early dynamic CT perfusion imaging with whole-brain MR diffusion and perfusion imaging in acute hemispheric stroke. AJNR Am J Neuroradiol 2003;24(9):1869–75.

65. Wintermark M, Flanders AE, Velthuis B, et al. Perfusion-CT assessment of infarct core and penumbra: receiver operating characteristic curve analysis in 130 patients suspected of acute hemispheric stroke. Stroke 2006;37(4):979–85.

66. Wintermark M, Reichhart M, Thiran JP, et al. Prognostic accuracy of cerebral blood flow measurement by perfusion computed tomography, at the time of emergency room admission, in acute stroke patients. Ann Neurol 2002;51(4):417–32.

67. Koenig M, Kraus M, Theek C, et al. Quantitative assessment of the ischemic brain by means of perfusion-related parameters derived from perfusion CT. Stroke 2001;32(2):431–7.

68. Schaefer PW, Roccatagliata L, Ledezma C, et al. First-pass quantitative CT perfusion identifies thresholds for salvageable penumbra in acute stroke patients treated with intra-arterial therapy. AJNR Am J Neuroradiol 2006;27(1):20–5.

69. Konstas AA, Goldmakher GV, Lee TY, et al. Theoretic basis and technical implementations of CT perfusion in acute ischemic stroke, part 2: technical implementations. AJNR Am J Neuroradiol 2009;30(5):885–92.

70. Lin K, Rapalino O, Law M, et al. Accuracy of the Alberta Stroke Program Early CT Score during the first 3 hours of middle cerebral artery stroke: comparison of noncontrast CT, CT angiography source images, and CT perfusion. AJNR Am J Neuroradiol 2008;29(5):931–6.

71. Ezzeddine MA, Lev MH, McDonald CT, et al. CT angiography with whole brain perfused blood volume imaging: added clinical value in the assessment of acute stroke. Stroke 2002;33(4):959–66.

72. Roberts HC, Roberts TP, Smith WS, et al. Multisection dynamic CT perfusion for acute cerebral ischemia: the "toggling-table" technique. AJNR Am J Neuroradiol 2001;22(6):1077–80.

73. Sorensen AG, Copen WA, Ostergaard L, et al. Hyperacute stroke: simultaneous measurement of relative cerebral blood volume, relative cerebral blood flow, and mean tissue transit time. Radiology 1999;210(2):519–27.

74. Karonen JO, Liu Y, Vanninen RL, et al. Combined perfusion- and diffusion-weighted MR imaging in acute ischemic stroke during the 1st week: a longitudinal study. Radiology 2000;217(3):886–94.

75. Schaefer PW, Hunter GJ, He J, et al. Predicting cerebral ischemic infarct volume with diffusion and perfusion MR imaging. AJNR Am J Neuroradiol 2002;23(10):1785–94.

76. Copen WA, Rezai Gharai L, Barak ER, et al. Existence of the diffusion-perfusion mismatch within 24 hours after onset of acute stroke: dependence on proximal arterial occlusion. Radiology 2009;250(3): 878–86.

77. Davis SM, Donnan GA, Parsons MW, et al. Effects of alteplase beyond 3 h after stroke in the Echoplanar Imaging Thrombolytic Evaluation Trial (EPITHET): a placebo-controlled randomised trial. Lancet Neurol 2008;7(4):299–309.

78. Janjua N, Brisman JL. Endovascular treatment of acute ischaemic stroke. Lancet Neurol 2007;6(12): 1086–93.

79. Nogueira RG, Schwamm LH, Hirsch JA. Endovascular approaches to acute stroke, part 1: drugs, devices, and data. AJNR Am J Neuroradiol 2009; 30(4):649–61.

80. Nogueira RG, Yoo AJ, Buonanno FS, et al. Endovascular approaches to acute stroke, part 2: a comprehensive review of studies and trials. AJNR Am J Neuroradiol 2009;30(5):859–75.

81. Smith WS, Sung G, Starkman S, et al. Safety and efficacy of mechanical embolectomy in acute ischemic stroke: results of the MERCI trial. Stroke 2005;36(7): 1432–8.

82. Qureshi AI, Janjua N, Kirmani JF, et al. Mechanical disruption of thrombus following intravenous tissue plasminogen activator for ischemic stroke. J Neuroimaging 2007;17(2):124–30.

83. del Zoppo GJ, Higashida RT, Furlan AJ, et al. PROACT: a phase II randomized trial of recombinant prourokinase by direct arterial delivery in acute middle cerebral artery stroke. PROACT investigators. Prolyse in acute cerebral thromboembolism. Stroke 1998;29(1):4–11.

84. Furlan A, Higashida R, Wechsler L, et al. Intra-arterial prourokinase for acute ischemic stroke. The PROACT II study: a randomized controlled trial. Prolyse in acute cerebral thromboembolism. JAMA 1999;282(21):2003–11.

85. Lewandowski CA, Frankel M, Tomsick TA, et al. Combined intravenous and intra-arterial r-TPA versus intra-arterial therapy of acute ischemic stroke: Emergency Management of Stroke (EMS) Bridging Trial. Stroke 1999;30(12):2598–605.

86. Gobin YP, Starkman S, Duckwiler GR, et al. MERCI 1: a phase 1 study of mechanical embolus removal in cerebral ischemia. Stroke 2004;35(12): 2848–54.

87. Smith WS. Safety of mechanical thrombectomy and intravenous tissue plasminogen activator in acute ischemic stroke. Results of the multi Mechanical Embolus Removal in Cerebral Ischemia (MERCI) trial, part I. AJNR Am J Neuroradiol 2006;27(6): 1177–82.

88. Wijdicks EF, Nichols DA, Thielen KR, et al. Intra-arterial thrombolysis in acute basilar artery thromboembolism: the initial Mayo Clinic experience. Mayo Clin Proc 1997;72(11):1005–13.

89. Brandt T, von Kummer R, Müller-Küppers M, et al. Thrombolytic therapy of acute basilar artery occlusion. Variables affecting recanalization and outcome. Stroke 1996;27(5):875–81.

90. Hacke W, Zeumer H, Ferbert A, et al. Intra-arterial thrombolytic therapy improves outcome in patients with acute vertebrobasilar occlusive disease. Stroke 1988;19(10):1216–22.

91. Ostrem JL, Saver JL, Alger JR, et al. Acute basilar artery occlusion: diffusion-perfusion MRI characterization of tissue salvage in patients receiving intra-arterial stroke therapies. Stroke 2004;35(2):e30–4.

Hemorrhagic Stroke

Scott D. Smith, MD[a], Clifford J. Eskey, MD, PhD[b],*

KEYWORDS

- Hemorrhagic stroke • Intracerebral hemorrhage
- Subarachnoid hemorrhage
- Susceptibility-weighted imaging • Vascular malformation
- Aneurysm

When patients present to the emergency room with sudden onset of focal neurologic symptoms or altered consciousness, hemorrhagic stroke is a major focus of emergency diagnostic evaluation. The entities that compose hemorrhagic stroke are readily diagnosed with advanced imaging. Emergency surgical or endovascular therapies may be life saving. Hemorrhagic stroke is defined as an acute neurologic injury occurring as a result of bleeding into the head. There are 2 distinct mechanisms: bleeding directly into the brain parenchyma (intracerebral hemorrhage [ICH]), or bleeding into the cerebrospinal fluid (CSF) containing sulci, fissures, and cisterns (subarachnoid hemorrhage [SAH]). Although both entities are less common than acute ischemia, they both convey greater morbidity and mortality. Hemorrhagic stroke has well-studied and characteristic imaging features. Treatment can be challenging and substantially different from ischemic forms of stroke. Some of the imaging principles relevant to ICH and SAH can be applied to other forms of intracranial hemorrhage, but the entities of subdural and epidural hemorrhage lie outside the scope of this discussion. Current imaging options for the detection of acute hemorrhage and the expected imaging findings for each modality are reviewed. Common and unusual causes for each entity with attention to their distinguishing imaging features are discussed. In addition, imaging strategies and recent work in specific imaging findings that may guide patient management in the future are discussed.

CLINICAL PRESENTATION

Rapid and accurate identification of hemorrhage is essential in acute stroke care, as the fundamental therapies for the management of ischemic and hemorrhagic stroke differ markedly. Both ischemic and hemorrhagic strokes are characterized by the relatively sudden onset of symptoms and neurologic deficits, the type and severity of which will vary according to lesion type, location, and size.

Classically described presentations do exist. For example, nearly all patients with SAH able to converse will describe "the worst headache of my life." One in 5 may report a less severe sentinel headache in the hours or days leading up to the event. The event may be accompanied by focal neurologic signs or other symptoms such as nausea/vomiting, loss of consciousness, or seizure. ICH, on the other hand, is classically described as a gradual process, with worsening of symptoms over minutes to hours. Headache and nausea/vomiting are more frequent in ICH than ischemic stroke. Despite these differences, there remains enough overlap in the clinical presentations that history and physical examination alone are unreliable in differentiating hemorrhagic from ischemic stroke, and current

[a] Department of Radiology, Dartmouth-Hitchcock Medical Center, One Medical Center Drive, Lebanon, NH 03756, USA
[b] Division of Neuroradiology, Department of Radiology, Dartmouth-Hitchcock Medical Center, One Medical Center Drive, Lebanon, NH 03756, USA
* Corresponding author.
E-mail address: Clifford.J.Eskey@Hitchcock.ORG

Radiol Clin N Am 49 (2011) 27–45
doi:10.1016/j.rcl.2010.07.011
0033-8389/11/$ — see front matter © 2011 Elsevier Inc. All rights reserved.

guidelines for each entity include brain imaging as an essential early component of the work-up.[1,2]

SELECTION OF IMAGING MODALITY

Contemporary options for acute stroke imaging include computed tomography (CT) and magnetic resonance (MR) imaging. As recently as 2003, un-enhanced head CT was considered the imaging modality of choice for the detection of acute intra-cranial hemorrhage.[3] Continuing advances in MR technology have addressed several perceived shortcomings and as a result MR is gaining increasing acceptance as a first-line modality.

CT remains in widespread use for both logistic and diagnostic reasons. It is widely available on a 24 hour basis. There are no absolute contraindi-cations to CT scanning, whereas approximately 10% of patients may be ineligible for MR imaging because of the presence of a pacemaker or ferro-magnetic foreign bodies. CT examination can be completed in minutes (rather than 10s of minutes for MR imaging). The speed of image acquisition and relative ease of patient monitoring maximize both patient safety and the chance of good quality results, whereas in 10% of patients undergoing MR imaging other medical factors such as hypo-tension, agitation, or otherwise altered level of consciousness preclude the acquisition of diag-nostic MR images.[4] The conspicuity of blood products is high on CT and their appearance is specific. For all these reasons, CT is better studied than MR imaging in the setting of acute stroke and has been the primary modality for the largest trials in acute stroke intervention. The immediate CT scanning of all patients with acute stroke has been shown to be a cost-effective policy that results in improved quality of life outcomes.[5]

Increasingly, however, MR imaging is gaining favor in the acute setting. Addressing some of the primary perceived deficiencies of the modality, faster sequences have been developed with the broader availability of higher field strengths, stronger and faster gradients, and the application of ever-improving computing power. Studies have shown that specific MR sequences are comparable with CT when used for the detection of acute and subacute blood products. MR has also been found to be more accurate in the detec-tion of chronic hemorrhage, the presence of which is believed to affect the risk of thrombolytic therapy. Other advantages of MR over CT in the acute stroke setting include the detection of small ischemic infarcts, the differentiation of acute from chronic ischemia, and the identification of satellite ischemic lesions that might better characterize the mechanism of stroke.[2] Unlike CT, to our

knowledge no outcomes or cost-effectiveness studies have yet been performed evaluating MR imaging as the initial imaging modality.

At our institution, CT remains the initial imaging modality of choice because of its proven sensitivity and specificity, availability, and speed. CT angiog-raphy (CTA) is performed soon thereafter in patients who are found to have ICH or SAH for which the cause is not immediately apparent from the clinical history. Digital subtraction angiog-raphy (DSA) and MR imaging are performed to evaluate for specific underlying causes (ie, aneu-rysm, vascular malformation, primary or secondary neoplasm, amyloid angiopathy, hemor-rhagic infarction, or venous sinus thrombosis).

INTRACRANIAL BLOOD PRODUCTS

One of the primary objectives of early stroke imaging is the identification and characterization of hemorrhage. In the ideal setting, imaging will have been obtained within less than 3 to 6 hours of symptom onset, so that blood products should be relatively fresh. However, this may not be the case in clinical practice. Hemorrhage evolution is a dynamic process with imaging findings that can change over time.

The molecular composition of extravasated blood changes as the blood products break down and are reabsorbed. Five stages are typi-cally referenced: blood consists primarily of intra-cellular oxyhemoglobin in the hyperacute stage; during the acute stage this gradually loses its oxygen to become deoxyhemoglobin; this is con-verted to intracellular methemoglobin by oxidative denaturation in the early subacute stage; in the late subacute stage, cell lysis occurs resulting in extra-cellular methemoglobin; this is converted to hemo-siderin and ferritin by macrophages in the chronic stage. Although there is good agreement in the naming of each stage and the molecular composi-tion of the associated blood products, discrep-ancies persist amongst investigators in delimiting the exact time interval of each stage.[6–8] This is a reflection of the dynamic nature of the break down of blood products, a process that can occur at different rates between patients or even within separate areas of a hematoma.

Hemorrhages into the various intracranial compartments demonstrate similar, although not always identical, progression over time. Subdural and epidural hematomas evolve similarly to ICH, although they progress through each stage more slowly because of the higher oxygen tension conveyed by the adjacent vascularized dura. Subarachnoid and intraventricular bleeds may differ in initial CT density and MR characteristics depending on the degree to which they mix with CSF. Their progression is also slow, again because of the relatively high local P_{O_2}.[6]

ICH
Epidemiology

ICH is the second most common cause of stroke, accounting for 10% to 15% of all strokes.[1,9] Although long term functional outcomes for stroke survivors are similar amongst hemorrhagic and ischemic cohorts,[10] ICH carries significantly higher mortality risks, with 30-day mortality estimates ranging from 35% to 52%, a rate approximately 5 times greater than the mortality for ischemic events.[1,9] The survival difference is most pronounced immediately after a stroke, with an initially 4-fold higher risk of death. This decreases to 2.5- and 1.5-fold at 1 and 3 weeks respectively, and the increased mortality risk of ICH continues to gradually decline such that no differences between the 2 groups of survivors are seen 3 months afterwards.[11]

CT Findings

The typical CT appearance of an acute hypertensive hemorrhage is a round or oval hyperattenuating mass (**Fig. 1**). In the hyperacute setting these typically measure 40 to 60 Hounsfield units (HU), and can appear heterogeneous. As the clot organizes it appears more homogeneous and hyperdense, increasing to 60 to 80 HU in hours to days and 80 to 100 HU over the course of a few days at which point it may be surrounded by a halo of hypoattenuation representing perihematomal edema.[6]

The conspicuity of a clot depends on several factors, including size, location, CT imaging parameters, and the window and level settings used for reading. Smaller bleeds may be more apparent on thin-slice imaging, and those located adjacent to the calvarium may be easier to detect with a wider (150–250 HU) window setting. In some cases it may be difficult to distinguish between focal calcification and blood. Usually this can be resolved with appropriate windowing and use of thin-section reconstructions. Alternatively, a dual kilovolt technique, which exploits the greater attenuation of calcium at lower tube voltage, can be used.[12] Caution must be used in the setting of extreme anemia, where blood may appear isodense to brain parenchyma because of low hematocrit. In the case of active extravasation, liquid blood products can appear hypodense relative to surrounding clot, resulting in the so-called swirl sign."[7] Similarly, acute hemorrhage in the setting of coagulopathy may appear isodense or may demonstrate a fluid/fluid level.[7]

As the hemorrhage ages, the CT density gradually decreases by an average of 0.7 to 1.5 HU per day. In a progression that begins at the periphery and continues to the center of the hematoma, hyperdense clot first becomes isodense, and progressively becomes hypodense until it is completely reabsorbed.[6] In the absence of rebleeding, the late sequelae of hemorrhage can include hypodense foci (37%), slit-like lesions (25%), calcification (10%), or no detectable abnormality (27%).[13]

MR Findings

The appearance of ICH similarly changes over time on MR imaging. Many variables influence the signal characteristics. These include factors intrinsic to the hematoma such as age, size, location, and episodes of recurrent hemorrhage; technical MR factors such as pulse sequence selection and parameters, magnetic field strength, and bandwidth; also biologic qualities such as P_{O_2}, pH, protein concentration, and integrity of a blood-brain barrier.[6] A detailed discussion of the technical factors determining signal properties at each stage is beyond the scope of this discussion, but the MR signal of blood products reliably correlates with each of the previously identified stages. The resultant MR appearance is summarized in **Table 1**.

Spin-echo T1- and T2-weighted imaging techniques are known to be adequate for the

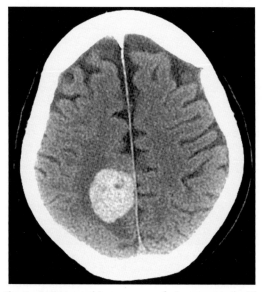

Fig. 1. A 73-year-old man on warfarin presented with balance problems and headache. Noncontrast head CT showed a 2.5×3.0 cm right parietal ICH.

Table 1
Evolution of intracranial blood products, CT and MR imaging appearance

Stage	Main Product	Time Frame[6]	CT	T1/T2
Hyperacute	Oxyhemoglobin	First few hours	Hyperdense	Isointense/hyperintense
Acute	Deoxyhemoglobin	1–3 d	Hyperdense	Isointense/hypointense
Early subacute	Intracellular methemoglobin	3–7 d	Hyperdense	Hyperintense/hypointense
Late subacute	Extracellular methemoglobin	4–7 d to 1 mo	Isodense	Hyperintense/hyperintense
Chronic	Hemosiderin, ferritin	>1 mo	Hypodense	Hypointense/hypointense

identification of subacute and chronic blood products, however their sensitivity is poor compared with CT for hyperacute hemorrhage. Gradient recalled-echo (GRE) imaging techniques with T2* weighting are substantially more sensitive to hyperacute hemorrhage.[14–16] Unlike spin-echo sequences, spin refocusing with gradient reversal does not refocus static magnetic field inhomogeneity. The paramagnetic properties of blood products induce local field inhomogeneity resulting in signal loss on T2*-weighted sequences. Several studies have evaluated the accuracy of T2*-weighted GRE imaging compared with CT in the detection of hyperacute ICH in all patients presenting with acute stroke (both excluded the evaluation of SAH.) MR was found to provide equal detection of acute ICH and to provide better detection of chronic hemorrhage.[17,18] Newer three-dimensional (3D) susceptibility-weighted imaging (SWI) sequences have also been developed which use a 3D fast low-angle shot (FLASH) technique with flow compensation. Although these were initially used as a tool for MR venography,[19] they are also useful in the evaluation of ICH

(**Fig. 2**). Studies have shown that such 3D SWI sequences are more sensitive than CT or even other T2*-GRE MR imaging in the detection of both chronic microhemorrhage and small volume hemorrhage within an acute infarct.[20,21]

Causes and Patterns of ICH

The presence of ICH alone is enough to alter the ongoing work-up and treatment plan of a patient with acute stroke. In most clinical scenarios, further characterization of the hemorrhage itself and adjacent structures helps to further shape diagnostic and therapeutic goals. There are numerous causes of ICH, and although several classic patterns of presentation have been described, there remains overlap among entities. The typical imaging appearance and potential distinguishing characteristics that can be of use in further directing care are reviewed.

Primary causes of ICH

Hypertension is the most common cause of spontaneous ICH in adults.[22] The underlying mechanism seems to be related to the effects of

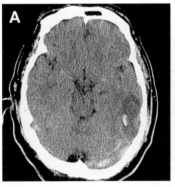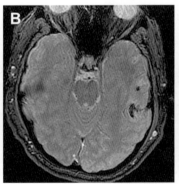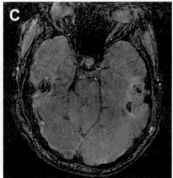

Fig. 2. A 44-year-old man with 2-week history of right frontotemporal headaches. (*A*) Noncontrast head CT (NCT) with a crescent-shaped hemorrhage within an area of hypoattenuation in the posterior left temporal lobe. The right transverse sinus contains high attenuation material (this hemorrhage was secondary to venous sinus thrombosis). (*B*) T2*-GRE MR with signal dropout at known crescent-shaped blood and smaller focus of blood anteriorly not visible on CT. (*C*) SWI MR demonstrates further signal dropout representing blood products not seen on T2*-GRE.

systemic blood pressure on small penetrating arteries that arise from major intracranial vessels. Specifically, these vessels are the lenticulostriate arteries arising from the middle cerebral arteries, thalamoperforating and thalamogeniculate arteries from the posterior cerebral arteries, and the pontine and brainstem perforators arising from the basilar artery. In response to hypertension, these small vessels can develop intimal hyperplasia, intimal hyalinization, and medial degeneration, which predispose them to focal necrosis and rupture.[23] Some investigators suggest that vessel injury can lead to microaneurysms, termed Charcot-Bouchard aneurysms, which are prone to subsequent rupture, resulting in micro- or macrohemorrhages.[24] The classic location of macroscopic hypertensive ICH also reflects the territories supplied by these small perforators, with 60% to 65% of bleeds in the putamen and internal capsule, 15% to 25% in the thalamus, and 5% to 10% in the pons.[7] Although the deep locations are most characteristic, hypertension remains a significant risk factor for lobar hemorrhage in the absence of other underlying causes.[25,26]

Hypertensive hemorrhages originating in the basal ganglia and brainstem have a propensity to extend into the nearby ventricular system (**Fig. 3**). Intraventricular blood characteristically appears hyperdense on CT, and can range in volume from a thin dependent layering to complete filling of one or all of the ventricles. The MR appearance of intraventricular hemorrhage

(IVH) at the various stages is similar to that of ICH, although the progression from stage to stage is typically slower.[6] Like ICH, IVH appears hypointense on SWI. Unlike ICH, IVH is readily identified on fluid-attenuated inversion recovery (FLAIR) sequences, because of its marked T2 hyperintensity relative to the adjacent dark CSF signal.

Another secondary finding that may be seen more often in the setting of hypertensive hemorrhage than other causes is the presence of microbleeds in the distribution of the small perforating vessels. These are the sequelae of hypertensive arteriopathy resulting in very small volume bleeding that is generally chronic and often multifocal. These microbleeds are not typically detected by CT. The characteristic MR appearance of a microbleed is that of a focal area of signal loss (<10 mm) on a susceptibility-weighted sequence. This finding has been pathologically correlated with the presence of hemosiderin-laden macrophages adjacent to small blood vessels.[27]

Cerebral amyloid angiopathy Cerebral amyloid angiopathy (CAA) is another common cause of spontaneous ICH. This is a disease with a strong predilection for advanced age, rarely seen in patients younger than 60 years and with progressively increasing incidence after the age of 65 years. CAA is characterized by the deposition of amyloid beta-peptide in the small- and medium-sized vessels of the leptomeninges and cortex, with relative sparing of vessels in the basal ganglia, white matter, and posterior fossa.[28] The exact mechanisms resulting in deposition are not well understood, although there seem to be associations with specific mutations in an amyloid precursor protein as well as specific alleles of the apolipoprotein E gene. Affected vessels undergo fibrinoid degeneration, necrosis, and microaneurysm formation. These weakened segments can subsequently rupture, resulting in either microbleeds or larger hematomas. In contrast to hypertensive ICH, CAA-related hemorrhages tend to occur in the cortex and subcortical white matter. Early descriptions suggested an equal distribution throughout the supratentorial brain,[28] although later series have suggested that bleeding occurs more often in the temporal and occipital lobes.[29] As in hypertensive ICH, the microbleeds associated with CAA are not visible on CT, and are best detected as focal areas of signal dropout on T2*-GRE or 3D SWI MR sequences (**Fig. 4**). The widely used Boston criteria for the diagnosis of CAA rely heavily on the imaging features of both macro- and microhemorrhages when pathologic evidence is not available (**Table 2**).

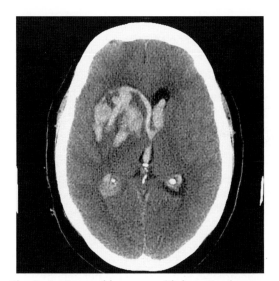

Fig. 3. A 48-year-old woman with hypertension presented with sudden onset of left hemiparesis and aphasia. There was ICH centered in the right lentiform nuclei with intraventricular extension.

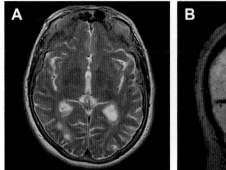 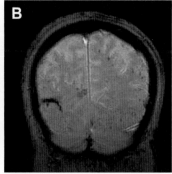

Fig. 4. A 69-year-old woman who had an episode of acute vision loss a few weeks previously. (*A*) Axial T2-weighted MR image shows subtle gyriform hypointense signal along the cortex of the right occipital lobe. (*B*) Coronal T2*-GRE reveals marked signal dropout at site of right occipital hemorrhage and many small foci of signal dropout compatible with amyloid microhemorrhage.

Secondary causes of ICH

In the setting of acute ICH, imaging becomes the primary tool for the detection or exclusion of many of the known secondary causes. Although some entities may have characteristic findings on unenhanced CT or MR according to a stroke protocol, multimodal evaluation including vascular evaluation and contrast enhancement can improve sensitivity for underlying lesions. The most common of the structural lesions that can result in ICH include vascular malformations, neoplasms, and hemorrhagic infarction.

Cerebral vascular malformations Four types of intracranial vascular malformations are classically described. In order from most to least common, these include developmental venous anomalies (DVA), arteriovenous malformations (AVM), capillary telangiectasias, and cavernous malformations (CM). Of these, AVMs and CMs have potential for hemorrhage, whereas DVA and capillary telangiectasia are generally considered benign.

AVM The prevalence of AVM in adults is about 0.2%, although they account for 4% of all primary

Table 2 Boston criteria for the diagnosis of CAA with ICH	
Definite CAA	Postmortem examination finding all 3 of 1. Lobar, cortical, or corticosubcortical hemorrhage, 2. Severe CAA 3. Absence of another causative lesion
Probable CAA with supporting pathologic evidence	Clinical data and pathologic specimen finding all 3 of 1. Lobar, cortical, or corticosubcortical hemorrhage 2. Some degree of vascular amyloid deposition in specimen 3. Absence of another causative lesion
Probable CAA	Clinical data and MR imaging finding all 3 of 1. Age ≥60 years 2. Multiple hemorrhages restricted to lobar, cortical, corticosubcortical regions 3. Absence of another causative lesion
Possible CAA	Clinical data and MR imaging findings: Age ≥60 years AND 1. Single lobar, cortical, or corticosubcortical hemorrhage without another cause OR 2. Multiple hemorrhages with possible but not definite cause or with some hemorrhages in atypical location

From Greenberg SM, Edgar MA. Case 22-1996- Cerebral hemorrhage in a 69-year-old woman receiving warfarin. N Engl J Med 1996;335(3):189–96; with permission.

ICH and up to one-third of all ICH in young adults. The risk of hemorrhage is about 2% per year in an unruptured AVM, and the risk for recurrent hemorrhage is as high as 18% in the first year.[30] AVMs are characterized by a connection between arterial and venous systems through a nidus of abnormal vascular channels without an intervening capillary bed. They typically consist of enlarged feeding arteries, a tightly packed vascular nidus consisting of shunt vessels with gliotic intervening brain parenchyma, and enlarged draining veins. Aneurysms may be present on feeding arteries or within the nidus. Pial arteriovenous fistulas are similar in many respects but lack the nidus present in AVM, and are much less common. Independent predictors for AVM hemorrhage include hemorrhagic presentation, advanced age, deep AVM location, and exclusively deep venous drainage.[31] Additional important features are those used by Spetzler and Martin in creating a 5-point grading system for the estimation of surgical resection risk (**Table 3**).

When hemorrhage is absent, CT reveals a mass lesion with the attenuation of the normal cerebral vessels, often accompanied by calcifications. However, after intracranial hemorrhage, the hematoma may obscure most or all of the AVM. Enlarged vessels nearby or calcifications within the hematoma are a clue to the presence of underlying AVM (**Fig. 5**). CTA typically reveals the vascular nidus and associated enlarged vessels. MR typically shows flow voids along the high-flow feeding and draining vessels as well as within the nidus itself. Recent advanced techniques using 3-T time-resolved MR angiography have shown 100% agreement with DSA in determining Spetzler-Martin grade.[32] Small AVMs or arteriovenous fistulae may not be visible on cross-sectional studies (**Fig. 6**) and DSA remains the gold standard for evaluation of underlying vascular anomaly in the setting of spontaneous ICH. Occasionally, delayed angiography can reveal vascular abnormalities that were not appreciable on initial imaging.[33] In the setting of a negative initial work-up in a young patient, a second evaluation should be undertaken once the mass effect from the hematoma has resolved.

CM The prevalence of CM is estimated to be between 0.3% and 0.6%.[34] The lesion is characterized by a cluster of thin-walled vessels without elastic fibers or smooth muscle, typically with a rim of hemosiderin-laden gliotic tissue. The latter is caused by chronic microhemorrhage, which is universal, although the risk of clinically significant de novo hemorrhage is relatively low, around 0.4% to 0.6% per year.[35,36] Most patients present with seizures or neurologic deficit.[34] In patients who have already presented with hemorrhage, the risk of rebleeding is increased, at 4.5% to 26% per year.[35,36] The hemorrhage of a CM has been found to be typically smaller in volume than AVM or dural arteriovenous fistula, and as a result these patients often present with less severe clinical symptoms[37] when the hemorrhage is not in the brainstem or spinal cord. The lesion itself typically appears isodense to slightly hyperdense on unenhanced CT and may contain calcifications. Faint or peripheral contrast enhancement is sometimes present, although not a reliable sign. MR imaging is the modality of choice for the detection of CM. Their classic appearance on T2-weighted imaging is that of a reticulated, or popcorn-like mass of variable signal intensity, caused by blood products in varying stages of evolution, with a hypointense hemosiderin rim (**Fig. 7**). Sequences with greater susceptibility weighting are more sensitive in detecting smaller lesions. In a population of patients with multiple CMs, 3D SWI detected 1.7 times as many lesions as T2*-GRE and 8 times as many as spin-echo T2 sequences.[38] Unlike the other vascular malformations, CMs are classically angiographically occult. If a CM is to be resected, contrast-enhanced CT or MR imaging should be performed to look for an associated DVA, which can be found in 8% to 33% of cases.[39] The inadvertent resection of all or part of a DVA along with a CM could result in venous infarction. The typical appearance of DVA on contrast-enhanced imaging is that of a stellate arrangement of tubular veins meeting in a collector vein that drains to a sinus or ependymal surface.[40]

Table 3 Spetzler-Martin grading scale for AVM[a]	
Graded Feature	**Points Assigned**
Size of AVM	
Small (<3 cm)	1
Medium (3–6 cm)	2
Large (>6 cm)	3
Eloquence of adjacent brain	
Noneloquent	0
Eloquent	1
Pattern of venous drainage	
Superficial only	0
Deep	1

[a] Grade = [size] + [eloquence] + [venous drainage]
From Spetzler RF, Martin NA. A proposed grading system for arteriovenous malformations. J Neurosurg 1986;65(4):476–83; with permission.

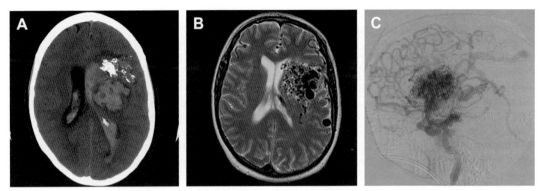

Fig. 5. A 59-year-old woman with known large AVM presented with dysarthria and ataxia. (*A*) NCT shows large left ICH with intraventricular extension. Irregular calcifications adjacent to blood suggest underlying vascular malformation. (*B*) Prehemorrhage T2-weighted MR shows many flow voids of varying sizes in the nidus of a large AVM. Large cortical and subependymal draining veins are present. (*C*) DSA with large left frontotemporal AVM and multiple large early draining veins.

Neoplasm Hemorrhage as a result of a primary or metastatic neoplasm accounts for 1% to 14% of ICH.[41] The propensity for bleeding varies by histologic tumor type; those most often presenting with macroscopic hemorrhage are listed in **Box 1**. The hemorrhage can be confined within the tumor or may extend into the brain parenchyma and other compartments. On unenhanced CT or MR imaging, the resultant hemorrhage appears similar to that from any other cause, although a few signs are believed to be suggestive of underlying neoplasm. Hematomas caused by tumor are

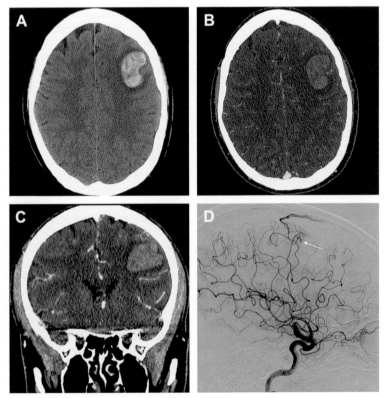

Fig. 6. A 45-year-old man with sudden onset of expressive aphasia. (*A*) NCT with left frontal ICH and small halo of surrounding edema. (*B, C*) Axial and coronal images from CTA were unrevealing for underlying vascular lesion. (*D*) DSA revealed a pial arteriovenous fistula fed by a tortuous middle cerebral artery branch with an early draining vein. A small aneurysm (*arrow*) is present near the fistulous site.

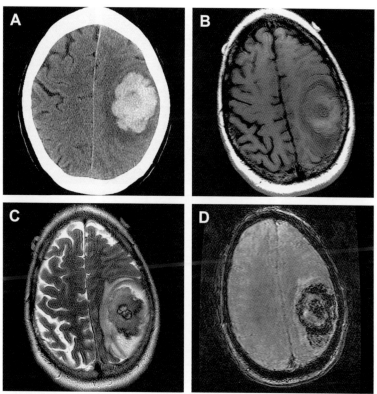

Fig. 7. A 47-year-old man with hypertension presents with 24 hours of headache, right-sided weakness, slurred speech and confusion. (*A*) NCT with large left frontal ICH and local mass effect. (*B*) T1-weighted MR with slightly hyperintense hematoma with relatively hypointense center. (*C*) T2-weighted MR with heterogeneous T2 prolongation and susceptibility-related signal loss. There is a central lobulated structure with peripheral rim and central popcorn hyperintensity, suspicious for cavernous malformation. (*D*) SWI MR with concentric areas of signal loss consistent with blood in different stages of evolution.

Box 1
Brain tumors likely to hemorrhage

Metastases (primary)
Melanoma
Lung
Kidney
Thyroid
Choriocarcinoma

Primary brain tumors
Pituitary adenoma
Glioblastoma/oligodendroglioma
Ependymoma/subependymoma
Peripheral neuroectodermal tumor
Epidermoid

Data From Osborn AG. Diagnostic neuroradiology. St Louis (MO): Mosby; 1994.

---

associated with a greater degree of surrounding vasogenic edema than nonneoplastic hematomas.[42] Neoplastic hematomas have been characterized as relatively more heterogeneous and have shown slower than expected degradation of blood products. An irregular or incomplete hemosiderin rim on MR may also be an indicator of underlying mass.[43] Complete evaluation should include contrast-enhanced imaging regardless of the imaging modality. Although minor enhancement may be present about subacute hematomas, it is rarely present acutely. The presence of any thick or nodular enhancement is suggestive of the presence of underlying neoplasm (**Fig. 8**). As in the case of vascular malformation, an underlying tumor can be obscured, particularly if it is small in relation to the hematoma size. Delayed imaging should be strongly considered in the case of a negative acute work-up.

Hemorrhagic infarction Hemorrhagic infarction (HI), also referred to as hemorrhagic transformation of an infarct, typically refers to bleeding into

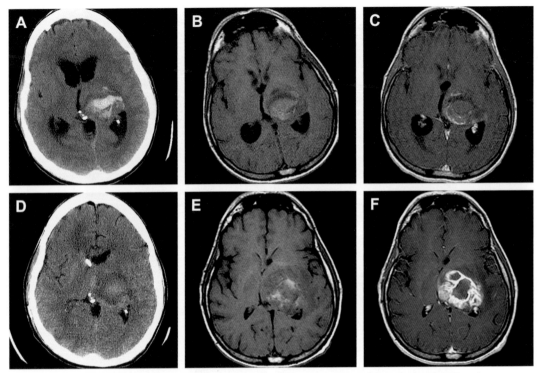

Fig. 8. A 42-year-old man with sudden onset right hemiparesis and slurring of speech. (*A, B*) NCT and noncontrast T1-weighted MR imaging with irregular left thalamic hematoma. (*C*) Post-Gd T1-weighted MR with incomplete peripheral enhancement that is nodular in areas. (*D*) 6-week follow-up NCT with decreasing density of blood products. (*E, F*) T1-weighted pre- and postcontrast MR revealed an irregular enhancing mass markedly increased in size. Pathology confirmed glioblastoma multiforme.

an area of preexisting arterial ischemia. An early prospective study identified HI in 43% of infarcts,[44] and depending on the investigative modality, incidence has been reported to be as high as 85%.[45] These hemorrhages tend to occur in 2 patterns: petechial hemorrhage and parenchymal hematoma.[46] Petechial hemorrhage is of little clinical significance by itself and whether it should alter plans for anticoagulation is questionable, whereas in parenchymal hematomas more than 30% of the ischemic area correlated with clinical deterioration and poor outcome.[47] HI usually occurs around the second week following infarct when presenting spontaneously; early hemorrhagic transformation is more common in the setting of thrombolysis and mechanical clot retrieval.

The CT appearance of petechial hemorrhage is that of subtle increased density with indistinct margins, with the density sometimes appearing speckled or punctate. Signal intensity may vary on spin-echo MR imaging, but characteristic signal dropout is seen on T2*-weighted sequences. On both CT and MR imaging there is a strong predilection for petechial hemorrhage to occur primarily in gray matter structures (**Fig. 9**). Parenchymal hematoma secondary to ischemia can be difficult to distinguish from other causes of ICH on CT and MR imaging. The distinction is most often made by history because the infarction usually precedes hemorrhagic transformation by at least a few days. This reinforces the need for timely initial imaging. In some cases it is possible to distinguish a larger area of cytotoxic edema affecting white matter and cortex outside the area of hematoma. As with other types of hemorrhage, MR performance is markedly improved with the inclusion of diffusion-weighted imaging and susceptibility-weighted sequences, which when used detect both infarction and hemorrhage with greater frequency than CT.[48] The clinical value of this improved sensitivity in the setting of ischemia remains as yet uncertain. Most treatment studies to date have used CT findings. HI in the setting of thrombolytic therapy for ischemia remains an area of great clinical interest. There have been significant efforts to identify pretreatment imaging characteristics that may help to predict the incidence or severity of treatment-related hemorrhage.[49–51]

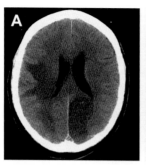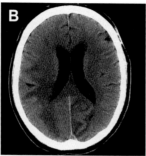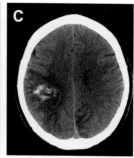

Fig. 9. A 56-year-old man status post trauma with known right parietal contusion, developed left gaze preference and right-sided neglect. (*A*) NCT with well-demarcated left occipital infarction. (*B*) NCT 5 days later with new hyperattenuation in cortical pattern, consistent with petechial hemorrhage. (*C*) NCT with known right parietal parenchymal contusion; note preservation of overlying cortical ribbon.

Other secondary causes of ICH

There are a large number of other rarer causes of acute ICH. These disorders include cerebral aneurysm, venous sinus thrombosis, septic embolism, bleeding dyscrasia, supratherapeutic anticoagulation, thrombolytic therapy, CNS infection, mycotic aneurysm, moyamoya, vasculitis, and vasoactive drugs. Often these entities are only suspected because of key features in the patients' clinical history. Sometimes they may be suspected from imaging findings.

Cerebral aneurysm Although most aneurysm ruptures result in SAH, up to 34% are associated with ICH,[52] and 1 series found that 1.6% of aneurysm ruptures result in ICH without SAH.[53] Such cases likely result from rupture of aneurysms that are pointed into or embedded in cerebral parenchyma. Ruptured aneurysm is a treatable cause of intracranial hemorrhage, and studies have shown that early treatment results in better outcomes. Furthermore, conservative management of ICH from a ruptured aneurysm has been associated with mortality of greater than 80%.[54] Whenever the hematoma extends from the base of the brain, and particularly when SAH is also present, rupture of a berry aneurysm should be considered in the differential diagnosis for ICH. In this setting, additional imaging to evaluate for aneurysm should be considered; both CTA and MR angiography (MRA) are reasonable alternatives. The imaging features specific to cerebral aneurysms are discussed in the section on subarachnoid hemorrhage.

Venous sinus thrombosis Thrombosis of the intracerebral veins or dural sinuses has an estimated incidence of 3 to 4 cases per 1 million adults, with 75% of cases presenting in women.[55] In the largest series to date, 39% were found to have associated hemorrhage.[56] The imaging appearance of the hematoma itself can be nonspecific, thus the identification of secondary signs is essential to making this diagnosis. A hyperattenuating cortical or deep vein adjacent to the hematoma had greater than 97% specificity in 1 retrospective study.[57] Contrast-enhanced CT may show the empty delta sign representing nonenhancing thrombus in involved sinuses.[58] Associated edema often precedes hemorrhage, follows venous rather than arterial distributions, and is generally greater than that seen with primary ICH.

MR sequences such as T2 or FLAIR may be better able to demonstrate parenchymal edema or ischemia. Venous thrombus has classically been described as T1 hyperintense, although the signal characteristics can vary considerably over time and may be confusing.[59] In the larger dural sinuses, the presence of uniform T1 isotense or T1 hyperintense signal is suggestive of thrombus, particularly when sinus expansion is present. Time-of-flight MR venography improves detection of sinus thrombus, although pitfalls in interpretation remain as a result of in-plane signal dropout mimicking thrombosis and T1 bright thrombus mimicking flow. Contrast-enhanced and four-dimensional MR venography techniques[60] as well as CT venography further improve diagnostic accuracy.

Dural arteriovenous fistula Dural arteriovenous fistulae (DAVFs) make up about 10% of all intracranial arteriovenous shunting malformations.[61] This lesion consists of a direct connection between dural arteries and dural veins without intervening vasculature. Unlike AVMs, they are believed to be acquired lesions secondary to trauma, surgery, infection, or venous sinus thrombosis. They produce intracranial venous hypertension and, when this becomes sufficiently severe, ICH.[62]

Male sex, posterior fossa location and advanced age are risk factors for hemorrhage.[63] These lesions are typically difficult to see on noncontrast CT, although enlarged veins or transosseous channels may be visible. Standard MR imaging also has poor sensitivity for this entity although dilated cortical veins and sinus thrombosis may be detected.[64] Time-of-flight MRA improves depiction of arterial feeders and fistula site.[65] One study using time-resolved contrast-enhanced MRA at 3 T yielded 100% concordance with DSA in identification of fistula site and venous collaterals although only 68% agreement for main arterial feeders.[66] As with AVM, DSA remains the gold standard for both detection and characterization of DAVF. In a young patient with ICH of uncertain cause, DAVF should be specifically sought with selective injection of vessels supplying the dural vasculature.

Specific Factors for Management Considerations

Hematoma size

There are imaging features of acute ICH that are helpful in managing patients and predicting neurologic outcomes. The location of hemorrhage and involvement of vital structures are strong predictors of outcome and influence the use of surgical decompression. For example, posterior fossa hemorrhage carries a worse prognosis and more often requires surgical decompression. The total volume of ICH is a strong predictor of 30-day mortality, particularly when combined with the presenting Glasgow Coma Scale score.[67] Hematoma volume can be quickly estimated on cross-sectional imaging by using the ABC/2 method, where A is the maximum hematoma diameter, B is the diameter measured at 90° to A, and C is the approximate number of slices containing hematoma multiplied by the slice thickness.[68]

Although outcomes generally worsen with increasing clot size, those measuring more than 60 cm^3 in particular have been found to correlate with poor outcomes.[67] The proximity of the clot to the cerebral surface does seem to influence the relative outcomes of nonsurgical management versus decompression; clots within 1 cm of the cerebral surface had better outcomes with surgical decompression.[69]

Hematoma expansion

In addition to size at presentation, the possibility of ongoing bleeding and hematoma expansion affects outcomes and may guide therapeutic intervention. The incidence of substantial enlargement of an ICH is controversial with some studies suggesting that it is relatively common, occurring in 38% of patients within the first 24 hours in 1 prospective series,[70] whereas other work has suggested that expansion after 24 hours is rare.[71] Early expansion of a hematoma has been shown to increase the risk of mortality and poor functional outcome, with each 10% increase in hematoma size resulting in a 5% increased hazard of death and 16% likelihood of worsening on the modified Rankin scale of functional outcomes.[72] These data suggest that repeat imaging is warranted for the detection of hematoma expansion. Imaging findings that predict expansion may also identify the patients most likely to benefit from such interventions as Factor VII infusion.

CTA spot sign

The presence of a 1- to 2-mm focus of intense enhancement within a hematoma on the CTA source images has been labeled the spot sign (Fig. 10). It is believed to represent the presence of a small pseudoaneurysm or active extravasation. This finding on CTA performed within 3 hours

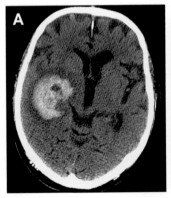 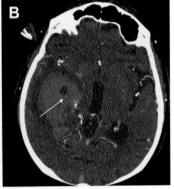

Fig. 10. A 98-year-old man on warfarin presented with confusion. (A) NCT with heterogeneous right basal ganglia hemorrhage extending to temporal lobe. (B) CTA with punctate focus of hyperattenuation within hematoma (arrow) not contiguous with another vessel: the spot sign.

of symptom onset was independently predictive of hematoma enlargement.[73] A contrast-enhanced head CT immediately after the CTA may demonstrate contrast leakage; that is, the delayed spot sign, and when this finding is added to the CTA spot sign, sensitivity and negative predictive value for predicting hematoma expansion are improved.[74]

Another study included CTAs obtained any time within 24 hours of admission and included both the spot sign and the delayed spot sign if an immediate contrast-enhanced CT was obtained. Three factors were found to be independent predictors of hematoma expansion, including the number of spot signs, the maximum axial dimension of the spot(s), and the maximum attenuation of the largest spot.[75] These were incorporated into a spot sign score, and although this has not yet been independently validated, it has the potential to serve as a predictor of hematoma expansion in ICH independent from other factors such as time of symptom onset and hematoma volume. A second review of the same cohort found that the spot sign score also served as an independent predictor of in-hospital mortality and poor functional outcome among survivors at 3 months.[76]

Intraventricular hemorrhage

A hematoma originating near a CSF space can spontaneously decompress into the adjacent intraventricular or subarachnoid space. The propensity for intraventricular spread is dependent on the size of the hematoma as well as its location.[77] Intraventricular extension of ICH has been correlated with poor functional outcome and increased mortality in several studies,[77,78] and has been incorporated into models for prediction of outcomes.[79,80] The association seems to be more robust when some measure of the volume or degree of IVH is used, as several studies using a binary variable for the presence or absence of intraventricular blood have failed to show a strong association with worsened outcomes.[79,81,82] The presence of hydrocephalus in the setting of intraventricular hematoma extension is a separate predictor of poor outcome.[83]

SAH
Epidemiology

Slightly less common than ICH, SAH accounts for between 3% and 5% of all strokes.[9,84] Much like ICH, outcomes following SAH are poor, with observed 30-day mortality in the range of 33% to 45%.[85,86] Most deaths caused by SAH occur early in the time course of the disease, with 61% of deaths occurring within 2 days of the initial event.[86]

Imaging Technique and Findings

Noncontrast CT is highly sensitive for SAH in the acute and subacute settings. The typical appearance of acute SAH is that of high attenuation material conforming to the subarachnoid space. It may be localized or diffuse and is present within the sulci, fissures, or basal cisterns. Initial sensitivity is 98% within 12 hours of symptom onset.[87] This decreases over time, dropping to 93% 24 hours after onset[88] and continuing to decline thereafter as a result of dilution and evolution of blood products that combine to result in decreasing density. A negative CT should reliably exclude larger volume SAH such as that from an aneurysm rupture, but lumbar puncture with CSF analysis remains the standard with which CT is compared, and is strongly recommended to exclude a CT-negative SAH such as might be seen from a sentinel bleed. Current guidelines recommend prompt CT scanning for the suspicion of SAH with strong consideration for lumbar puncture to follow if the CT is negative.[84]

MR has demonstrated added value in the diagnosis of subacute SAH. Hyperacute blood products in the subarachnoid space should appear hyperintense on T1- and proton density–weighted images as a result of the increased protein content. Similarly, the signal in blood-containing CSF fails to null on FLAIR sequences resulting in hyperintense signal in the affected CSF spaces (**Fig. 11**). When compared against CT, FLAIR and proton density–weighted sequences have been found equally sensitive for the detection of SAH less than 12 hours from symptom onset.[89] The sensitivity of FLAIR imaging does not seem to drop off nearly as quickly as CT, and FLAIR remains more sensitive than CT in the first 2 weeks.[90,91] The use of FLAIR in the diagnosis of SAH is limited by its low specificity (other CSF alterations from infection or increased protein content produce similar signal changes) and the presence of flow-related artifacts about the brainstem. Like CT, negative MR does not reliably exclude low volume or dilute SAH, because a review of patients with SAH who had negative CT and positive lumbar puncture showed FLAIR sensitivity of less than 20%.[92]

Causes of SAH

Aneurysm rupture

The most common cause of spontaneous SAH is the rupture of a cerebral aneurysm, accounting for about 85% of SAHs.[93] Cerebral aneurysms are present in about 2% of asymptomatic adults.[94] Saccular aneurysms tend to occur at branch points along cerebral vessels, whether at

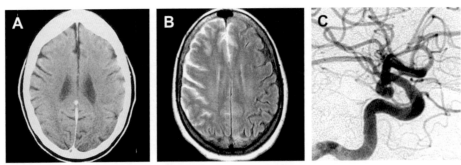

Fig. 11. A 69-year-old woman with intermittent severe headache of several days duration. (*A*) NCT was read as normal with no evidence of increased density in the subarachnoid space. (*B*) FLAIR MR imaging with marked hyperintensity of the CSF in the anterior interhemispheric fissure and sulci over the right cerebral convexity. (*C*) DSA with lobulated right posterior communicating artery aneurysm.

a bifurcation or the origin of a side branch.[95] Most aneurysms (80%–85%) are located in the anterior circulation, commonly at the origins of the posterior or anterior communicating arteries or the middle cerebral artery bifurcation; posterior circulation aneurysms are most often seen at the basilar tip or posterior-inferior cerebellar artery origin.[96] The annual risk of rupture for any given aneurysm is about 0.7%. Rupture risk is predicted by aneurysm size and location, with risk increasing significantly for aneurysms greater than 7 mm in diameter, and an increased rupture risk for those arising from the posterior communicating arteries or posterior cerebral circulation.[97]

When spontaneous SAH is detected, the next steps of the imaging work-up are directed toward detecting a ruptured aneurysm or other underlying cause. The pattern of SAH at presentation can be of predictive value in localizing an aneurysm. For example, a ruptured anterior cerebral artery aneurysm is associated with a substantial amount of blood in the interhemispheric fissure. Hemorrhage pattern may be less helpful for other aneurysm locations.[98] In some cases the aneurysm can be identified directly on unenhanced imaging (**Fig. 12**). On CT an aneurysm may appear as a rounded or lobulated mass within the hematoma. The presence of mural calcification can help to locate an underlying aneurysm, and portions may be of high attenuation when there is intra-aneurysmal thrombus. Some aneurysms may be detected on MR as a flow void or a mass with flow-related artifact in the phase-encoding direction.

Aneurysm detection is markedly improved with the use of dedicated vascular imaging in either modality. Review articles quote a sensitivity and specificity of CTA in the range of 77% to 100%.[84,93] Sensitivity nears 100% for aneurysm greater than 3 mm in size, although accuracy is reduced in the case of small aneurysms or

tortuous vessels. MRA has shown similar sensitivities (85%–100%) for aneurysms greater than 5 mm, although dropping to 56% less than that size.[84] MRA at 3 T has shown promising results with 100% sensitivity and greater than 95% accuracy compared with rotational DSA.[99] DSA has been the gold standard for vascular evaluation for some time, although recent studies have shown further improvements in aneurysm detection with the addition of planar and 3D reconstructions derived from a 3D rotational acquisition.[100]

In the patient presenting to the emergency room, the most common cause of SAH is

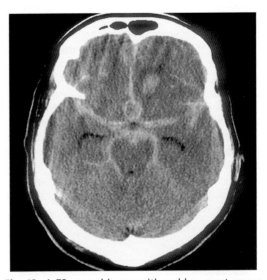

Fig. 12. A 72-year-old man with sudden onset severe headache and confusion. NCT reveals diffuse subarachnoid hemorrhage filling the basal cisterns, interhemispheric fissure, and Sylvian fissures. A filling defect at the posterior aspect of the interhemispheric fissure was found to be an anterior communicating artery aneurysm. Also note the small intraparenchymal hematoma in the inferior left frontal lobe.

craniospinal trauma. In most cases, the history is clear and the extent of SAH is small. In cases where SAH is prominent and the history of the injury suggests the possibility that the SAH may have occurred first (and caused the trauma), a full evaluation for aneurysm is necessary.

Nonaneurysmal SAH

There are a variety of other conditions that can result in nontraumatic SAH, all of which are rare compared with aneurysmal SAH. There is some overlap with lesions that can result in ICH, and entities include intracranial or spinal vascular malformations, neoplasm, primary vasculopathy, drug abuse, sickle cell anemia, coagulopathies, and pituitary apoplexy. Relevant clinical history can be helpful in establishing the correct diagnosis in many of these settings.

An important entity not included in this list is non-aneurysmal perimesencephalic SAH. Accounting for between 21% and 68% of angiography-negative SAH,[101] this is a specific entity first described in 1985, with a characteristic distribution of subarachnoid blood, negative angiographic work-up, and a generally benign clinical course. The pattern of blood seen by CT or MR imaging is SAH centered immediately anterior to the midbrain. This may or may not extend to the anterior part of the ambient cistern or the basal portions of the Sylvian fissure.[102] Furthermore, there can be no other identifiable source of hemorrhage on cross-sectional or angiographic imaging. The presentation of this subgroup is typically indistinguishable from other types of SAH, but their prognosis is excellent. Rates of recurrent hemorrhage, hydrocephalus, and vasospasm are low and good outcomes were seen in 100%, compared with 88% of other patients with SAH who were angiography negative and 64% of patients with aneurysmal SAH.[101]

Prognostic Indicators

There are several factors that can be evaluated at the time of SAH presentation and used to direct immediate management or predict clinical outcomes. Acute hydrocephalus, usually in the setting of IVH, is a surgical emergency requiring ventriculostomy decompression. Aneurysm location and morphology are used to guide the treatment algorithm; each aneurysm requires careful review by an experienced cerebrovascular team to determine optimum treatment. Features such as branches arising from the aneurysm dome and difficult endovascular access favor surgical clipping, whereas difficult surgical access, presence of nearby perforating arteries, and neck calcification favor endovascular treatment. The

Hunt and Hess grading scale is based on neurologic status at presentation and underlying medical comorbidities, and is used to estimate the mortality of aneurysmal SAH.[103] A grading scale developed by Fisher and colleagues[104] uses findings on the noncontrast CT at presentation, such as thickness of SAH, the presence of subarachnoid blood clots, and intraventricular or intracerebral extension to predict the likelihood of cerebral vasospasm.

SUMMARY

The timely and accurate identification of hemorrhagic stroke is essential in the clinical management of patients presenting with acute stroke symptoms. Cross-sectional imaging should be readily available and initial protocols should include unenhanced head CT or dedicated stroke protocol MR imaging including blood-sensitive T2* or 3D SWI and FLAIR sequences. When detected, the appearance and location of hemorrhage can help to narrow the differential diagnosis, direct additional advanced imaging, guide immediate management, and provide early prognostic information with regard to patient outcomes.

REFERENCES

1. Broderick J, Connolly S, Feldmann E, et al. Guidelines for the management of spontaneous intracerebral hemorrhage in adults: 2007 update: a guideline from the American Heart Association/American Stroke Association Stroke Council, High Blood Pressure Research Council, and the Quality of Care and Outcomes in Research Interdisciplinary Working Group: The American Academy of Neurology affirms the value of this guideline as an educational tool for neurologists. Stroke 2007; 38(6):2001–23.

2. Adams HP, del Zoppo G, Alberts MJ, et al. Guidelines for the early management of adults with ischemic stroke: a guideline from the American Heart Association/American Stroke Association Stroke Council, Clinical Cardiology Council, Cardiovascular Radiology and Intervention Council, and the Atherosclerotic Peripheral Vascular Disease and Quality of Care Outcomes in Research Interdisciplinary Working Groups: The American Academy of Neurology affirms the value of this guideline as an educational tool for neurologists. Stroke 2007;38(5):1655–711.

3. Adams HP, Adams RJ, Brott T, et al. Guidelines for the early management of patients with ischemic stroke: a scientific statement from the Stroke Council of the American Stroke Association. Stroke 2003;34(4):1056–83.

4. Singer OC, Sitzer M, du Mesnil de Rochemont R, et al. Practical limitations of acute stroke MRI due to patient-related problems. Neurology 2004;62(10): 1848–9.

5. Wardlaw JM, Seymour J, Cairns J, et al. Immediate computed tomography scanning of acute stroke is cost-effective and improves quality of life. Stroke 2004;35(11):2477–83.

6. Parizel PM, Makkat S, Miert EV, et al. Intracranial hemorrhage: principles of CT and MRI interpretation. Eur Radiol 2001;11(9):1770–83.

7. Osborn AG. Diagnostic neuroradiology. St. Louis (MO): Mosby; 1994.

8. Alemany Ripoll M, Stenborg A, Sonninen P, et al. Detection and appearance of intraparenchymal haematomas of the brain at 1.5 T with spin-echo, FLAIR and GE sequences: poor relationship to the age of the haematoma. Neuroradiology 2004; 46(6):435–43.

9. Lloyd-Jones D, Adams RJ, Brown TM, et al. Heart disease and stroke statistics—2010 update. A report from the American Heart Association. Circulation 2010;121:e46–215.

10. Counsell C, Boonyakarnkul S, Dennis M, et al. Primary intracerebral haemorrhage in the Oxford-shire Community Stroke Project. Cerebrovasc Dis 1995;5(1):26–34.

11. Andersen KK, Olsen TS, Dehlendorff C, et al. Hemorrhagic and ischemic strokes compared: stroke severity, mortality, and risk factors. Stroke 2009;40(6):2068–72.

12. Marshall WH, Easter W, Zatz LM. Analysis of the dense lesion at computed tomography with dual kVp scans. Radiology 1977;124(1):87–9.

13. Kreel L, Kay R, Woo J, et al. The radiological (CT) and clinical sequelae of primary intracerebral haemorrhage. Br J Radiol 1991;64(768):1096–100.

14. Liang L, Korogi Y, Sugahara T, et al. Detection of intracranial hemorrhage with susceptibility-weighted MR sequences. AJNR Am J Neuroradiol 1999;20(8):1527–34.

15. Patel MR, Edelman RR, Warach S. Detection of hyperacute primary intraparenchymal hemorrhage by magnetic resonance imaging. Stroke 1996;27(12):2321–4.

16. Schellinger PD, Jansen O, Fiebach JB, et al. A standardized MRI stroke protocol: comparison with CT in hyperacute intracerebral hemorrhage. Stroke 1999;30(4):765–8.

17. Kidwell CS, Chalela JA, Saver JL, et al. Comparison of MRI and CT for detection of acute intracerebral hemorrhage. JAMA 2004;292(15):1823–30.

18. Fiebach JB, Schellinger PD, Gass A, et al. Stroke magnetic resonance imaging is accurate in hyperacute intracerebral hemorrhage: a multicenter study on the validity of stroke imaging. Stroke 2004;35(2):502–6.

19. Reichenbach JR, Venkatesan R, Schillinger DJ, et al. Small vessels in the human brain: MR venography with deoxyhemoglobin as an intrinsic contrast agent. Radiology 1997;204(1):272–7.

20. Nandigam R, Viswanathan A, Delgado P, et al. MR imaging detection of cerebral microbleeds: effect of susceptibility-weighted imaging, section thickness, and field strength. AJNR Am J Neuroradiol 2009;30(2):338–43.

21. Wycliffe ND, Choe J, Holshouser B, et al. Reliability in detection of hemorrhage in acute stroke by a new three-dimensional gradient recalled echo susceptibility-weighted imaging technique compared to computed tomography: a retrospective study. J Magn Reson Imaging 2004;20(3):372–7.

22. Bozzola FG, Gorelick PB, Jensen JM. Epidemiology of intracranial hemorrhage. Neuroimaging Clin N Am 1992;2(1):1–10.

23. Ellison D, Love S. Hemorrhage. In: Ellison D, Love S, Chimelli L, et al, editors. Neuropathology. London: Mosby; 1998. p. 10–3.

24. Wakai S, Kumakura N, Nagai M. Lobar intracerebral hemorrhage. J Neurosurg 1992;76(2):231–8.

25. Broderick J, Brott T, Tomsick T, et al. Lobar hemorrhage in the elderly. The undiminishing importance of hypertension. Stroke 1993;24(1):49–51.

26. Jackson CA, Sudlow CL. Is hypertension a more frequent risk factor for deep than for lobar supratentorial intracerebral haemorrhage? J Neurol Neurosurg Psychiatry 2006;77(11):1244–52.

27. Fazekas F, Kleinert R, Roob G, et al. Histopathologic analysis of foci of signal loss on gradient-echo T2*-weighted MR images in patients with spontaneous intracerebral hemorrhage: evidence of microangiopathy-related microbleeds. AJNR Am J Neuroradiol 1999;20(4):637–42.

28. Vinters H. Cerebral amyloid angiopathy. A critical review. Stroke 1987;18(2):311–24.

29. Rosand J, Muzikansky A, Kumar A, et al. Spatial clustering of hemorrhages in probable cerebral amyloid angiopathy. Ann Neurol 2005;58(3): 459–62.

30. Al-Shahi R, Warlow C. A systematic review of the frequency and prognosis of arteriovenous malformations of the brain in adults. Brain 2001;124(10): 1900–26.

31. Stapf C, Mast H, Sciacca R, et al. Predictors of hemorrhage in patients with untreated brain arteriovenous malformation. Neurology 2006;66(9):1350–5.

32. Hadizadeh DR, von Falkenhausen M, Gieseke J, et al. Cerebral arteriovenous malformation: Spetzler-Martin classification at subsecond-temporal-resolution four-dimensional MR angiography compared with that at DSA1. Radiology 2008;246(1):205–13.

33. Willinsky RA, Fitzgerald M, TerBrugge K, et al. Delayed angiography in the investigation of

intracerebral hematomas caused by small arteriovenous malformations. Neuroradiology 1993;35(4):307–11.

34. Raychaudhuri R, Batjer HH, Awad IA. Intracranial cavernous angioma: a practical review of clinical and biological aspects. Surg Neurol 2005;63(4):319–28.

35. Aiba T, Tanaka R, Koike T, et al. Natural history of intracranial cavernous malformations. J Neurosurg 1995;83(1):56–9.

36. Kondziolka D, Lunsford LD, Kestle JR. The natural history of cerebral cavernous malformations. J Neurosurg 1995;83(5):820–4.

37. Cordonnier C, Salman RA, Bhattacharya JJ, et al. Differences between intracranial vascular malformation types in the characteristics of their presenting haemorrhages: prospective, population-based study. J Neurol Neurosurg Psychiatry 2008;79(1):47–51.

38. de Souza J, Domingues R, Cruz L, et al. Susceptibility-weighted imaging for the evaluation of patients with familial cerebral cavernous malformations: a comparison with T2-weighted fast spin-echo and gradient-echo sequences. AJNR Am J Neuroradiol 2008;29(1):154–8.

39. Rammos S, Maina R, Lanzino G. Developmental venous anomalies: current concepts and implications for management. Neurosurgery 2009;65(1):20–9 [Review] [100 refs].

40. Lee C, Pennington M, Kenney C. MR evaluation of developmental venous anomalies: medullary venous anatomy of venous angiomas. AJNR Am J Neuroradiol 1996;17(1):61–70.

41. Destian S, Sze G, Krol G, et al. MR imaging of hemorrhagic intracranial neoplasms. AJR Am J Roentgenol 1989;152(1):137–44.

42. Tung GA, Julius BD, Rogg JM. MRI of intracerebral hematoma: value of vasogenic edema ratio for predicting the cause. Neuroradiology 2003;45(6):357–62.

43. Atlas SW, Grossman RI, Gomori JM, et al. Hemorrhagic intracranial malignant neoplasms: spin-echo MR imaging. Radiology 1987;164(1):71–7.

44. Hornig C, Dorndorf W, Agnoli A. Hemorrhagic cerebral infarction—a prospective study. Stroke 1986;17(2):179–85.

45. Mayer TE, Schulte-Altedorneburg G, Droste DW, et al. Serial CT and MRI of ischaemic cerebral infarcts: frequency and clinical impact of haemorrhagic transformation. Neuroradiology 2000;42(4):233–9.

46. Wolpert S, Bruckmann H, Greenlee R, et al. Neuroradiologic evaluation of patients with acute stroke treated with recombinant tissue plasminogen activator. The rt-PA Acute Stroke Study Group. AJNR Am J Neuroradiol 1993;14(1):3–13.

47. Berger C, Fiorelli M, Steiner T, et al. Hemorrhagic transformation of ischemic brain tissue: asymptomatic or symptomatic? Stroke 2001;32(6):1330–5.

48. Arnould M, Grandin CB, Peeters A, et al. Comparison of CT and three MR sequences for detecting and categorizing early (48 hours) hemorrhagic transformation in hyperacute ischemic stroke. AJNR Am J Neuroradiol 2004;25(6):939–44.

49. The National Institute of Neurological Disorders and Stroke rt-PA Stroke Study Group. Tissue plasminogen activator for acute ischemic stroke. N Engl J Med 1995;333(24):1581–8.

50. Hacke W, Kaste M, Fieschi C, et al. Randomised double-blind placebo-controlled trial of thrombolytic therapy with intravenous alteplase in acute ischaemic stroke (ECASS II). Lancet 1998;352(9136):1245–51.

51. Furlan A, Higashida R, Wechsler L, et al. Intra-arterial prourokinase for acute ischemic stroke: the PROACT II Study: a randomized controlled trial. JAMA 1999;282(21):2003–11.

52. Pasqualin A, Bazzan A, Cavazzani P, et al. Intracranial hematomas following aneurysmal rupture: experience with 309 cases. Surg Neurol 1986;25(1):6–17.

53. Thai Q, Raza SM, Pradilla G, et al. Aneurysmal rupture without subarachnoid hemorrhage: case series and literature review. Neurosurgery 2005;57(2):225–9.

54. Niemann DB, Wills AD, Maartens NF, et al. Treatment of intracerebral hematomas caused by aneurysm rupture: coil placement followed by clot evacuation. J Neurosurg 2003;99(5):843–7.

55. Stam J. Thrombosis of the cerebral veins and sinuses. N Engl J Med 2005;352(17):1791–8.

56. Ferro JM, Canhao P, Stam J, et al. Prognosis of cerebral vein and dural sinus thrombosis: results of the International Study on Cerebral Vein and Dural Sinus Thrombosis (ISCVT). Stroke 2004;35(3):664–70.

57. Linn J, Pfefferkorn T, Ivanicova K, et al. Noncontrast CT in deep cerebral venous thrombosis and sinus thrombosis: comparison of its diagnostic value for both entities. AJNR Am J Neuroradiol 2009;30(4):728–35.

58. Virapongse C, Cazenave C, Quisling R, et al. The empty delta sign: frequency and significance in 76 cases of dural sinus thrombosis. Radiology 1987;162(3):779–85.

59. Leach JL, Fortuna RB, Jones BV, et al. Imaging of cerebral venous thrombosis: current techniques, spectrum of findings, and diagnostic pitfalls1. Radiographics 2006;26(Suppl 1):S19–41.

60. Meckel S, Reisinger C, Bremerich J, et al. Cerebral venous thrombosis: diagnostic accuracy of combined, dynamic and static, contrast-enhanced

4D MR venography. AJNR Am J Neuroradiol 2010; 31(3):527–35.

61. Newton TH, Cronqvist S. Involvement of dural arteries in intracranial arteriovenous malformations. Radiology 1969;93(5):1071–8.

62. Cognard C, Gobin YP, Pierot L, et al. Cerebral dural arteriovenous fistulas: clinical and angiographic correlation with a revised classification of venous drainage. Radiology 1995;194(3):671–80.

63. Singh V, Smith WS, Lawton MT, et al. Risk factors for hemorrhagic presentation in patients with dural arteriovenous fistulae. Neurosurgery 2008;62(3): 628–35.

64. De Marco JK, Dillon WP, Halback VV, et al. Dural arteriovenous fistulas: evaluation with MR imaging. Radiology 1990;175(1):193–9.

65. Chen JC, Tsuruda JS, Halbach VV. Suspected dural arteriovenous fistula: results with screening MR angiography in seven patients. Radiology 1992; 183(1):265–71.

66. Nishimura S, Hirai T, Sasao A, et al. Evaluation of dural arteriovenous fistulas with 4D contrast-enhanced MR angiography at 3T. AJNR Am J Neuroradiol 2010;31(1):80–5.

67. Broderick J, Brott T, Duldner J, et al. Volume of intracerebral hemorrhage. A powerful and easy-to-use predictor of 30-day mortality. Stroke 1993; 24(7):987–93.

68. Kothari RU, Brott T, Broderick JP, et al. The ABCs of measuring intracerebral hemorrhage volumes. Stroke 1996;27(8):1304–5.

69. Mendelow AD, Gregson BA, Fernandes HM, et al. Early surgery versus initial conservative treatment in patients with spontaneous supratentorial intracerebral haematomas in the International Surgical Trial in Intracerebral Haemorrhage (STICH): a randomised trial. Lancet 2005;365(9457):387–97.

70. Brott T, Broderick J, Kothari R, et al. Early hemorrhage growth in patients with intracerebral hemorrhage. Stroke 1997;28(1):1–5.

71. Kazui S, Naritomi H, Yamamoto H, et al. Enlargement of spontaneous intracerebral hemorrhage: incidence and time course. Stroke 1996;27(10):1783–7.

72. Davis SM. Hematoma growth is a determinant of mortality and poor outcome after intracerebral hemorrhage. Neurology 2006;66(8):1175–81.

73. Wada R, Aviv RI, Fox AJ, et al. CT angiography "spot sign" predicts hematoma expansion in acute intracerebral hemorrhage. Stroke 2007;38(4):1257–62.

74. Ederies A, Demchuk A, Chia T, et al. Postcontrast CT extravasation is associated with hematoma expansion in CTA spot negative patients. Stroke 2009;40(5):1672–6.

75. Delgado Almandoz JE, Yoo AJ, Stone MJ, et al. Systematic characterization of the computed tomography angiography spot sign in primary intracerebral hemorrhage identifies patients at highest risk for hematoma expansion: the spot sign score. Stroke 2009;40(9):2994–3000.

76. Delgado Almandoz JE, Yoo AJ, Stone MJ, et al. The spot sign score in primary intracerebral hemorrhage identifies patients at highest risk of in-hospital mortality and poor outcome among survivors. Stroke 2010;41(1):54–60.

77. Hallevi H, Albright KC, Aronowski J, et al. Intraventricular hemorrhage: anatomic relationships and clinical implications. Neurology 2008;70(11):848–52.

78. Tuhrim S, Horowitz DR, Sacher M, et al. Volume of ventricular blood is an important determinant of outcome in supratentorial intracerebral hemorrhage. Crit Care Med 1999;27(3):617–21.

79. Lisk DR, Pasteur W, Rhoades H, et al. Early presentation of hemispheric intracerebral hemorrhage: prediction of outcome and guidelines for treatment allocation. Neurology 1994;44(1):133.

80. Portenoy RK, Lipton RB, Berger AR, et al. Intracerebral haemorrhage: a model for the prediction of outcome. J Neurol Neurosurg Psychiatry 1987;50(8):976–9.

81. Rost NS, Smith EE, Chang Y, et al. Prediction of functional outcome in patients with primary intracerebral hemorrhage: the FUNC score. Stroke 2008; 39(8):2304–9.

82. Tuhrim S, Horowitz DR, Sacher M, et al. Validation and comparison of models predicting survival following intracerebral hemorrhage. Crit Care Med 1995;23(5):950–4.

83. Diringer MN, Edwards DF, Zazulia AR. Hydrocephalus: a previously unrecognized predictor of poor outcome from supratentorial intracerebral hemorrhage. Stroke 1998;29(7):1352–7.

84. Bederson JB, Connolly ES, Batjer HH, et al. Guidelines for the management of aneurysmal subarachnoid hemorrhage: a statement for healthcare professionals from a Special Writing Group of the Stroke Council, American Heart Association. Stroke 2009;40(3):994–1025.

85. Cross DT, Tirschwell DL, Clark MA, et al. Mortality rates after subarachnoid hemorrhage: variations according to hospital case volume in 18 states. J Neurosurg 2003;99(5):810–7.

86. Broderick J, Brott T, Duldner J, et al. Initial and recurrent bleeding are the major causes of death following subarachnoid hemorrhage. Stroke 1994; 25(7):1342–7.

87. van der Wee N, Rinkel GJ, Hasan D, et al. Detection of subarachnoid haemorrhage on early CT: is lumbar puncture still needed after a negative scan? J Neurol Neurosurg Psychiatry 1995;58(3): 357–9.

88. Sames TA, Storrow AB, Finkelstein JA, et al. Sensitivity of new-generation computed tomography in subarachnoid hemorrhage. Acad Emerg Med 1996;3(1):16–20.

89. Wiesmann M, Mayer TE, Yousry I, et al. Detection of hyperacute subarachnoid hemorrhage of the brain by using magnetic resonance imaging. J Neurosurg 2002;96(4):684–9.

90. Noguchi K, Ogawa T, Seto H, et al. Subacute and chronic subarachnoid hemorrhage: diagnosis with fluid-attenuated inversion-recovery MR imaging. Radiology 1997;203(1):257–62.

91. da Rocha AJ, da Silva CJ, Gama HP, et al. Comparison of magnetic resonance imaging sequences with computed tomography to detect low-grade subarachnoid hemorrhage: role of fluid-attenuated inversion recovery sequence. J Comput Assist Tomogr 2006;30(2):295–303.

92. Mohamed M, Heasely DC, Yagmurlu B, et al. Fluid-attenuated inversion recovery MR imaging and subarachnoid hemorrhage: not a panacea. AJNR Am J Neuroradiol 2004;25(4):545–50.

93. van Gijn J, Rinkel GJ. Subarachnoid haemorrhage: diagnosis, causes and management. Brain 2001; 124(2):249–78.

94. Rinkel GJE, Djibuti M, Algra A, et al. Prevalence and risk of rupture of intracranial aneurysms: a systematic review. Stroke 1998;29(1):251–6.

95. Rhoton AL. Aneurysms. Neurosurgery 2002;51(4): 1–121.

96. Schievink WI. Intracranial aneurysms. N Engl J Med 1997;336(1):28–40.

97. Wiebers DO. Unruptured intracranial aneurysms: natural history, clinical outcome, and risks of surgical and endovascular treatment. Lancet 2003;362(9378):103–10.

98. van der Jagt M, Hasan D, Bijvoet H, et al. Validity of prediction of the site of ruptured intracranial aneurysms with CT. Neurology 1999;52(1): 34–9.

99. Li M, Cheng Y, Li Y, et al. Large-cohort comparison between three-dimensional time-of-flight magnetic resonance and rotational digital subtraction angiographies in intracranial aneurysm detection. Stroke 2009;40(9):3127–9.

100. van Rooij W, Sprengers M, de Gast A, et al. 3D Rotational angiography: the new gold standard in the detection of additional intracranial aneurysms. AJNR Am J Neuroradiol 2008;29(5):976–9.

101. Schwartz TH, Solomon RA. Perimesencephalic nonaneurysmal subarachnoid hemorrhage: review of the literature. Neurosurgery 1996;39(3):433–40.

102. Rinkel G, Wijdicks E, Vermeulen M, et al. Nonaneurysmal perimesencephalic subarachnoid hemorrhage: CT and MR patterns that differ from aneurysmal rupture. AJNR Am J Neuroradiol 1991;12(5):829–34.

103. Hunt WE, Hess RM. Surgical risk as related to time of intervention in the repair of intracranial aneurysms. J Neurosurg 1968;28(1):14–20.

104. Fisher CM, Kistler JP, Davis JM. Relation of cerebral vasospasm to subarachnoid hemorrhage visualized by computerized tomographic scanning. Neurosurgery 1980;6(1):1–9.

Emergent Neuroimaging of Intracranial Infection/ Inflammation

Mark E. Mullins, MD, PhD

KEYWORDS
- CNS • CT • Infection • Inflammation • Intracranial
- MR imaging • Review

In neuroimaging, the expression inflammation may be confusing. For the purposes of this article, the reader should assume this process characteristically induces edema (through leaky vessels) and involves infiltration by leukocytes. One would presume that this accompanies second messenger abnormalities, related to each of these. Purists might point out that this description describes acuity, which is not in conflict with the proposed paradigm. This acuity seems to be the most likely characteristic of the underlying pathology and an emergent/urgent presentation. The scope of this article has been limited to fit the space provided and to increase focus. In the author's opinion, these are some of the most interesting and, unfortunately, occasionally confounding processes in neuroimaging.

Generally speaking, any structure in the human body may become inflamed or infected. These conditions can coexist and are therefore not mutually exclusive. The same is true of some other pathologic processes that are discussed elsewhere in this issue, such as cerebral infarction, traumatic injury, and the posterior reversible encephalopathy syndrome. Inflammation or infection is a classic, albeit not pathognomonic, process to invoke when more than one anatomic space is involved on neuroimaging. The spaces involved are important to characterize and document for many reasons, including that it might help with the diagnosis, differential diagnosis, and clinical correlation. Although simplistic, a useful paradigm is to consider that the human body only has a limited and relatively generic way to respond to an acute irritant such as an infection: it becomes inflamed and swells.

Infection/inflammation of the space containing cerebrospinal fluid is called *meningitis*, of the brain is called *cerebritis* (technically *encephalitis* is a clinical diagnosis but some use this interchangeably or to describe different diagnoses), of the lining of the ventricles is called *ventriculitis* (or *ependymitis*), and of the bones is called *osteomyelitis*. An encapsulated pyogenic collection in the brain or subarachnoid space is an *abscess* and in the extra-axial space may be called an *empyema*.

Because of the characteristic derangements at the cellular level that lead to the aforementioned processes (eg, edema), neuroimaging may identify several characteristic findings. As per usual in neuroimaging, recognition of the patterns in the scan should assist in the summarization. For example, contrast material enhancement is predicated on the lack of a blood–brain barrier, or at least one that is not normal. Therefore, it is nonspecific. Infectious and noninfectious inflammatory lesions characteristically show low density change (CT) or high signal change (T2 MR imaging) consistent with edema, and associated swelling, mass effect, and shift may be present. Thus, acuity on neuroimaging is variable; it may wax and wane. It may be a one-time manifestation or it may be chronic, and it may vary with treatment.

In addition to conventional CT and MR imaging, advanced neuroimaging techniques such as MR spectroscopy (metabolites), CT and MR perfusion

Department of Radiology, Emory University School of Medicine, 1364 Clifton Road NE, Room D125A, Atlanta, GA 30322, USA
E-mail address: memulli@emory.edu

Radiol Clin N Am 49 (2011) 47–62
doi:10.1016/j.rcl.2010.08.002
0033-8389/11/$ — see front matter © 2011 Elsevier Inc. All rights reserved.

(cerebral blood flow and cerebral blood volume), and positron emission tomography (glucose use) may provide additional information about the pathophysiologic process being interrogated. This information may be of use, even in the acute/emergent setting. A detailed discussion of these methodologies is beyond the scope of this article.

PROTOCOLLING

Please note that the following are the author's own personal opinions, so…caveat emptor. CT scan[1] is best used when time is of the essence[2] or screening is clinically indicated. In general, the author begins with a noncontrast head CT scan and then proceeds from there. If the patient is unlikely to have an MR imaging scan, one may want to consider a head CT with or without contrast from the beginning. Under most circumstances, a noncontrast head CT may be expected to screen for large, acute intracranial pathologies, such as large mass lesions, and may also screen for postinflammatory changes. If mastoiditis or sinusitis is clinically suspected, the initial CT can be tailored or optimized to evaluate the temporal bones/skull base or maxillofacial structures. A discussion of contrast material is provided later.

MR imaging scans offer several possibilities[3–7] in terms of a la carte tailoring, but unless a good reason exists to do so on the initial scans (eg, prior MR imaging of the brain that suggested a specific protocol on follow-up), the author suggests tailoring the scan based on the clinical scenario.[8,9] For example, does the clinical scenario suggest the suprasellar space? If so, one should consider a pituitary protocol MR imaging scan. Does the clinical scenario suggest the cranial nerves of the posterior fossa? If so, an internal auditory canal protocol MR imaging scan should be considered. Initial imaging with MR imaging may be preferable in some situations, but many times the head CT scan is performed initially and then an MR imaging scan follows. Therefore, the author prefers to not give contrast material on the initial head CT scan unless the MR image is not expected to be performed or there is some other extenuating circumstance.

In general, contrast material[10,11] will be a prime consideration[12] whenever inflammation and/or infection within a patient's head is known or suspected. Except in the presence of a contraindication, gadolinium should be included in any protocol assessing for intracranial infection/inflammation. If MR imaging is contraindicated and the patient is not known to have any risk factors for receiving iodinated contrast material, consider adding postcontrast head CT following initial noncontrast head CT.

INTRACRANIAL INFECTION

The author was the neuroradiologist at a multidisciplinary conference at which the guest speaker was an expert in central nervous system (CNS) infections, and who made some very sobering points that had a long-lasting impression. He said that at least a couple hundred types of infectious pathogens exist that can reside in the intracranial compartment…that are known. Almost assuredly more exist that are not known. For those that are known, only a few have reliable methods for their diagnosis and even fewer have effective treatments. Many times the pathogen is ultimately identifiable and potentially treatable.[13] The archetype of this is bacterial infection.[14–16]

Intracranial Bacterial Infection

The formation of pus and a mature rim of an abscess is an evolutionary process that takes time to develop. Thus, a bacterial (or other) infection may be present on a scan even though the classical findings are not well identified.

Bacterial meningitis may be invisible on neuroimaging (and thus a motivating factor for considering cerebrospinal fluid [CSF] sampling when meningitis is suspected), but it could also manifest as lack of the normal CSF signal on MR imaging (especially when the abnormal signal seems to be sedimentary and restricts diffusion) or as intermediate to high density on CT (classically, hyperdensity, which could potentially appear similar to hemorrhage). Hydrocephalus may be a manifestation of meningitis caused by disturbance of the normal CSF resorptive process or through blocking the normal flow of CSF through the ventricular system. Leptomeningeal prominence[17] may be present secondary to leptomeningeal enhancement. Cerebral swelling may be found in meningitis, especially in pediatric patients.

The author prefers to differentiate cerebral edema (obscuration of the gray–white matter interface) and brain swelling, but these may coexist. Bacterial infection of the intraventricular space may result in ventriculitis[18,19] and can result in hydrocephalus. Periventricular edema may be seen, especially in the setting of acute, uncompensated hydrocephalus. When the ependymal lining is inflamed (ependymitis), it also can enhance. Bacterial infection of the brain may result in cerebritis, which could progress to pyogenic abscess (**Fig. 1**). The appearance of cerebritis on neuroimaging may be variable, but the most characteristic appearance to the author is that of parenchymal edema, swelling, and ill-defined enhancement in a distribution that does not fit well into an arterial distribution. Characteristically,

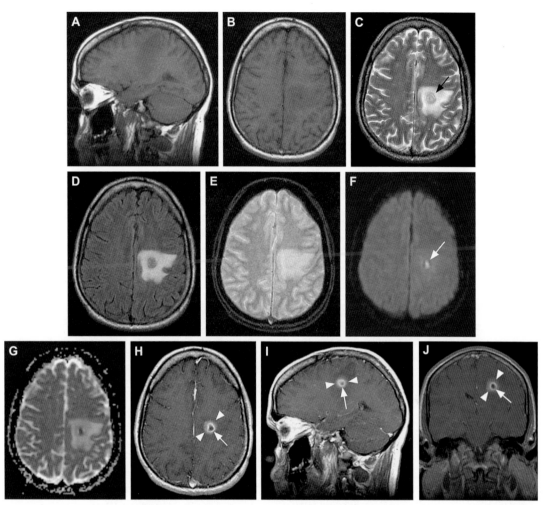

Fig. 1. Adult patient with fungal brain abscess. An intra-axial mass is evident within the dorsal left frontal lobe, manifest by heterogeneous signal on T1-weighted imaging (*A, B*) including peripheral edema, surrounding a rounded central lesion that is readily identified on T2-weighted imaging (*C, arrow*) and fluid attenuation inversion recovery (*D*). No abnormally decreased signal is noted on the susceptibility-sensitive image (*E*) to suggest associated bleeding or overt mineralization. The central portion of the mass restricts diffusion (*arrow, F* and *G*), suggesting pyogenic contents (pus). Triplane postcontrast T1-weighted imaging (*H, I, J*) shows an irregular contour of ring enhancement that contains a central portion of more uniform and thickened ring enhancement (*arrow*) and more peripheral ill-defined enhancement (between *arrowheads*). This constellation of findings suggests an atypical pyogenic abscess such as one related to fungal infection, as in this instance.

a relatively smooth rim-enhancing intra-axial mass is present and the portion of the enhancing margin closest to the ventricle would be thinnest (perhaps because of differences in blood supply), the central nonenhancing portion most classically restricts diffusion,[20] and the rim of the mass may have decreased signal on T2-weighted imaging (T2WI; possibly from paramagnetism presumably related to unpaired electrons).

Intracranial Fungal Infection

Although fungal infections are somewhat unusual, they can be extremely dangerous in terms of morbidity and mortality.[21–23] Moreover, empiric antibiotics may not cover a potential fungal infection. Therefore, it may be prudent to consider this pathogen when interpreting a case of suspected infection that has atypical imaging features. Characteristically, the fungus would have decreased signal on T2WI, perhaps even appearing as a signal void (like air). The appearance on T1WI may be iso- to hyperintense, which in concert with hypointensity on T2WI is worrisome for fungus. The hypointensity on T2WI is presumed to be related to heavy metals in the oxidative pathways of the fungi. The hyperintensity on T1WI is believed to be from an elevated amount of protein, although some of this signal may also be related to the metals.

Intracranial fungal infection may have findings similar to bacterial infection, including formation of a classical-appearing pyogenic cerebral abscess. Findings of tropism favoring the paranasal sinuses,[24–29] orbits, and arterial vasculature[30,31] especially prompt the author to consider this diagnosis. In the author's experience, small "tendrils" of enhancement extending from the outer margins of a ring-enhancing mass suggest a fungal origin. If a patient is immunocompromised, consideration of fungal infection on neuroimaging has increased relevance; one of the archetypes of this situation includes patients with diabetes and suspected or known Mucor. Accurate and timely diagnosis is essential in mitigating morbidity and mortality in this setting.

Intracranial Viral Infection

The list of possible viral infections is legion, many of which may infect the intracranial compartment.[32–37] This section concentrates on a couple of instructive situations.

Viral meningitis[38] may have similar findings to bacterial meningitis but for it to manifest with restricted diffusion would be unusual. Patients

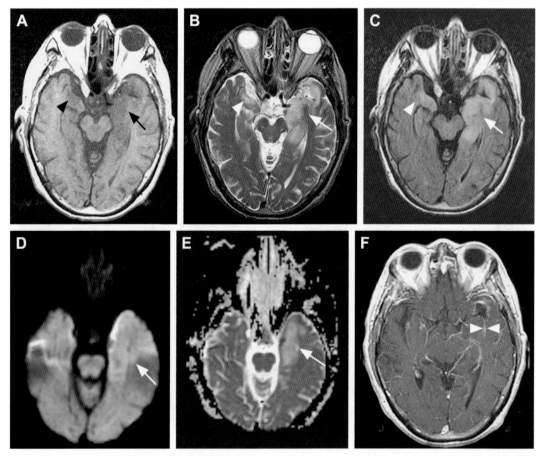

Fig. 2. Adult patient with herpes encephalitis/cerebritis. Bilateral temporal lobe abnormalities are identified, manifesting hypointensity on T1-weighted imaging (*A, arrows*), hyperintensity on T2-weighted imaging (*2B, arrows*) and hyperintensity on fluid attenuation inversion recovery (*C, arrows*). Intrinsic hyperintensity on diffusion-weighted imaging is noted within the left temporal lobe (*D, arrow*) with associated hyperintensity on the ADC map (*E, arrow*), consistent with T2 shine-through. A leading edge of enhancement is seen along the lateral margin of the left temporal lobe lesion (*F, between arrows*), indicative of an inflammatory component to this pathologic process. Note that the involvement of the temporal lobes is bilateral but asymmetric.

could theoretically have superinfections and thus may have coexistent viral and nonviral intracranial infections.

Herpes simplex virus (HSV) may result in a cerebritis (**Fig. 2**) that characteristically has tropism for the limbic system and, in particular, the mesial temporal lobes, cingulate gyrus, and insular cortices. Involvement of the temporal lobes is usually bilateral, although it can be asymmetric. Other findings include ill-defined partial enhancement and intralesional hemorrhage, with the latter a common finding microscopically. Restricted diffusion is variably present secondary to an exuberant cytotoxic response to the pathogen and inclusion of DWI and ADC maps should be strongly considered in any infection/inflammation MR imaging protocol.

HIV infection of the intracranial compartment[39,40] may result in direct manifestations within the brain, so-called HIV encephalopathy (**Fig. 3**), which is typically a diagnosis of exclusion. When findings are present, patchy/confluent white-matter T2 hyperintensity and central volume loss are characteristic.

One potentially associated diagnosis of interest in this section is progressive multifocal leukoencephalopathy (PML). The JC virus, combined with a low CD4 count, is the typical clinical combination that results in a pattern of demyelination, which has a nonspecific and variable appearance on neuroimaging. PML characteristically appears as patchy or mass-like foci of T2 hyperintensity in the cerebral or cerebellar white matter, with swelling and a leading edge of feathery enhancement. Ernst and colleagues[41] have suggested that magnetization transfer MR imaging may be useful in this setting.

A lengthy description of the neuroimaging manifestations of HIV,[42] related superinfections,[43–47] and AIDS[48] are beyond the scope of this article. However, the author would like to suggest that there is a related, and potentially useful, "thought construct" in trying to differentiate two potentially inflammatory processes: intracranial infection and

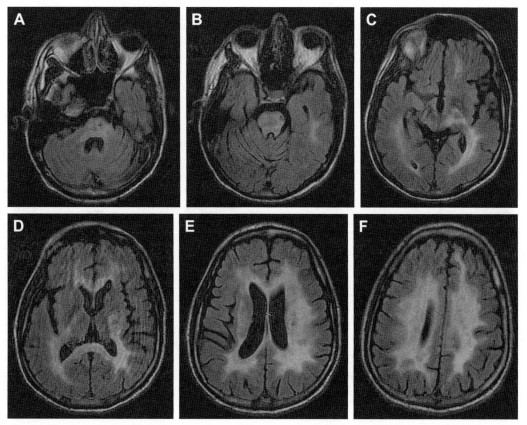

Fig. 3. Adult patient with HIV encephalopathy. A series of six (*A–F*) fluid attenuation inversion recovery images illustrates marked severe white matter hyperintensity superimposed on diffuse brain volume loss. There is remarkable involvement of the brainstem and asymmetric preferential involvement of the central more than peripheral white matter abnormal signal. There is also apparent multifocal sparing of the subcortical U-fibers. Although strictly nonspecific, this pattern in the proper clinical context is suggestive of this particular diagnosis, usually a diagnosis of exclusion.

neoplasia. In patients with AIDS and an intra-axial enhancing mass, a classical primary differential diagnosis may be evoked, with top considerations of CNS lymphoma[49] or toxoplasmosis.[50–52] The author suggests that this is a good construct to think through in terms of factors such as pathophysiology, clinical aspects, imaging aspects, and management options in comparing and contrasting intracranial inflammation and infection.

Many other intracranial viral infections exist, but space constraints prevent their discussion. Many of these receive much attention in the popular press and neuroimaging literature.[53–55] A recent example is West Nile virus. Although the neuroimaging appearance is typically nonspecific and variable, characteristic of this infection (West Nile virus infection with possible meningoencephalitis), one may visualize inflammatory changes centered within the deep brain, including the thalami and adjacent structures.[56,57]

Intracranial Parasitic Infection

Although a lengthy discussion of the many potential intracranial parasitic infections is beyond the scope of this article, a couple of the archetypes are discussed in this section.

Neurocysticercosis[58,59] is one if not the only leading cause of seizure in endemic parts of the world. Regardless of practice location, one could potentially identify a manifestation of this infection on emergent neuroimaging. Although the most characteristic finding on head CT scan for this infection is multifocal peripherally located calcification indicating chronic/remote infection, different stages of infection may manifest in different imaging findings. Different stages commonly coexist. One of the classification schemes that is used is the Escobar classification and includes primarily active, transitional, and inactive forms.[60] The most characteristic findings on MR imaging scan include rounded/oval cystic lesions with partial or complete marginal enhancement (**Fig. 4**). Recent advances regarding this infection include testing of not only CSF but also blood and urine,[61] may be helpful if neurocysticercosis is on the differential diagnosis, and also illustrates how medicine evolves.

Intracranial Prion Infection

One of the more provocative and unnerving diagnoses that has become infamous in the last couple of decades is that of prion infection of the intracranial compartment. The archetype for this infection is Creutzfeldt-Jakob disease (CJD), which is a relentless progressive neurodegenerative process that results in dementia and ultimately death (**Fig. 5**).[62–64] Four types of CJD exist, each reflecting different mechanisms of disease: sporadic, variant, iatrogenic, and genetic, with sporadic the most common.[62–64] One of the most characteristic patterns of abnormal signal on MR imaging scan is restricted diffusion in the cerebral cortex and caudate/lentiform nuclei.[62–64] A tropism occurs toward the ventral caudate and lentiform nuclei, with progression dorsally as the disease progresses. The diffusion restriction may precede clear T2 signal changes, swelling is mild at most, and enhancement is distinctly uncommon.[62,64] An additional sign described in the neuroimaging literature is the *pulvinar sign*,

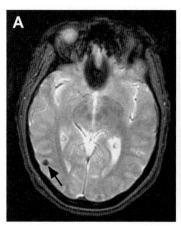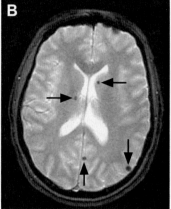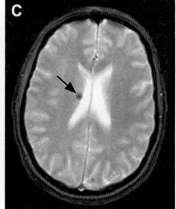

Fig. 4. Adult patient with neurocysticercosis. A series of three (*A–C*) susceptibility-weighted images illustrates focal hypointensities (*arrows*) consistent with calcifications. The compartmentalization of these lesions is most likely a combination of intra-axial and leptomeningeal. No edema is noted in associated with any of the calcifications. Although a differential diagnosis exists for this appearance, the appearance is most consistent with neurocysticercosis in the proper clinical context.

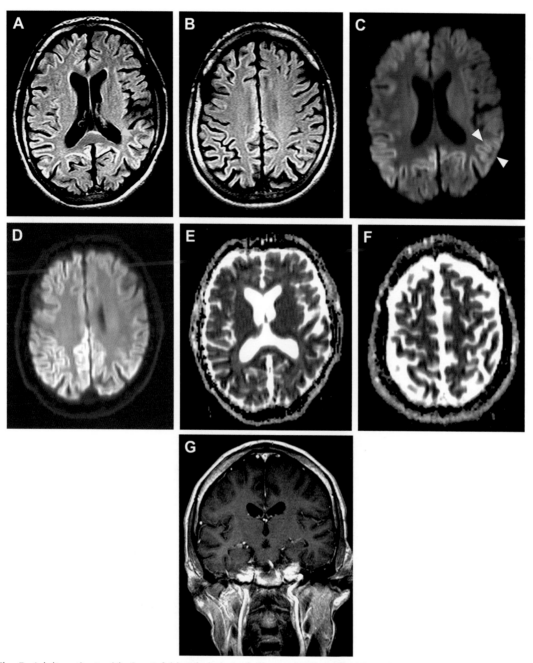

Fig. 5. Adult patient with Creutzfeldt-Jakob (prion) disease (CJD) cortical hyperintensity on fluid attenuation inversion recovery (FLAIR) imaging (*A, B*) is noted multifocally within the bilateral frontal and parietal lobes, albeit somewhat asymmetric. Note that these cortical regions do not appear particularly swollen. These areas of abnormal signal on FLAIR (between *arrows, A*) exhibit hyperintensity on the diffusion-weighted images (between *arrows, C; D*) and corresponding hypointensity on the apparent diffusion coefficient (ADC) map (*E, F*), most consistent with restricted diffusion. On postcontrast coronal T1-weighted imaging (*G*), no abnormal enhancement is identified. The appearance on FLAIR and diffusion-weighted imaging may be so diffuse that one may be inclined to window down this "super scan equivalent" and perhaps not notice it until the ADC map is reviewed. This constellation of imaging findings is highly suggestive of CJD.

which is described in variant CJD[62,64] and includes symmetric T2 hyperintensity with the medial thalami and pulvinar.

A potential diagnostic pitfall concerning brain MR imaging performed in patients relatively early in the infection may be that diffusion abnormalities may precede abnormality on T2WI.[63] Therefore, the history of progressive dementia, as opposed to acute neurologic symptoms relating to a cortical stroke, is an important clue to the diagnosis.

Other Notable Intracranial Infections

Tuberculous infection of the intracranial compartment may manifest with a nonspecific and variable appearance on neuroimaging.[22] Focusing on *Mycobacteria tuberculosis* infection in this context, one of the more characteristic appearances is a nodulolinear leptomeningeal thickening and enhancement that is centered within the basilar cisterns.[22] This condition may manifest as isodensity filling/obscuring the basal cisterns on CT, isointense signal in the basal cisterns on MR imaging, and thick subarachnoid enhancement. Tuberculous abscess, called *tuberculomas*, may also form.[65] Coinfections such as HIV may complicate diagnosis.[66]

An example of a rare intracranial infection that may present in the acute setting is *Histoplasma capsulatum* (histoplasmosis) infection of the CNS.[67] Findings on neuroimaging are nonspecific

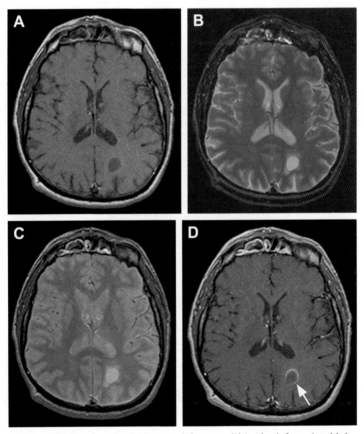

Fig. 6. Adult patient with multiple sclerosis. An intra-axial mass within the left parietal lobe exhibits central hypointensity and a slightly hyperintense rim on T1-weighted imaging (*A*); central robust hyperintensity and less prominent hyperintense rim on T2-weighted imaging (*B*); no abnormal hypointensity on the susceptibility-weighted image (*C*) to suggest blood products or mineralization; and ill-defined and probably incomplete rim-enhancement on axial T1-weighted postcontrast imaging (*D, arrow*). The enhancement characteristics are nonspecific. No restricted diffusion was identified (not shown). This lesion has an extensive differential diagnosis. In this instance, the lesion was a plaque of multiple sclerosis with some radiographic acuity. Some may consider this isolated mass within the spectrum of tumefactive multiple sclerosis.

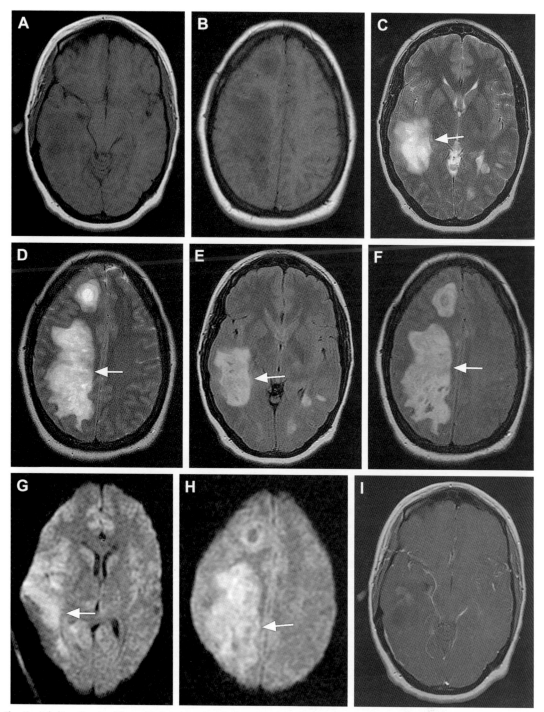

Fig. 7. Adult patient with multiple sclerosis, Marburg variant. Multiple intra-axial masses within the right frontal and parietal lobes exhibit predominant hypointensity on T1-weighted imaging (*A, B*); central robust hyperintensity and less prominent hyperintense rim on T2-weighted imaging (*arrow, C, D*), and similar findings on fluid attenuation inversion recovery (*arrow, E, F*); associated hyperintensity on diffusion-weighted imaging (*arrow, G, H*); associated hypointensity on the apparent diffusion coefficient map (not shown); and partial rim-enhancement on axial T1-weighted postcontrast imaging (*I;* between *arrows, J, K;* adjacent to *arrow, L*). This constellation of findings has an extensive differential diagnosis. In this instance, the diagnosis was multiple sclerosis with multifocal radiographic acuity. Some may consider this within the spectrum of tumefactive multiple sclerosis.

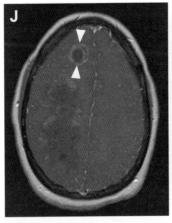
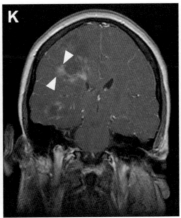
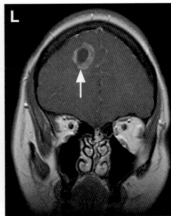

Fig. 7. (*continued*)

and variable, including parenchymal abnormalities (not otherwise specified), infarctions, and meningitis.[67]

INTRACRANIAL INFLAMMATION

For the sake of brevity and focus, discussion in this section is limited to a couple of examples of inflammatory intracranial processes. A lot of potential exists for overlap[68–71] with many other disease processes, depending on how one categorizes intracranial anatomy and pathology.[72,73] For example, both neoplastic[74] and ischemic brain disorders may result in a superimposed inflammatory response by adjacent tissues. To further complicate categorization, some classical inflammatory brain pathologies may be related to infections (eg, acute disseminated encephalomyelitis).

Multiple Sclerosis

Multiple sclerosis may result in acute clinical presentations and robust abnormalities on imaging that may suggest more sinister disease processes (**Figs. 6–8**).[75,76] For example, Balo's concentric sclerosis may not only result in significant mass effect but also incite considerable adjacent edema. The most characteristic appearance for this diagnosis is an intra-axial mass with the appearance of an enhancing lesion, and a cross-sectional appearance that is reminiscent of an onion in cross-section. Findings most consistent with radiographic acuity of multiple sclerosis plaques are peripheral leading edge contrast enhancement and restricted diffusion.[77] In the author's experience, multiple sclerosis plaques usually lack significant mass effect, even when tumefactive, and this may be useful in suggesting tumefactive multiple sclerosis over other diagnoses, including high-grade primary brain tumors.[77,78] It

is also in this context that a leading edge of enhancement may be of differential diagnostic interest, disfavoring neoplasia and favoring a predominantly inflammatory process.[77,78] Associated edema may be prominent, and this characteristic is not pathognemonic.[78] However, although neuroimaging may contribute, the diagnosis of multiple sclerosis remains a clinical diagnosis.

Neuromyelitis optica

Depending on what reference is used, neuromyelitis optica (NMO), or Devic disease, may be generally considered to be a specific diagnosis or a variant of multiple sclerosis.[79,80] The classical presentation may be acute and typically involves a transverse myelitis and painful vision loss in one eye.[79,80] Corresponding neuroimaging findings of transverse myelitis or brainstem involvement with optic neuritis may occur.[79,80] Concordant nonspecific white matter lesions within the brain are common in this setting, and therefore one of the prime differential diagnostic considerations is multiple sclerosis.[79,80]

Acute Disseminated Encephalomalacia

Although nonspecific and variable, characteristic brain parenchymal lesions in acute disseminated encephalomalacia (ADEM) are centered within the white matter and are typically manifestations of acute severe demyelination involving any age, but favoring children over adults.[81] Involvement of the deep gray structures is not uncommon and may dissuade others from considering this diagnosis. This involvement may be related to crossing white matter fiber involvement. Classically patients have a history of recent vaccination or presumed viral systemic infection.[81] Imaging

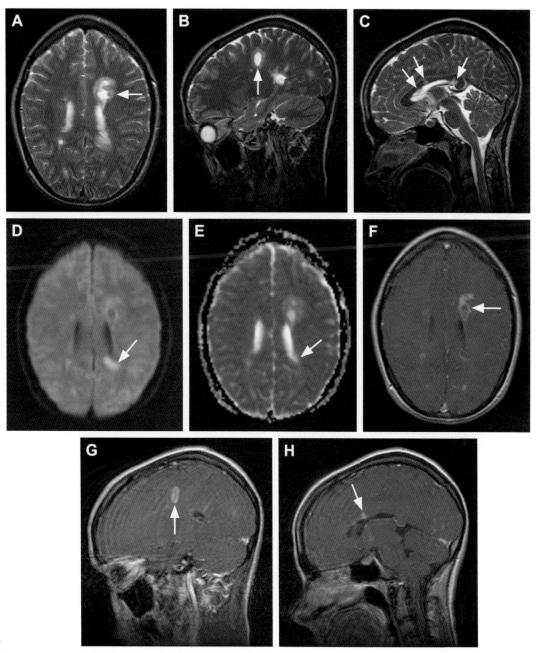

Fig. 8. Adult patient with multiple sclerosis. Multiple intra-axial masses within the bilateral frontal and parietal lobes with prominent involvement of the corpus callosum and morphology suggestive of Dawson fingers exhibit central hyperintensity and a slightly less hyperintense rim on T2-weighted imaging (*arrows, A, B, C*). One of these lesions manifests hyperintensity on diffusion-weighted imaging (*arrow, D*) and hyperintensity on the apparent diffusion coefficient map (*arrow, E*) most consistent with so-called T2 shine-through. A different lesion manifests nodulolinear enhancement on T1 postcontrast imaging (*arrows, F–H*). This constellation of findings has an extensive differential diagnosis. In this instance, the diagnosis was multiple sclerosis with radiographic acuity.

characteristics, such as enhancement patterns and diffusion signal, are most characteristically similar to those of multiple sclerosis, which is usually one of the primary differential diagnostic considerations when ADEM is contemplated.[81] The presence of lesions of multiple ages favors a monophasic process such as ADEM over the more typical multiphasic multiple sclerosis, with

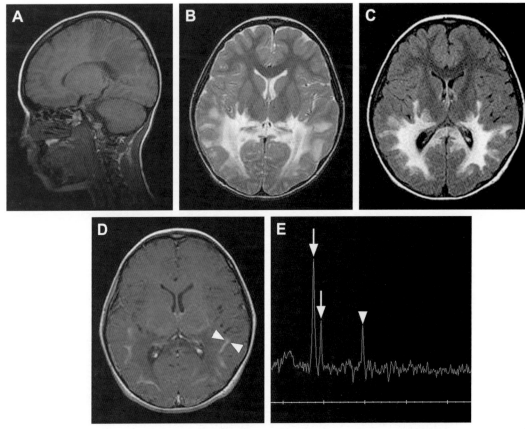

Fig. 9. Pediatric patient with adrenoleukodystrophy. Intra-axial fronto-parieto-occipital hypointensity with expansion also involving the corpus callosum is noted on axial T1-weighted imaging (*A*). This region manifests associated robust T2 hyperintensity on T2-weighted imaging (*B*) and fluid attenuation inversion recovery (FLAIR) (*C*). Axial T1 postcontrast imaging (*D*) shows ill-defined enhancement (between *arrows*) along the margins of this parenchymal abnormality. This enhancement pattern suggests a leading edge of enhancement and a prominent component of inflammation. Single-voxel MR spectroscopy (MRS) was performed (*E*); voxel placement not shown but centered at the edge of the T2/FLAIR abnormal signal. From left-to-right, the arrows (*E*) point to peaks for choline and creatine and the arrowhead (*E*) points to N-acetylaspartate (NAA). The MRS appearance is most suggestive of a neoplasia, with an elevated choline:creatine ratio and decreased NAA. The diagnosis in this instance was adrenoleukodystrophy. If interpreted in the absence of so-called conventional neuroimaging, MRS may be potentially misleading. MRS of inflammatory masses within the brain may manifest with similar results.

the caveat that monophasic ADEM and the first episode of multiple sclerosis may appear identical on neuroimaging.

PEARLS AND (POTENTIAL) PITFALLS

- Intracranial infection/inflammation covers a broad range of pathologies with many overlapping findings on neuroimaging. These studies should be interpreted with the maximal amount of history, laboratory findings, and clinical context to increase diagnostic acumen and improve patient outcomes.

- A noncontrast head CT is almost always indicated in this setting to help exclude other causes and assess for significant changes. MR imaging with or without gadolinium is critical to further refine the diagnosis and assess for complications of infection/inflammation.

- In patients with an intracranial infection, one should try to ascertain the pathway for how the infection accessed the intracranial compartment (eg, hematogenous, direct extension). This information may help management decisions. For example, cerebritis may be related to a nearby sinusitis or mastoiditis.

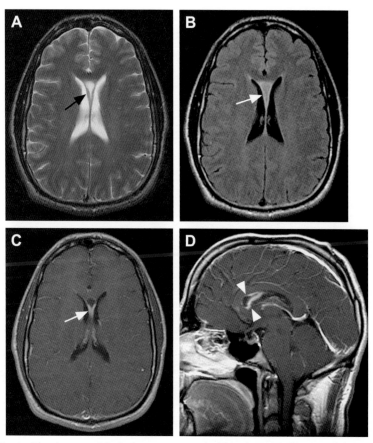

Fig. 10. Adult patient with neurosarcoidosis. A mass centered within the ventral aspect of the septum pellucidum is noted to be hyperintense on T2-weighted imaging (*arrow, A*) and fluid attenuation inversion recovery (*arrow, B*). Axial (*arrow, C*) and sagittal (between *arrows, D*) T1 postcontrast imaging show ill-defined enhancement along the margins of this parenchymal abnormality. This enhancement pattern suggests a leading edge of enhancement and a prominent component of inflammation. This constellation of findings has an extensive differential diagnosis, including neoplasia. In this instance, the diagnosis was neurosarcoidosis.

- Acute complications of intracranial infectious and inflammatory processes should be actively sought out, especially in patients with an acute clinical presentation. For example, does a patient have acute, obstructive hydrocephalus subsequent to a ventriculitis or transverse sinus thrombosis with mastoiditis?
- When formulating a differential diagnosis, questions to ask are: could this be a primary infectious or inflammatory disease? For example, is a mass tumefactive multiple sclerosis and not tumor?
- Consider infectious or inflammatory intracranial processes when the neuroimaging results appear nonspecific or confusing. The author suggests that an infectious or inflammatory process should not be excluded unless it can be ruled out with certainty. One should realize one's "limits."

- Ill-defined enhancement that is most prominent or isolated at the margins of an intra-axial mass suggests a leading edge of enhancement (**Figs. 9** and **10**) and is one of the findings that suggest an inflammatory pathophysiology.
- Advanced neuroimaging techniques such as MR spectroscopy and MR perfusion can be helpful in problematic cases but are not typically used as front-line techniques in the acute setting.

SUMMARY

Infectious and inflammatory processes of the intracranial compartment are common, have varied clinical presentations, protean imaging manifestations, and significant neuroimaging overlap. Although many of the patterns indicate a general category (ie, bacterial infection), careful scrutiny and thought can reveal specific patterns of involvement and specific diagnoses (ie, sporadic CJD, HSV encephalitis, neurocysticercosis). Contemporaneous historical and laboratory information in combination with appropriate neuroimaging studies provides radiologists with the tools to have significant added value and hopefully positively influence patient outcomes.

REFERENCES

1. Zimmerman RA, Patel S, Bilaniuk LT. Demonstration of purulent bacterial intracranial infections by computed tomography. AJR Am J Roentgenol 1976;127(1):155–65.
2. Mafee MF, Singleton EL, Valvassori GE, et al. Acute otomastoiditis and its complications: role of CT. Radiology 1985;155(2):391–7.
3. Weingarten K, Zimmerman RD, Becker RD, et al. Subdural and epidural empyemas: MR imaging. AJR Am J Roentgenol 1989;152(3):615–21.
4. Simonson TM, Magnotta VA, Ehrhardt JC, et al. Echo-planar FLAIR imaging in evaluation of intracranial lesions. Radiographics 1996;16(3):575–84.
5. Tsuchiya K, Inaoka S, Mizutani Y, et al. Fast fluid-attenuated inversion-recovery MR of intracranial infections. AJNR Am J Neuroradiol 1997;18(5):909–13.
6. Schaefer PW, Grant PE, Gonzalez RG. Diffusion-weighted MR imaging of the brain. Radiology 2000;217(2):331–45.
7. van der Knaap MS, Vermeulen G, Barkhof F, et al. Pattern of white matter abnormalities at MR imaging: use of polymerase chain reaction testing of Guthrie cards to link pattern with congenital cytomegalovirus infection.[erratum appears in Radiology 2004 May;231(2):605]. Radiology 2004;230(2):529–36.
8. Chang KH, Han MH, Roh JK, et al. Gd-DTPA-enhanced MR imaging of the brain in patients with meningitis: comparison with CT. AJR Am J Roentgenol 1990;154(4):809–16.
9. Cha S, Knopp EA, Johnson G, et al. Intracranial mass lesions: dynamic contrast-enhanced susceptibility-weighted echo-planar perfusion MR imaging. Radiology 2002;223(1):11–29.
10. Runge VM, Carollo BR, Wolf CR, et al. A review of clinical indications in central nervous system magnetic resonance imaging. Radiographics 1989;9(5):929–58.
11. Smirniotopoulos JG, Murphy FM, Rushing EJ, et al. Patterns of contrast enhancement in the brain and meninges. Radiographics 2007;27(2):525–51.
12. Hurley MC, Heran MK. Imaging studies for head and neck infections. Infect Dis Clin North Am 2007;21(2):305–53.
13. Ziai WC, Lewin JJ III. Update in the diagnosis and management of central nervous system infections. Neurol Clin 2008;26(2):427–68.
14. Ferris EJ, Rudikoff JC, Shapiro JH. Cerebral angiography of bacterial infection. Radiology 1968;90(4):727–34.
15. Lam AH, Berry A, deSilva M, Williams G. Intracranial Serratia infection in preterm newborn infants. AJNR Am J Neuroradiol 1984;5(4):447–51.
16. Vazquez E, Castellote A, Piqueras J, et al. Imaging of complications of acute mastoiditis in children. Radiographics 2003;23(2):359–72.
17. Sze G. Diseases of the intracranial meninges: MR imaging features. AJR Am J Roentgenol 1993;160(4):727–33.
18. Fukui MB, Williams RL, Mudigonda S. CT and MR imaging features of pyogenic ventriculitis. AJNR Am J Neuroradiol 2001;22(8):1510–6.
19. Fujikawa A, Tsuchiya K, Honya K, et al. Comparison of MRI sequences to detect ventriculitis. AJR Am J Roentgenol 2006;187(4):1048–53.
20. Gupta RK, Hasan KM, Mishra AM, et al. High fractional anisotropy in brain abscesses versus other cystic intracranial lesions. AJNR Am J Neuroradiol 2005;26(5):1107–14.
21. Lai PH, Lin SM, Pan HB, et al. Disseminated miliary cerebral candidiasis. AJNR Am J Neuroradiol 1997;18(7):1303–6.
22. Harisinghani MG, McLoud TC, Shepard JA, et al. Tuberculosis from head to toe. Radiographics 2000;20(2):449–70, quiz 528–9, 32.
23. Rumboldt Z, Castillo M. Indolent intracranial mucormycosis: case report. AJNR Am J Neuroradiol 2002;23(6):932–4.
24. Whelan MA, Stern J, deNapoli RA. The computed tomographic spectrum of intracranial mycosis: correlation with histopathology. Radiology 1981;141(3):703–7.
25. Gamba JL, Woodruff WW, Djang WT, et al. Craniofacial mucormycosis: assessment with CT. Radiology 1986;160(1):207–12.
26. Ashdown BC, Tien RD, Felsberg GJ. Aspergillosis of the brain and paranasal sinuses in immunocompromised patients: CT and MR imaging findings. AJR Am J Roentgenol 1994;162(1):155–9.
27. Schnipper D, Spiegel JH. Management of intracranial complications of sinus surgery. Otolaryngol Clin North Am 2004;37(2):453–72.
28. Aribandi M, McCoy VA, Bazan C III. Imaging features of invasive and noninvasive fungal sinusitis: a review. Radiographics 2007;27(5):1283–96.
29. Cho YS, Lee DK, Hong SD, et al. Intracranial aspergillosis involving the internal auditory canal and inner ear in an immunocompetent patient. AJNR Am J Neuroradiol 2007;28(1):138–40.
30. Wynne PJ, Younger DS, Khandji A, et al. Radiographic features of central nervous system vasculitis. Neurol Clin 1997;15(4):779–804.
31. Laupland KB. Vascular and parameningeal infections of the head and neck. Infect Dis Clin North Am 2007;21(2):577–90.

32. Rowen M, Singer MJ, Moran ET. Intracranial calcification in the congenital rubella syndrome. Am J Roentgenol Radium Ther Nucl Med 1972;115(1): 86–91.

33. Drose JA, Dennis MA, Thickman D. Infection in utero: US findings in 19 cases. Radiology 1991; 178(2):369–74.

34. Bale JF Jr, Murph JR. Congenital infections and the nervous system. Pediatr Clin North Am 1992;39(4): 669–90.

35. Jain R, Deveikis J, Hickenbottom S, et al. Varicella-zoster vasculitis presenting with intracranial hemorrhage. AJNR Am J Neuroradiol 2003;24(5):971–4.

36. Malinger G, Lev D, Zahalka N, et al. Fetal cytomegalovirus infection of the brain: the spectrum of sonographic findings. AJNR Am J Neuroradiol 2003; 24(1):28–32.

37. Weeks JK, Helton KJ, Conley ME, et al. Diffuse CNS vasculopathy with chronic Epstein-Barr virus infection in X-linked lymphoproliferative disease. AJNR Am J Neuroradiol 2006;27(4):884–6.

38. Bonthius DJ, Karacay B. Meningitis and encephalitis in children. An update. Neurol Clin 2002;20(4): 1013–38.

39. Kauffman WM, Sivit CJ, Fitz CR, et al. CT and MR evaluation of intracranial involvement in pediatric HIV infection: a clinical-imaging correlation. AJNR Am J Neuroradiol 1992;13(3):949–57.

40. Smith AB, Smirniotopoulos JG, Rushing EJ. From the archives of the AFIP: central nervous system infections associated with human immunodeficiency virus infection: radiologic-pathologic correlation. [erratum appears in Radiographics 2009 Mar–Apr; 29(2):638]. Radiographics 2008;28(7):2033–58.

41. Ernst T, Chang L, Witt M, et al. Progressive multifocal leukoencephalopathy and human immunodeficiency virus-associated white matter lesions in AIDS: magnetization transfer MR imaging. Radiology 1999;210(2):539–43.

42. Letendre S, Ances B, Gibson S, et al. Neurologic complications of HIV disease and their treatment. Top HIV Med 2007;15(2):32–9.

43. Cornell SH, Jacoby CG. The varied computed tomographic appearance of intracranial cryptococcosis. Radiology 1982;143(3):703–7.

44. Popovich MJ, Arthur RH, Helmer E. CT of intracranial cryptococcosis. AJR Am J Roentgenol 1990;154(3): 603–6.

45. Tien RD, Chu PK, Hesselink JR, et al. Intracranial cryptococcosis in immunocompromised patients: CT and MR findings in 29 cases. AJNR Am J Neuroradiol 1991;12(2):283–9.

46. Caldemeyer KS, Mathews VP, Edwards-Brown MK, et al. Central nervous system cryptococcosis: parenchymal calcification and large gelatinous pseudocysts. AJNR Am J Neuroradiol 1997;18(1): 107–9.

47. Chayakulkeeree M, Perfect JR. Cryptococcosis. Infect Dis Clin North Am 2006;20(3):507–44.

48. Whelan MA, Kricheff II, Handler M, et al. Acquired immunodeficiency syndrome: cerebral computed tomographic manifestations. Radiology 1983; 149(2):477–84.

49. O'Malley JP, Ziessman HA, Kumar PN, et al. Diagnosis of intracranial lymphoma in patients with AIDS: value of 201TI single-photon emission computed tomography. AJR Am J Roentgenol 1994;163(2):417–21.

50. Post MJ, Chan JC, Hensley GT, et al. Toxoplasma encephalitis in Haitian adults with acquired immunodeficiency syndrome: a clinical-pathologic-CT correlation. AJR Am J Roentgenol 1983;140(5):861–8.

51. Chinn RJ, Wilkinson ID, Hall-Craggs MA, et al. Toxoplasmosis and primary central nervous system lymphoma in HIV infection: diagnosis with MR spectroscopy. Radiology 1995;197(3):649–54.

52. Lee GT, Antelo F, Mlikotic AA. Best cases from the AFIP: cerebral toxoplasmosis. Radiographics 2009; 29(4):1200–5.

53. Maschke M, Kastrup O, Forsting M, et al. Update on neuroimaging in infectious central nervous system disease. Curr Opin Neurol 2004;17(4):475–80.

54. Kastrup O, Wanke I, Maschke M. Neuroimaging of infections. NeuroRx 2005;2(2):324–32. PMCID: 1064994.

55. Kastrup O, Wanke I, Maschke M. Neuroimaging of infections of the central nervous system. Semin Neurol 2008;28(4):511–22.

56. Petropoulou KA, Gordon SM, Prayson RA, et al. West Nile virus meningoencephalitis: MR imaging findings. AJNR Am J Neuroradiol 2005;26(8): 1986–95.

57. Kramer LD, Li J, Shi PY. West Nile virus. Lancet Neurol 2007;6(2):171–81.

58. Leite CC, Jinkins JR, Escobar BE, et al. MR imaging of intramedullary and intradural-extramedullary spinal cysticercosis. AJR Am J Roentgenol 1997; 169(6):1713–7.

59. Litt AW, Mohuchy T. Case 10: neurocysticercosis. Radiology 1999;211(2):472–6.

60. Carpio A, Placencia M, Santillan F, et al. A proposal for classification of neurocysticercosis. Can J Neurol Sci 1994;21(1):43–7.

61. Castillo Y, Rodriguez S, Garcia HH, et al. Urine antigen detection for the diagnosis of human neurocysticercosis. Am J Trop Med Hyg 2009;80(3): 379–83.

62. Mendonca RA, Martins G, Lugokenski R, et al. Subacute spongiform encephalopathies. Top Magn Reson Imaging 2005;16(2):213–9.

63. Ukisu R, Kushihashi T, Tanaka E, et al. Diffusion-weighted MR imaging of early-stage Creutzfeldt-Jakob disease: typical and atypical manifestations. Radiographics 2006;26(Suppl 1):S191–204.

64. Tschampa HJ, Zerr I, Urbach H. Radiological assessment of Creutzfeldt-Jakob disease. Eur Radiol 2007;17(5):1200–11.

65. Luthra G, Parihar A, Nath K, et al. Comparative evaluation of fungal, tubercular, and pyogenic brain abscesses with conventional and diffusion MR imaging and proton MR spectroscopy. AJNR Am J Neuroradiol 2007;28(7):1332–8.

66. Whiteman M, Espinoza L, Post MJ, et al. Central nervous system tuberculosis in HIV-infected patients: clinical and radiographic findings. AJNR Am J Neuroradiol 1995;16(6):1319–27.

67. Saccente M. Central nervous system histoplasmosis. Curr Treat Options Neurol 2008;10(3):161–7.

68. Hayes WS, Sherman JL, Stern BJ, et al. MR and CT evaluation of intracranial sarcoidosis. AJR Am J Roentgenol 1987;149(5):1043–9.

69. Mafee MF, Dorodi S, Pai E. Sarcoidosis of the eye, orbit, and central nervous system. Role of MR imaging. Radiol Clin North Am 1999;37(1):73–87.

70. Lalani TA, Kanne JP, Hatfield GA, et al. Imaging findings in systemic lupus erythematosus. Radiographics 2004;24(4):1069–86.

71. Hagan IG, Burney K. Radiology of recreational drug abuse. Radiographics 2007;27(4):919–40.

72. Rabin BM, Meyer JR, Berlin JW, et al. Radiation-induced changes in the central nervous system and head and neck. Radiographics 1996;16(5):1055–72.

73. Osborn AG, Preece MT. Intracranial cysts: radiologic-pathologic correlation and imaging approach. Radiology 2006;239(3):650–64.

74. Mehta RC, Pike GB, Haros SP, et al. Central nervous system tumor, infection, and infarction: detection with gadolinium-enhanced magnetization transfer MR imaging. Radiology 1995;195(1):41–6.

75. Ge Y, Grossman RI, Udupa JK, et al. Brain atrophy in relapsing-remitting multiple sclerosis and secondary progressive multiple sclerosis: longitudinal quantitative analysis. Radiology 2000;214(3):665–70.

76. Ge Y, Grossman RI, Udupa JK, et al. Brain atrophy in relapsing-remitting multiple sclerosis: fractional volumetric analysis of gray matter and white matter. Radiology 2001;220(3):606–10.

77. Enzinger C, Strasser-Fuchs S, Ropele S, et al. Tumefactive demyelinating lesions: conventional and advanced magnetic resonance imaging. Mult Scler 2005;11(2):135–9.

78. Lucchinetti CF, Gavrilova RH, Metz I, et al. Clinical and radiographic spectrum of pathologically confirmed tumefactive multiple sclerosis. Brain 2008;131(Pt 7):1759–75.

79. Filippi M, Rocca MA. MR imaging of Devic's neuromyelitis optica. Neurol Sci 2004;25(Suppl 4):S371–3.

80. Simon JH, Kleinschmidt-DeMasters BK. Variants of multiple sclerosis. Neuroimaging Clin N Am 2008;18(4):703–16, xi.

81. Young NP, Weinshenker BG, Lucchinetti CF. Acute disseminated encephalomyelitis: current understanding and controversies. Semin Neurol 2008;28(1):84–94.

Posterior Reversible Encephalopathy Syndrome and Venous Thrombosis

Bojan D. Petrovic, MD[a],*, Alexander J. Nemeth, MD[b], Erin N. McComb, MD[b], Matthew T. Walker, MD[b]

KEYWORDS

- Posterior • Reversible • Encephalopathy • Syndrome
- Venous • Thrombosis

Posterior reversible encephalopathy syndrome (PRES) and venous thrombosis are frequently encountered first in the emergency setting and share some common characteristics. The clinical presentation of both is vague, and the brain parenchymal findings of PRES may resemble those of venous thrombosis in some ways. Both entities often occur in a bilateral posterior distribution and may be associated with reversible parenchymal findings if the inciting factor is treated. These diagnoses should be at the forefront of differential diagnosis when confronted with otherwise unexplained brain edema, among other findings described in this article.

PRES

PRES is a clinicoradiologic entity with characteristic symptoms and imaging features.[1,2] It is classically associated with a distinct pattern of edema that is primarily posterior, including the parietal and occipital lobes (**Fig. 1**).[1] PRES occurs in the setting of neurotoxicity, and the accompanying brain edema is reversible if the underlying cause is addressed.[2]

Although these statements are true for classic cases of PRES, it is important to recognize that the term PRES is, in many ways, a misnomer for this entity. PRES is not always posterior and may occur primarily in the frontal lobes. In addition, PRES is not always reversible if the cause is not treated. Again, these factors are of prime importance when considering an unusual pattern of brain edema not otherwise explained. Also, the patient may not always present with an encephalopathy, which is usually understood as altered mental status; instead, the patient may have various clinical presentations as described later. Also, the patient may not present with a syndrome.

Clinical Presentation and Demographics

Patients with PRES often develop headaches, visual disturbances (eg, blurry vision, hemianopsia, visual neglect, cortical blindness), seizures, and/or altered mental status.[3–5] Occasionally, these patients may develop focal neurologic deficits such as paresis or hemianopsia.[1,5] Because the symptoms are nonspecific, PRES can be a diagnostic dilemma from a clinical standpoint unless one maintains a high clinical suspicion in patients with risk factors for the disease. Symptoms associated with PRES may develop acutely or over several days.[1]

PRES is more prevalent in women.[6] It can occur over a wide age range and has been reported in patients aged 2 to 90 years.[6] The overall incidence of PRES has not been established.[6] The incidence of PRES in the setting of solid-organ transplant

[a] Neuroradiology Section, Department of Radiology, NorthShore University HealthSystem, 2650 Ridge Avenue, Evanston, IL 60201, USA
[b] Neuroradiology Section, Radiology Department, Northwestern Memorial Hospital, Feinberg School of Medicine, Northwestern University, 676 North Saint Clair Street, Suite 1400, Chicago, IL 60611, USA
* Corresponding author.
E-mail address: BPetrovic2@northshore.org

Radiol Clin N Am 49 (2011) 63–80
doi:10.1016/j.rcl.2010.07.016
0033-8389/11/$ – see front matter © 2011 Elsevier Inc. All rights reserved.

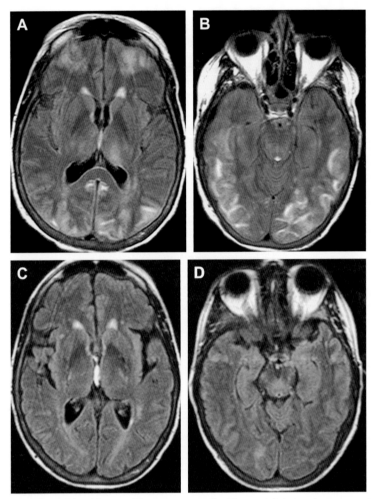

Fig. 1. A 59-year-old woman with a history of lupus presented with mental status changes and sepsis. Axial fluid-attenuated inversion recovery (FLAIR) MR images (*A*, *B*) show increased signal intensity in the cortex and subcortical white matter of the parietal and occipital lobes bilaterally and, to a lesser extent, in the bilateral frontal lobes and left thalamus. Axial FLAIR images obtained on follow-up several months later (*C*, *D*) demonstrate resolution of the findings without parenchymal sequelae such as encephalomalacia. The findings are consistent with PRES.

ranges from 0.4% to 6%.[1] In the setting of allogeneic bone marrow transplant with myeloablative marrow preconditioning and cyclosporine therapy, the incidence of PRES is 7% to 9%, although it may be as high as 16% with higher-dose myeloablative preconditioning and as low as 3% with nonmyeloablative therapy.[1]

Risk Factors and Causes of PRES

There are many conditions associated with the development of PRES. Frequently seen in the setting of moderate or severe hypertension, PRES was formerly referred to as hypertensive encephalopathy.[1] PRES, as it is now understood as a distinct clinical entity, was first described in patients with eclampsia and renal disease and in

those receiving immunosuppressant therapy.[4,5] Immunosuppressive agents most commonly associated with PRES include calcineurin inhibitors such as cyclosporine A and tacrolimus (FK-506).[5] PRES is now also known to occur in patients on antineoplastic chemotherapy (especially high-dose multidrug therapy), patients with certain autoimmune diseases (eg, lupus), and in the setting of infection, sepsis, or shock.[2,5]

The pathophysiology of PRES is not well understood. Because most patients with PRES (70%–80%)[1] have moderate to severe hypertension that developed either acutely or subacutely, one of the most commonly accepted theories is that severe hypertension exceeds the compensatory ability of the autoregulatory mechanisms of cerebral blood flow, ultimately resulting in vasodilation and edema.[5] Some investigators have asserted that the degree of hypertension required to induce PRES depends on the patient's baseline blood pressure.[5] Patients with baseline low-normal blood pressure may develop PRES if they experience a substantial increase in blood pressure, even if that elevated blood pressure is considered to be within the broad range of normal blood pressure.[5] In fact, 20% to 30% of patients with PRES may be normotensive or only minimally hypertensive.[1] Also, the upper limit of autoregulation may be increased in a chronically hypertensive patient.[7]

The major failing of the theory that is based on the collapse of the autoregulation of cerebral blood flow is that it cannot account for cases of PRES that occur in absence of severe or acute hypertension (20%–30%). Furthermore, by imaging studies, normotensive patients with PRES have been shown to develop greater edema than patients with severe hypertension.[1] Other known causes of PRES, such as cyclosporine A neurotoxicity, are also not readily explained by this theory. An alternative theory that has been proposed is that of an exaggerated cerebral autoregulatory response leading to potentially reversible vasospasm and ischemia.[8–10] More recently, the concept of a neurotoxic state has been introduced, in which circulating toxic substances induce endothelial injury or dysfunction, resulting in the breakdown of the blood-brain barrier and development of edema.[5]

Imaging Features

Although the causes of PRES are diverse, the imaging appearance is fundamentally the same regardless of the cause.[7] Typically, PRES is first encountered on computed tomography (CT) in the emergency setting; however, MR imaging is a more sensitive modality in the detection of PRES.[11] The characteristic findings in PRES are cortical and subcortical areas of hypoattenuation on CT or T2 hyperintensity on MR imaging with a predominantly posterior distribution in the parietal and occipital lobes.[5] On MR imaging, the findings are most apparent on fluid-attenuated inversion recovery (FLAIR) images.[11] The imaging hallmark of PRES is that the findings are potentially reversible. Resolution of findings on follow-up imaging often confirms the diagnosis.[6]

The reason why PRES is predisposed to involve the territory of the posterior circulation is uncertain but is thought to be related to the limited sympathetic innervation of the vertebrobasilar circulation.[12] This sympathetic innervation assists in the defense of the brain against marked increases in intravascular pressure, as might be seen with severe hypertension.[11] There is an inversely proportional relationship between the amount of sympathetic innervation and the degree of parenchymal involvement in PRES. The posterior aspects of the cerebral hemispheres are more commonly involved in PRES because there is relatively less protection via sympathetic innervation. However, in some cases, the protective efforts of sympathetic innervation in the anterior aspects of the cerebral hemispheres can also be overcome and involvement of the frontal and/or temporal lobes may be seen.[1,5] Thus, Narbone and colleagues[13] have suggested that potentially reversible encephalopathy syndrome may actually be a more appropriate term for PRES.

When areas of the brain apart from the parietal and occipital lobes are involved, it is sometimes referred to as atypical PRES.[12] However, Bartynski and Boardman[14] demonstrated that frontal lobe involvement was common as seen in 68% of patients (see **Fig. 1**). A posterior predominance can also be seen within each lobe.[11] For example, in a study by McKinney and colleagues,[11] when the frontal lobe was involved, the posterior portion of the superior frontal gyrus and the precentral gyrus were most commonly affected. The orbitofrontal region was affected only in the most severe cases.[11] Other structures that may be involved in PRES include the basal ganglia, brainstem, or cerebellum (**Figs. 2** and **3**).[1,5] The deep white matter may also be affected, including the corona radiata, splenium of the corpus callosum, or internal or external capsules.[14] In descending order, PRES most commonly involves the parietal and occipital lobes, frontal lobes, inferior temporo-occipital junction, and cerebellum.[1]

Earlier, PRES was referred to as posterior reversible leukoencephalopathy syndrome. This term has fallen out of favor because it suggests that there is a destructive process of the white matter, which is not usually the case.[10] The pathology of PRES in acute toxicity has shown nonspecific edema in the white matter but without overt inflammation, demyelination, or neuronal damage.[2] Although parenchymal changes in PRES primarily affect white matter, the cortex can also be involved.[12] In fact, FLAIR images show that the involvement of the gray matter is more extensive than was initially appreciated and that the development of edema may even commence in the cortex.[3,10] Up to 94% of patients with PRES have cortical involvement.[3]

Cerebral hemisphere involvement tends to be bilateral and symmetric. The lesions become confluent as the disease progresses.[1] Although typically bilateral, in a series by McKinney and

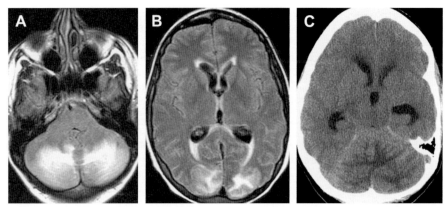

Fig. 2. A 22-year-old woman with a history of acute lymphocytic leukemia and mental status changes. Axial FLAIR MR images (*A, B*) show cortical and subcortical FLAIR hyperintensity bilaterally in the occipital lobes and the superior cerebellar hemispheres. FLAIR images also show mild hydrocephalus with dilatation of the lateral ventricles and periventricular FLAIR hyperintensity consistent with transependymal flow of cerebrospinal fluid. An axial CT image (*C*) also shows hypoattenuation in the superior cerebellum and mild hydrocephalus with dilatation of the lateral and third ventricles. After 2 months, follow-up MR image (not shown) demonstrated resolution of the findings that were attributed to PRES.

colleagues,[11] PRES was unilateral in 2.6% of patients. This unilateral involvement creates a diagnostic difficulty because differential considerations in this setting include neoplasms as well as infectious and inflammatory causes.

Although severe hypertension is a major risk factor for PRES, it should be noted that the degree

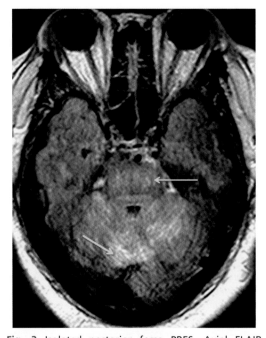

Fig. 3. Isolated posterior fossa PRES. Axial FLAIR image shows FLAIR hyperintensity in the cerebellar hemispheres, cerebellar vermis, and pons (*arrows*). The remainder of the brain (not shown) was unremarkable.

of hypertension in patients with PRES does not correlate with the distribution of the imaging findings.[14] Furthermore, in a study by Mueller-Mang and colleagues,[5] there was no statistically significant difference in the location of PRES parenchymal signal abnormalities between hypertensive and nonhypertensive patients with PRES related to cytotoxic or immunosuppressive drugs.[5] In fact, there is no way to distinguish between the varied causes of PRES based on the imaging findings.[10]

If there is marked involvement of the brainstem or cerebellum, the edema may result in hydrocephalus or even brainstem compression (see **Fig. 2**).[1] This condition is particularly true if there is localized mass effect on the cerebral aqueduct.

Slight enhancement may also be seen in PRES (**Figs. 4** and **5**), although this is not consistently present.[12] The enhancement most commonly occurs as mild, gyriform, leptomeningeal, or stippled (see **Fig. 5**) cortical enhancement. However, some reported cases have shown enhancement in the deep white matter or dura in addition to the leptomeningeal or cortical enhancement.[11] McKinney and colleagues[11] found no correlation between the presence of enhancement and the extent of FLAIR signal edema.

Diffusion-weighted MR imaging is useful in PRES because it can distinguish between vasogenic and cytotoxic edema.[12] Restricted diffusion seen with infarction or cytotoxic edema is uncommon in PRES but has been reported in 11% to 26% of patients (see **Fig. 5**).[1] When present, the typical pattern is to have small, patchy, or punctate areas of restricted diffusion,

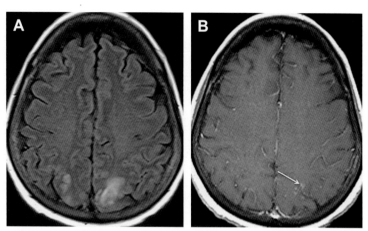

Fig. 4. PRES with enhancement. Axial FLAIR image (*A*) demonstrates FLAIR hyperintensity in the cortex and subcortical white matter of the parietal lobes bilaterally. Postgadolinium axial T1-weighted image (*B*) shows stippled cortical and subcortical enhancement (*arrow*) in the area of FLAIR hyperintensity in the left parietal lobe.

which correspond to areas of cytotoxic edema. The cytotoxic edema is considerably less extensive than the surrounding vasogenic edema.[11]

Hemorrhage is not often associated with PRES. However, intraparenchymal or subarachnoid hemorrhage can be seen in up to 15% of patients with PRES (**Fig. 6**).[1,15] In a study conducted by Aranas and colleagues,[2] most patients with PRES who developed intracranial hemorrhage had an underlying bleeding diathesis or coagulopathy. The incidence of hemorrhage does not correlate with the blood pressure at toxicity.[15]

PRES may result in vasculopathy that is demonstrable on MR angiography. The vasculopathy can appear as vessel irregularity, with focal areas of vasoconstriction and vasodilation, diffuse areas of vasoconstriction, or vessel pruning (see **Fig. 6**).[1] On catheter angiography, the vasculopathy of PRES may even result in a string of beads appearance that mimics fibromuscular dysplasia when PRES involves the internal carotid arteries or vertebral arteries.[1] Bartynski and Boardman[8] found evidence of vasculopathy in patients with PRES on 30 of 43 MR angiograms and 8 of 9 catheter angiograms. Follow-up MR angiography after treatment of PRES may demonstrate reversal of the vasculopathy.[1]

Potential Pitfalls

Accurately diagnosing PRES is important to avoid unnecessary brain biopsies or complications of PRES related to delayed treatment.[10] When the distribution of the imaging findings is archetypal and the clinical history is consistent with PRES, the diagnosis is straightforward. However, there may be isolated involvement in uncharacteristic locations (atypical PRES) such as the basal

ganglia, brainstem, and deep white matter, making diagnosis difficult.[1] When atypical imaging features of PRES (eg, an uncommon distribution of parenchymal changes, contrast enhancement, or hemorrhage) are found, clinical history is indispensable in making the diagnosis. Follow-up imaging demonstrating resolution of the findings after appropriate therapy is confirmatory.

Although CT is often used in the evaluation of patients in the emergency setting, the radiologist should be cognizant that subtle or atypical lesions may be missed in patients with PRES who undergo only CT evaluation.[14] MR imaging should be considered for patients in whom there is a clinical concern for PRES without diagnostic CT findings or when there is difficulty in differentiating PRES from other conditions that can mimic its appearance. For instance, vasogenic edema from PRES and cytotoxic edema from infarction have an identical CT appearance but are readily distinguished with diffusion-weighted MR imaging.

A particularly good mimic of PRES is dural sinus thrombosis. The edema pattern of both conditions may be identical. For instance, biparietal vasogenic edema can be seen in both PRES and superior sagittal sinus thrombosis. Dural sinus thrombosis is easily excluded with CT or MR venography.

Prognosis and Treatment

The prognosis in patients with PRES is variable but is typically considered to be favorable.[2] In many patients, the clinical and imaging findings are completely reversible with appropriate therapy.[5] However, in some patients, PRES progresses to ischemia, infarction, or death.[5,16] Patients whose MR images demonstrate extensive T2 parenchymal signal abnormalities are at a greater risk

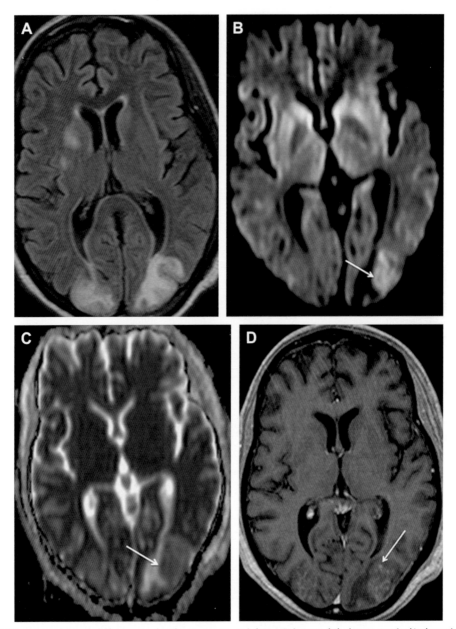

Fig. 5. PRES with restricted diffusion and enhancement. Axial FLAIR image (*A*) shows cortical/subcortical FLAIR hyperintensity in the occipital lobes bilaterally as well as within the right basal ganglia. Axial diffusion-weighted image (*B*) shows an area of increased signal intensity in the left occipital lobe (*arrow*). Axial apparent diffusion coefficient map image (*C*) shows punctate focus of low signal (*arrow*) along the medial margin of the diffusion abnormality in the left occipital lobe consistent with a small focus of restricted diffusion next to a larger area of vasogenic edema with increased signal. Axial postgadolinium T1-weighted image (*D*) shows stippled enhancement (*arrow*) in the areas of FLAIR signal abnormality in the occipital lobes.

for a poor outcome than patients whose MR images show minimal parenchymal T2 changes.[12] Prognosis for patients with PRES associated with intracranial hemorrhage may be worse than in patients without hemorrhage, with increased morbidity and mortality.[2] In a small series by Aranas and colleagues,[2] only 28% of patients with PRES and intracranial hemorrhage attained a favorable functional outcome. It is indeterminate whether the poor outcome is caused by the hemorrhage itself or it reflects the severity of the disease in these patients.[2]

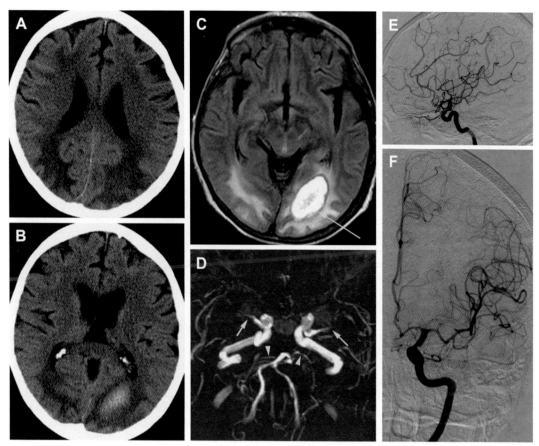

Fig. 6. A 56-year-old woman with septic shock, renal failure, and thrombocytopenia developed mental status changes. Axial noncontrast CT images (*A, B*) demonstrate confluent cortical/subcortical hypoattenuation involving more of the parietal and occipital lobes than the frontal lobes, in a pattern consistent with PRES. Intraparenchymal hemorrhage in the left occipital lobe is also present. Axial FLAIR MR image (*C*) demonstrates confluent cortical/subcortical FLAIR hyperintensity in the occipital lobes as well as the intraparenchymal hemorrhage in the left occipital lobe (*arrow*). Collapsed 3-dimensional time-of-flight MR angiographic image (*D*) demonstrates spasm with cutoff of the middle cerebral arteries bilaterally (*arrows*) as well as irregularity of the posterior cerebral arteries bilaterally (*arrowheads*) consistent with the vasculopathy of PRES. Follow-up catheter angiograms (*E, F*) display a normal left middle cerebral artery, consistent with resolution of the vasculopathy of PRES.

Timely treatment is necessary to minimize the risk of complications in PRES.[12] Treatment is aimed at the underlying causes. For example, in patients with hypertension, maintaining adequate blood pressure is a mainstay of therapy. In eclamptic patients who are refractory to medical therapy, delivery by cesarean section may be necessary.[6] In patients on tacrolimus, symptoms can often be reversed by reducing the dosage of the medication or withholding the medication for a few days.[12] Some physicians may also consider adding antiepileptic drugs or magnesium sulfate because of the risk of developing status epilepticus.[6]

CEREBRAL VENOUS THROMBOSIS

Cerebral venous thrombosis is an uncommon but serious condition first described in the early nineteenth century.[17,18] The estimated annual incidence is 2 to 7 cases per million population per year.[19] The myriad causes of cerebral venous thrombosis and the broad spectrum of clinical manifestations make diagnosis difficult.[20–22] However, rapid diagnosis is vital because appropriate therapy can significantly curtail the risk of serious complications including intracranial stroke or death.[23]

Causes and Risk Factors

The causes of cerebral venous thrombosis are protean. Cerebral venous thrombosis may be related to local conditions that directly affect the cerebral veins and dural sinuses or a systemic process leading to a hypercoagulable state. Examples of local conditions affecting the cerebral veins and dural sinuses include trauma to the dural sinuses, infection in structures adjacent to the dural sinuses, or invasion or compression of the sinuses by neoplastic processes.[21,24] Hypercoagulable states such as protein C or protein S deficiency, presence of lupus anticoagulant, oral contraceptive use, pregnancy, or malignancy may also predispose to cerebral venous thrombosis.[21,24] Dural arteriovenous fistula is also associated with cerebral venous thrombosis,[25] although it is unclear whether this is the cause or result of cerebral venous thrombosis. In a study by Tsai and colleagues,[26] 39% of patients with dural arteriovenous fistula also had dural sinus thrombosis. In most cases, the dural sinus thrombosis was near the site of the dural arteriovenous fistula.[26]

Risk factors for cerebral venous thrombosis in children often differ from those seen in adults.[27] Perinatal complications, such as hypoxic ischemic encephalopathy, are the most common risk factors in neonates.[27] In young children, head and neck infections (eg, otitis media, mastoiditis, sinusitis) are the most frequent risk factors for cerebral venous thrombosis.[27] In older children, chronic diseases, such as connective tissue diseases, are more common causes.[27]

Demographics and Clinical Presentation

Cerebral venous thrombosis occurs in all age groups, although it chiefly occurs in patients aged 20 to 35 years.[28] Cerebral venous thrombosis is the cause of approximately 1% to 2% of strokes in young adults.[29] Among children with cerebral venous thrombosis, neonates are the most commonly affected group.[27]

Clinical signs and symptoms of cerebral venous thrombosis are often vague. Most patients with cerebral venous thrombosis develop generalized neurologic symptoms with headache, seen in 75% to 95% of patients,[21] as a common first clinical symptom[30]; nausea is also seen.[30] Papilledema may be noted on physical examination, indicating elevated intracranial pressure.[31] Some patients develop seizures or focal sensory or motor deficits (such as vision changes[30] or hemiparesis).[21] Cranial nerve palsies may occur,[30] particularly when there is involvement of the petrous sinuses.[32] In some cases, cerebral venous thrombosis may even lead to coma or death.[32]

Cerebral venous thrombosis results in elevated venous pressure.[21,31] In some instances, a robust collateral venous drainage network may mitigate against venous hypertension.[21] However, if adequate collateral venous drainage fails to materialize, the venous pressure increases. As venous pressure increases, venous congestion develops with an accompanying decline in arterial perfusion pressure[21] and a reversible compromise of oxygen and glucose consumption.[32] If reduction of arterial perfusion pressure is severe enough and prolonged enough, venous infarction occurs[21] and hemorrhage may ensue.[18] Again, if collateral venous drainage develops or recanalization occurs before cell death, the parenchymal changes identified on imaging (including vasogenic and cytotoxic edema) may partially or even completely resolve.[21,33]

Unlike arterial thrombosis, symptoms in cerebral venous thrombosis tend to develop slowly or subacutely.[30] The clinical manifestations of cerebral venous thrombosis are determined by the extent, site, and acuity of thrombosis.[21] The clinical scenario may also vary over time because of thrombosis and concurrent endogenous thrombolysis and recanalization.[21]

Imaging Modalities and Imaging Features

In patients with cerebral venous thrombosis, the superior sagittal sinus is most commonly involved, seen in approximately two-thirds of patients.[17] Many patients with superior sagittal sinus thrombosis also have thrombus extending into the transverse and sigmoid sinuses (**Fig. 7**).[17] Deep venous system thrombosis (eg, thrombosis of the internal cerebral veins, vein of Galen, or straight sinus) is seen in approximately 16% of patients with cerebral venous thrombosis (**Figs. 8 and 9**).[21] Most of these patients present with symptoms of intracranial hypertension and may rapidly deteriorate to a comatose state.[21]

Imaging of the cerebral venous structures may be performed with MR or CT venography (CTV). With time-of-flight (TOF) MR venography, normal flow results in high signal, whereas absence of flow yields low signal.[17] CTV demonstrates thrombus as a filling defect within a contrast-enhanced dural sinus or nonopacification of a cerebral vein.

The most common MR venography techniques are 2-dimensional TOF (2D-TOF) MR venography and contrast-enhanced MR venography. TOF MR venography displays flowing blood as high signal. The background is dark secondary to the suppression of signal from stationary tissues. The 2D-TOF techniques are most sensitive to the flow that is perpendicular to the plane of acquisition.[21] In areas where venous flow is parallel to the plane of acquisition, saturation effects can lead to loss of signal, which must not be mistaken for venous thrombosis.[17,21] With contrast-enhanced MR venography, the paramagnetic

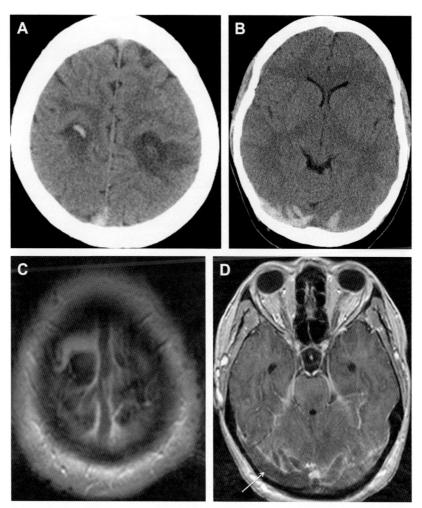

Fig. 7. Venous hemorrhagic infarction. Axial noncontrast CT image (*A*) shows biparietal intraparenchymal hemorrhages with surrounding hypoattenuation consistent with vasogenic edema. Hyperattenuation within the superior sagittal sinus suggesting hemorrhagic infarcts secondary to dural sinus thrombosis. A more caudal noncontrast axial CT image (*B*) demonstrates linear hyperattenuation along the transverse sinuses and cortical veins consistent with dural sinus and cortical venous thromboses. Postgadolinium axial 3-dimensional magnetized-prepared rapid gradient echo images (*C, D*) confirm the presence of superior sagittal sinus, transverse sinus (*arrow*), and cortical venous thrombosis with filling defects found in those locations.

effect of gadolinium shortens T1, resulting in intravascular contrast enhancement.[21] When compared with TOF MR venography, contrast-enhanced MR venography offers superior visualization of smaller vessels with fewer problematic effects of turbulent flow.[21] There are several methods for performing contrast-enhanced MR venography. Among the more common methods are the magnetized-prepared rapid gradient echo and volumetric interpolated brain examination pulse sequences. A particular advantage of these techniques is that the signal is not affected by the angle between the vessels and the scan plane.[34] This advantage is especially helpful in the evaluation of the sigmoid sinuses and jugular bulb, which are often problematic with other techniques because of artifacts and turbulent flow.

CTV is commonly used in the emergency setting because it can be performed swiftly and offers improved visualization of small vessels when compared with MR venography (eg, the inferior sagittal sinus, basal veins of Rosenthal, and nondominant transverse sinus).[30,35] In addition, CTV is not affected by the flow-related artifacts that are sometimes problematic with MR venography.[17] In the assessment of cerebral venous thrombosis, CTV has been shown to be at least as accurate as TOF MR venography.[17,21,35] One of the disadvantages of this technique is the complexity of generation of maximum intensity

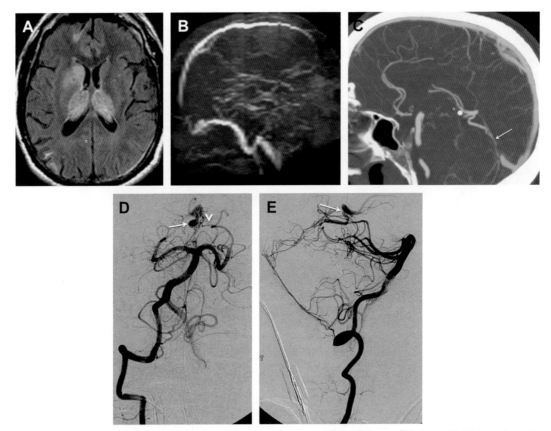

Fig. 8. Deep venous thrombosis and dural arteriovenous fistula. Axial FLAIR image (*A*) shows FLAIR hyperintensity in the right basal ganglia and bilateral thalami. Maximum intensity projection image from 2-dimensional time-of-flight MR venography (*B*) demonstrates lack of flow-related enhancement in the straight sinus consistent with dural sinus thrombosis. On the sagittal CT angiographic image (*C*), there is no visualization of most of the straight sinus (*arrow*), compatible with thrombosis. Anteroposterior and lateral catheter angiograms with right vertebral injection (*D, E*) show a dural arteriovenous fistula within the straight sinus with a left posterior cerebral artery branch arterial feeder (*arrowheads*) and early filling of deep veins including the vein of Galen (*arrows*). On more delayed images (not shown), there was nonvisualization of the straight sinus, compatible with dural sinus thrombosis.

projection (MIP) images from the source data secondary to the care that must be taken not to omit part of the sinus when subtracting the bone.[21] However, Wetzel and colleagues[36] showed that CTV with multiplanar reformations has increased sensitivity in depiction of the venous anatomy compared with CTV with MIP images.[30] Sensitivity and specificity of CTV for cerebral venous thrombosis approach 100%.[30] Nevertheless, a hyperdense venous thrombus can be mistaken for normal enhancing sinus, referred to as the "cord sign." Therefore, it is imperative that CTV be reviewed in conjunction with an unenhanced head CT.[30] Occasionally, chronic thrombus may also be difficult to detect on CTV because the clot may enhance, thereby failing to manifest as a filling defect.[30]

Unenhanced CT examinations can sometimes demonstrate findings that raise the possibility of cerebral venous thrombosis. Chief among these findings is a hyperdense dural venous sinus or a dense cortical vein (**Fig. 10**). However, a hyperdense sinus is seen only in 25% of patients with dural venous sinus thrombosis. Other potential causes of increased dural sinus attenuation include dehydration and polycythemia.[16,21] Comparison of the density of dural venous sinus with that of the arteries can be helpful in differentiating dural venous sinus thrombosis from physiologic causes of increased attenuation. If venous sinus hyperdensity is identified on unenhanced CT, this should be further evaluated with CTV or MR venography. Nonspecific findings, such as edema or parenchymal hemorrhage, not

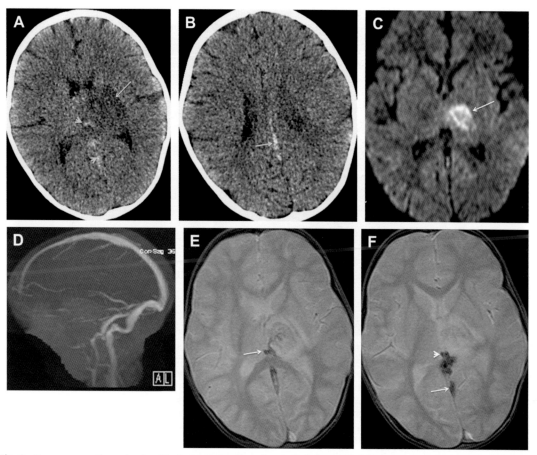

Fig. 9. Deep venous thrombosis with thalamic and basal ganglia infarcts. Axial noncontrast CT images (*A, B*) show confluent hypoattenuation in the left thalamus and left basal ganglia (*arrow in A*) as well as subtle hyperattenuation along the deep veins (*arrowheads on A* and *arrow on B*), suggesting thrombosis. Axial diffusion-weighted image (*C*) shows restricted diffusion in the left thalamus (*arrow*) consistent with acute infarction. Maximum intensity projection MR venographic image (*D*) demonstrates lack of flow-related enhancement in the internal cerebral veins, vein of Galen, and straight sinus, consistent with thrombosis. Axial gradient echo images (*E, F*) demonstrate blooming of susceptibility artifact within the deep veins (*arrow in E* and *arrowhead in F*) and straight sinus (*arrow in F*) caused by deep venous thrombosis.

conforming to an arterial territory can sometimes suggest the diagnosis of venous thrombosis and/or venous infarction. Rarely, subarchnoid hemorrhage may be the sole finding in cerebral venous thrombosis[18] and should be considered in patients without an identifiable cause for subarachnoid hemorrhage.

Unenhanced conventional MR imaging can sometimes raise the specter of cerebral venous thrombosis and is more sensitive than noncontrast CT in the identification of cerebral venous thrombosis.[21] Thrombosis should be considered when there is loss of an expected dural venous sinus flow void.[17,21] With careful review, this finding may be seen in 80% of patients with cerebral venous thrombosis.[17] However, turbulent or slow flow can also affect dural venous sinus signal

and is a potential pitfall, particularly at the jugular bulb.[21] When dural venous sinus thrombosis is present, venous sinus signal abnormalities are typically seen on multiple sequences. The appearance of a venous thrombus on T1- and T2-weighted images varies with the age of the thrombus (**Table 1**). On gradient echo MR images, magnetic susceptibility artifact related to deoxyhemoglobin or methemoglobin may sometimes be a helpful diagnostic adjunct in the detection of dural venous sinus thrombosis (**Fig. 11**).[21] However, chronic thrombus may not be associated much with gradient susceptibility artifact.[19] The reason for this is unclear but may be because of elimination of blood breakdown products by macrophages during the process of thrombus organization.[19] In some cases, a dural venous

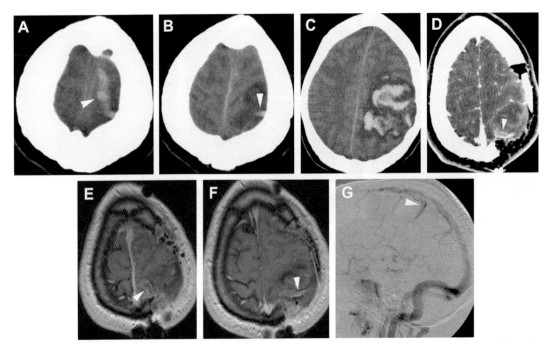

Fig. 10. Isolated cortical vein thrombosis. Axial noncontrast CT images (*A, B,* and *C*) demonstrate a curvilinear hyperdense structure (*arrowheads*) along the left parietal lobe consistent with a thrombosed cortical vein. A large intraparenchymal hemorrhage with surrounding hypoattenuation consistent with vasogenic edema is seen in the left parietal lobe in image C, compatible with a venous hemorrhagic infarct. Axial CT angiographic image after left parietal craniectomy for decompression (*D*) shows a filling defect (*arrowhead*) within an enlarged left parietal cortical vein consistent with thrombus. Axial postgadolinium 3D magnetized-prepared rapid gradient echo images after left parietal craniectomy for decompression (*E, F*) confirm the filling defect (*arrowheads*) in the left parietal cortical vein consistent with thrombus. Lateral view of a catheter angiogram in the venous phase (*G*) also shows the filling defect in the parietal vein (*arrowhead*), confirming the venous thrombosis.

sinus thrombus may demonstrate restricted diffusion.[21]

Conventional contrast-enhanced CT or MR imaging of the brain can sometimes provide clues to the diagnosis of dural venous sinus thrombosis. The empty delta sign is characterized by the presence of a central intraluminal filling defect surrounded by contrast-enhanced dural collateral venous channels and cavernous spaces in the sinus wall. This sign is diagnostic of dural venous sinus thrombosis.[21,37] Although the empty delta sign is very specific for the diagnosis of dural venous thrombosis, its sensitivity is only approximately 30%.[37] Subacute thrombus on postcontrast T1-weighted MR images may display increased signal intensity that may occasionally simulate the signal of flow.[35] However, subacute thrombus rarely achieves the very bright signal intensity of normal flow.[24,35] But chronic organized dural venous sinus thrombus may enhance.[21] As a thrombus ages, it is invaded by fibroblasts and endothelial-lined channels, converting it to a vascularized tissue that enhances.[19,21,37] Contrast enhancement in the dural venous sinuses does

not definitely exclude thrombosis, and even contrast-enhanced MR venography may have a decreased sensitivity for chronic thrombus.[21,37] Because the length of time required for chronic

| Table 1 |
| MR signal characteristics of thrombus versus thrombus age |

Age of Thrombus	Signal Characteristics
Acute (0–5 d)	Isointense on T1-weighted images Hypointense on T2-weighted images
Subacute (6–15 d)	Hyperintense on T1- and T2-weighted images
Chronic (>15 d)	Variable signal characteristics but typically isointense on T1-weighted images and isointense to hyperintense on T2-weighted images

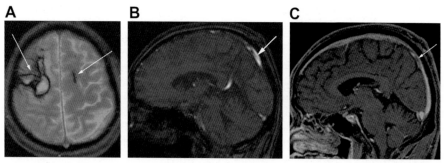

Fig. 11. Chronic superior sagittal sinus thrombus on 2D-TOF MR venography and postgadolinium volumetric interpolated brain examination (VIBE) MR venography. Axial gradient echo image (A) shows susceptibility artifact (arrows) in the frontal lobes bilaterally consistent with intraparenchymal hemorrhages. MIP image from 2D-TOF MR venography (B) shows subtle nonocclusive filling defect (arrow) within the superior sagittal sinus consistent with chronic thrombus. Postgadolinium VIBE MR venographic image (C) in the same patient demonstrates thrombus (arrow) in the superior sagittal sinus to better advantage.

thrombus to begin to demonstrate significant enhancement is unclear, it is helpful to perform both contrast-enhanced and TOF MR venography.[19]

Parenchymal abnormalities are seen in many patients with cerebral venous thrombosis. Parenchymal abnormalities include edema (vasogenic or cytotoxic), hemorrhage, or enhancement. Edema may manifest as areas of hypoattenuation (on CT) or T2 hyperintensity (on MR imaging) involving cortex, white matter, or both. Unlike arterial infarcts that are typically transcortical, intraparenchymal changes in cerebral venous thrombosis are often subcortical.[29] Mass effect is also seen in most patients,[33] but it should be noted that the edema leading to parenchymal swelling does not always manifest as parenchymal attenuation or signal abnormalities. In fact, there may be evidence of parenchymal swelling with sulcal or ventricular effacement in up to 42% of patients without associated parenchymal attenuation or signal abnormalities.[21]

Approximately one-third of patients with cerebral venous thrombosis develop intraparenchymal hemorrhages (see **Fig. 11**).[21] This development may be related to continued arterial perfusion in areas of infarction or venous hypertension beyond a critical limit.[21] The hemorrhages are typically cortical with subcortical extension.[21] Cerebral venous thrombosis may also result in subarachnoid hemorrhage[22] related to rupture of dilated cortical veins.[22]

Enhancement patterns that have been described in patients with cerebral venous thrombosis include parenchymal enhancement (often gyral in location), tentorial enhancement, leptomeningeal enhancement, and prominent cortical venous enhancement.[21]

The location of the parenchymal abnormalities usually reflects the site of thrombosis. For instance, edema or hemorrhage in the bilateral frontal, parietal, and occipital lobes is typical of superior sagittal sinus thrombosis,[23] whereas deep venous thrombosis often affects the thalami that have primary venous pathways draining into the internal cerebral veins.[21] The characteristic parenchymal finding in patients with deep cerebral venous thrombosis is thalamic hemorrhage or bilateral thalamic edema, with occasional involvement of the caudate nuclei and deep white matter.[21] Unilateral thalamic parenchymal findings in deep cerebral venous thrombosis are rare.[21] Although the distribution of parenchymal abnormalities may suggest the site of thrombosis, there are some atypical cases.[21] For example, dural sinus thrombosis may result in edema or hemorrhage in the supratentorium as well as in the cerebellum and brainstem.[23]

Isolated cortical venous thrombosis without associated dural sinus thrombosis is rare because both the thromboses are usually related, with the thrombus extending in a retrograde manner from the thrombosed sinus.[29] Many patients with isolated cortical venous thrombosis either have a coagulopathy or a chronic inflammatory disease such as inflammatory bowel disease.[21] The typical finding in cortical venous thrombosis is a hyperdense or hyperintense cortical vein that shows blooming on gradient echo images.[21] There may or may not be associated edema or hemorrhage in the parenchyma drained by the vein. Occasionally, cortical venous thrombosis may be detected on MR venography as loss of flow-related or contrast-related enhancement within the thrombosed cortical vein. The thrombosis of the main draining vein of a developmental venous anomaly associated with a thrombosed venous varix and thrombosed cortical vein is shown in **Fig. 12**.[21]

Potential Pitfalls

With cerebral venous thrombosis, the average delay from onset of symptoms to diagnosis is 7 days.[30] Many clinical conditions including arterial stroke, brain tumors, encephalitis, and benign intracranial hypertension may mimic cerebral venous thrombosis.[18] Clinical diagnosis of cerebral venous thrombosis is further complicated by vague nonspecific symptoms. If a high index of suspicion is not maintained in such patients without a clear alternate diagnosis, then diagnosis of cerebral venous thrombosis is often missed. Cerebral venous sinus thrombosis should always be considered in young or middle-aged patients with atypical or severe headache or with strokelike symptoms in patients without the usual risk factors for stroke.[30] The diagnosis should also be suspected when imaging demonstrates localized cerebral edema or infarction that does not conform to an arterial vascular territory.[29]

Although positive findings of cerebral venous thrombosis (eg, hemorrhagic venous infarcts, the dense vein sign on unenhanced CT, and the empty delta sign on contrast-enhanced CT) are helpful, it must be kept in mind that positive findings on screening examinations are only seen in a minority of patients with cerebral venous thrombosis.[17] When there is concern for cerebral venous thrombosis, CTV or MR venography must be performed.

When evaluating for cerebral venous sinus thrombosis, the radiologist must be aware of several potential pitfalls, including dural venous sinus asymmetry, slow flow in a hypoplastic sinus on TOF MR venography, variant sinus confluence anatomy, arachnoid granulations, intrinsic thrombus signal on TOF MR venography, and sinus signal intensity variations. Dural venous sinus asymmetry is relatively common, with the right transverse sinus typically larger than the left. Furthermore, a dural venous sinus may be hypoplastic or atretic. With 2D-TOF MR venography, the radiologist may not be able to differentiate a hypoplastic or atretic sinus from dural venous sinus thrombosis.[34] Slow flow in hypoplastic dural venous sinuses may manifest as

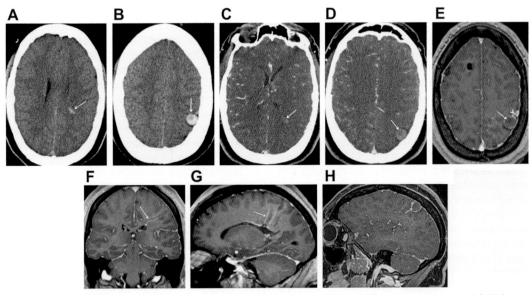

Fig. 12. A 27-year-old woman with new-onset right-sided seizures. (*A*) and (*B*) are noncontrast axial CT images demonstrating hyperdense material (*arrows*) in the left parietal lobe. CT angiographic images (*C, D*) show that this hyperdensity corresponds to a filling defect within the main draining vein of a large left parietal developmental venous anomaly (*arrow in C*) and an associated venous varix (*arrow in D*). The filling defect is consistent with thrombus. Axial postgadolinium 3D magnetized-prepared rapid gradient echo (MP-RAGE) image (*E*) shows thrombus extending into a cortical vein (*arrowhead*) associated with the left parietal venous varix (*arrow*). The left parietal developmental venous anomaly (*arrows*) is well demonstrated on coronal and sagittal postgadolinium 3D MP-RAGE images (*F, G*). Postgadolinium sagittal volumetric interpolated brain examination MR venographic image (*H*) confirms the filling defect (*arrow*) in the venous varix associated with the developmental venous anomaly.

flow gaps on TOF MR venography because the flow-related enhancement may be insufficient to distinguish it from stationary tissue.[35]

TOF MR venography is prone to signal loss from saturation effects when the direction of blood flow is parallel rather than perpendicular to the acquisition plane.[19,21] This signal loss may cause a flow gap simulating thrombosis.[19,35] Misdiagnosis of cerebral venous thrombosis can often be averted in these settings by referring to the source images as well as TOF MR venographic images obtained in an orthogonal plane.

A high or asymmetric bifurcation at the torcular Herophili can be mistaken for thrombus (pseudoempty delta sign). This pitfall can be avoided by careful evaluation of the source and reformatted images.

Lesions that protrude into or invade a dural venous sinus may mimic a thrombus. Arachnoid granulations, which normally extend into the dural venous sinuses, can cause defects that may be misdiagnosed as thrombi, particularly if they are large (Fig. 13). Arachnoid granulations are typically focal round defects with a signal intensity or attenuation similar to that of the cerebrospinal fluid.[21] Although the granulations may occur anywhere in the dural venous sinus system, they are most commonly seen in the transverse sinus or superior sagittal sinus. In the transverse sinus, they are commonly seen in the lateral transverse sinus, the drainage site for the vein of Labbé, and lateral tentorial sinus.[21] A tumor such as a meningioma may also invade or cause mass effects on a dural venous sinus, simulating a thrombus.[35]

Increased signal intensity associated with subacute thrombus can sometimes simulate normal flow on T1-weighted TOF or contrast-enhanced MR venography. Review of the source images usually helps in differentiation.[21,30] Also, the signal of subacute thrombus is rarely as high in signal intensity as normal flow. Organized chronic thrombus is also a potential pitfall on T1-weighted images, because enhancement related to chronic thrombus may simulate the contrast-enhanced MR venography of a patent sinus.[19] Small flow voids may be seen within chronic thrombus on T2-weighted images.

CT venograms and MR venograms are often displayed with an MIP algorithm. This technique displays the highest intensity pixel in the volume along a ray perpendicular to the viewing screen.[35] The advantage of this technique is that it enables the viewing of the high-density or high signal intensity vessels through the relative low-density or low signal intensity brain parenchyma.[35] However, because MIP images emphasize the brightest voxels in a vessel, the thrombus may be obscured by the surrounding high-density contrast on CTV or high signal intensity flow on MR venography.[35] Thus, the source images should always be consulted when reviewing MIP images.[35]

Subdural hematoma along a dural venous sinus may be mistaken for acute dural venous thrombosis on unenhanced CT or MR.[17]

Spin-echo imaging can sometimes demonstrate artifactual loss of the expected dural venous sinus flow void because of flow-related enhancement or echo rephrasing.[17] Venous signal abnormalities caused by turbulent flow are especially problematic at the level of the jugular bulb.

Prognosis and Treatment

The most severe complications of cerebral venous thrombosis include intracranial hemorrhage, venous infarct, and death. Reported mortality rates of cerebral venous thrombosis range from 5% to 30%.[18,28,29] Factors associated with a poor prognosis of cerebral venous thrombosis include infancy, advanced age, thrombus largely affecting the deep venous system or cerebellar veins, and rapid onset of coma and focal neurologic deficits.[28]

Treatment option for cerebral venous thrombosis includes intravenous heparin or intradural thrombolysis.[20,31] Anticoagulation and/or thrombolytic therapy can improve clinical outcome in cerebral venous thrombosis.[18] Anticoagulation with intravenous heparin halts the progression of thrombosis and allows the body's endogenous thrombolytic process to achieve partial or complete recanalization.[28] With heparin therapy, approximately 70% of patients achieve complete recovery.[28] Even in the presence of hemorrhage, heparin therapy can greatly improve outcome and reduce mortality.[24]

Thrombolysis is most commonly used in patients whose clinical status worsens while on anticoagulation.[20] Thrombolysis is most often accomplished with a pharmacologic agent such as tissue plasminogen activator. Hemorrhage or massive venous infarction is not a contraindication to thrombolysis in the setting of cerebral venous thrombosis, unlike with arterial occlusion.[23] In patients with poor response to intradural thrombolysis, rapid neurologic deterioration, or contraindication to pharmacologic thrombolysis, mechanical thrombectomy with a rheolytic catheter may be attempted.[28] Mechanical thrombectomy may also be considered as an adjunctive therapy in patients undergoing pharmacologic thrombolysis.[31]

Treatment of chronic thrombus is controversial because it may not respond as well to anticoagulation as acute thrombus.[19]

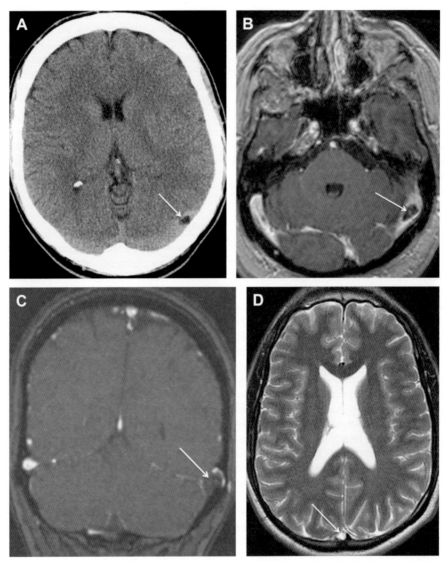

Fig. 13. Arachnoid granulations. Noncontrast axial CT image (*A*) demonstrates a focus of cerebrospinal fluid (CSF) attenuation (*arrow*) within the left transverse sinus consistent with an arachnoid granulation. Axial postgadolinium 3D magnetized-prepared rapid gradient echo (MP-RAGE) image (*B*) shows a filling defect (*arrow*) in the distal left transverse sinus with a typical location and appearance of an arachnoid granulation. Coronal postgadolinium 3D MP-RAGE image (*C*) shows an unusually large arachnoid granulation (*arrow*) as a filling defect in the distal left transverse sinus. Axial T2-weighted image (*D*) depicts a round T2 hyperintense structure (*arrow*) in the superior sagittal sinus demonstrating CSF signal and is compatible with an arachnoid granulation.

SUMMARY

PRES and venous thrombosis are discussed together in this article because both these entities have vague clinical presentations and similar imaging findings and radiologists may be the first to suggest the diagnosis. When brain edema and intraparenchymal hemorrhage occur without respecting vascular territories, or are above and below the tentorium, both entities should be considered in the differential diagnosis. It is crucial to be familiar with these entities when reading emergency neuroradiology studies.

REFERENCES

1. Bartynski WS. Posterior reversible encephalopathy syndrome, part 1: fundamental imaging and clinical features. AJNR Am J Neuroradiol 2008;29(6): 1036–42.

2. Aranas RM, Prabhakaran S, Lee VH. Posterior reversible encephalopathy syndrome associated with hemorrhage. Neurocrit Care 2009;10(3): 306–12.

3. Finocchi V, Bozzao A, Bonamini M, et al. Magnetic resonance imaging in posterior reversible encephalopathy syndrome: report of three cases and review of literature. Arch Gynecol Obstet 2005;271(1): 79–85.

4. Hinchey J, Chaves C, Appignani B, et al. A reversible posterior leukoencephalopathy syndrome. N Engl J Med 1996;334(8):494–500.

5. Mueller-Mang C, Mang T, Pirker A, et al. Posterior reversible encephalopathy syndrome: do predisposing risk factors make a difference in MRI appearance? Neuroradiology 2009;51(6):373–83.

6. O'Hara McCoy H. Posterior reversible encephalopathy syndrome: an emerging clinical entity in adult, pediatric, and obstetric critical care. J Am Acad Nurse Pract 2008;20(2):100–6.

7. Bartynski WS. Posterior reversible encephalopathy syndrome, part 2: controversies surrounding pathophysiology of vasogenic edema. AJNR Am J Neuroradiol 2008;29(6):1043–9.

8. Bartynski WS, Boardman JF. Catheter angiography, MR angiography, and MR perfusion in posterior reversible encephalopathy syndrome. AJNR Am J Neuroradiol 2008;29(3):447–55.

9. Bartynski WS, Boardman JF, Zeigler ZR, et al. Posterior reversible encephalopathy syndrome in infection, sepsis, and shock. AJNR Am J Neuroradiol 2006;27(10):2179–90.

10. Casey SO, Sampaio RC, Michel E, et al. Posterior reversible encephalopathy syndrome: utility of fluid-attenuated inversion recovery MR imaging in the detection of cortical and subcortical lesions. AJNR Am J Neuroradiol 2000;21(7):1199–206.

11. McKinney AM, Short J, Truwit CL, et al. Posterior reversible encephalopathy syndrome: incidence of atypical regions of involvement and imaging findings. AJR Am J Roentgenol 2007;189(4): 904–12.

12. Hodnett P, Coyle J, O'Regan K, et al. PRES (posterior reversible encephalopathy syndrome), a rare complication of tacrolimus therapy. Emerg Radiol 2009;16(6):493–6.

13. Narbone MC, Musolino R, Granata F, et al. Posterior or potentially reversible encephalopathy syndrome? Neurol Sci 2006;27(3):187–9.

14. Bartynski WS, Boardman JF. Distinct imaging patterns and lesion distribution in posterior reversible encephalopathy syndrome. AJNR Am J Neuroradiol 2007;28(7):1320–7.

15. Hefzy HM, Bartynski WS, Boardman JF, et al. Hemorrhage in posterior reversible encephalopathy syndrome: imaging and clinical features. AJNR Am J Neuroradiol 2009;30(7):1371–9.

16. Healy JF, Nichols C. Polycythemia mimicking venous sinus thrombosis. AJNR Am J Neuroradiol 2002;23(8):1402–3.

17. Khandelwal N, Agarwal A, Kochhar R, et al. Comparison of CT venography with MR venography in cerebral sinovenous thrombosis. AJR Am J Roentgenol 2006;187(6):1637–43.

18. Tang PH, Chai J, Chan YH, et al. Superior sagittal sinus thrombosis: subtle signs on neuroimaging. Ann Acad Med Singap 2008;37(5): 397–401.

19. Leach JL, Wolujewicz M, Strub WM. Partially recanalized chronic dural sinus thrombosis: findings on MR imaging, time-of-flight MR venography, and contrast-enhanced MR venography. AJNR Am J Neuroradiol 2007;28(4):782–9.

20. Manzione J, Newman GC, Shapiro A, et al. Diffusion- and perfusion-weighted MR imaging of dural sinus thrombosis. AJNR Am J Neuroradiol 2000;21(1): 68–73.

21. Leach JL, Fortuna RB, Jones BV, et al. Imaging of cerebral venous thrombosis: current techniques, spectrum of findings, and diagnostic pitfalls. Radiographics 2006;26(Suppl 1):S19–41 [discussion: S42–3].

22. Oppenheim C, Domigo V, Gauvrit JY, et al. Subarachnoid hemorrhage as the initial presentation of dural sinus thrombosis. AJNR Am J Neuroradiol 2005;26(3):614–7.

23. Tsai FY, Wang AM, Matovich VB, et al. MR staging of acute dural sinus thrombosis: correlation with venous pressure measurements and implications for treatment and prognosis. AJNR Am J Neuroradiol 1995;16(5):1021–9.

24. Vogl TJ, Bergman C, Villringer A, et al. Dural sinus thrombosis: value of venous MR angiography for diagnosis and follow-up. AJR Am J Roentgenol 1994;162(5):1191–8.

25. Morales H, Jones BV, Leach JL, et al. Documented development of a dural arteriovenous fistula in an infant subsequent to sinus thrombosis: case report and review of the literature. Neuroradiology 2010; 52(3):225–9.

26. Tsai LK, Jeng JS, Liu HM, et al. Intracranial dural arteriovenous fistulas with or without cerebral sinus thrombosis: analysis of 69 patients. J Neurol Neurosurg Psychiatr 2004;75(11):1639–41.

27. deVeber G, Andrew M, Adams C, et al. Cerebral sinovenous thrombosis in children. N Engl J Med 2001;345(6):417–23.

28. Peeters E, Stadnik T, Bissay F, et al. Diffusion-weighted MR imaging of an acute venous stroke: case report. AJNR Am J Neuroradiol 2001;22(10): 1949–52.

29. Chang R, Friedman DP. Isolated cortical venous thrombosis presenting as subarachnoid hemorrhage: a report of three cases. AJNR Am J Neuroradiol 2004;25(10):1676–9.

30. Linn J, Ertl-Wagner B, Seelos KC, et al. Diagnostic value of multidetector-row CT angiography in the evaluation of thrombosis of the cerebral venous sinuses. AJNR Am J Neuroradiol 2007;28(5): 946–52.

31. Dowd CF, Malek AM, Phatouros CC, et al. Application of a rheolytic thrombectomy device in the treatment of dural sinus thrombosis: a new technique. AJNR Am J Neuroradiol 1999;20(4):568–70.

32. Kuehnen J, Schwartz A, Neff W, et al. Cranial nerve syndrome in thrombosis of the transverse/sigmoid sinuses. Brain 1998;121(Pt 2):381–8.

33. Mullins ME, Grant PE, Wang B, et al. Parenchymal abnormalities associated with cerebral venous sinus thrombosis: assessment with diffusion-weighted MR imaging. AJNR Am J Neuroradiol 2004;25(10): 1666–75.

34. Liang L, Korogi Y, Sugahara T, et al. Evaluation of the intracranial dural sinuses with a 3D contrast-enhanced MP-RAGE sequence: prospective comparison with 2D-TOF MR venography and digital subtraction angiography. AJNR Am J Neuroradiol 2001;22(3):481–92.

35. Ozsvath RR, Casey SO, Lustrin ES, et al. Cerebral venography: comparison of CT and MR projection venography. AJR Am J Roentgenol 1997;169(6): 1699–707.

36. Wetzel SG, Kirsch E, Stock KW, et al. Cerebral veins: comparative study of CT venography with intraarterial digital subtraction angiography. AJNR Am J Neuroradiol 1999;20(2):249–55.

37. Dormont D, Sag K, Biondi A, et al. Gadolinium-enhanced MR of chronic dural sinus thrombosis. AJNR Am J Neuroradiol 1995;16(6):1347–52.

Imaging of Head Trauma

Tarek A. Hijaz, MD[a],*, Enzo A. Cento, MD[b],
Matthew T. Walker, MD[a]

KEYWORDS

- Head trauma • CT • MR imaging • Intracranial hemorrhage
- Diffuse axonal injury • Cerebral contusion

Traumatic head injury results in a substantial number of deaths and permanent disabilities around the world. According to the Centers for Disease Control (CDC), approximately 1.4 million people suffer traumatic brain injury annually in the United States alone. Of those, approximately 50,000 people die, and 235,000 are hospitalized.[1]

The CDC data reveal that almost half of cases of traumatic brain injury are caused by falls (28%) and motor vehicle accidents (20%). Other common causes include collisions with moving or stationary objects (19%), which includes sports-related injuries and assaults (11%).[1] Most deaths as a result of traumatic brain injury involve the use of a firearm, and approximately 90% of patient's with traumatic brain injury due to this mechanism die.[1]

The costs related to traumatic brain injury are substantial. In 2000, the combination of direct medical expenditures and indirect costs, including lost productivity, was an estimated $60 billion.[2] These costs have increased a great deal over the past few years given the injuries sustained by military personnel in the Afghanistan and Iraq wars. One should also not forget the immeasurable human toll, in the form of psychological and emotional trauma, borne by patients and their families and friends as a consequence of traumatic brain injury.

The usefulness of imaging in the setting of head trauma is indisputable. Imaging has become a virtually indispensable part of the initial assessment and subsequent management of these patients. Trauma patients routinely undergo computed tomography (CT) imaging on their arrival in the emergency department. Imaging can be particularly useful in patients in whom a neurologic examination is limited by their decreased level of consciousness. With current scanner technology, in seconds, a tremendous amount of invaluable information, including the presence or absence of fractures, penetrating foreign bodies, contusions, and intra- or extraaxial hemorrhage is available to the physicians administering care. During a hospital admission, sequelae of trauma, such as intracranial hemorrhage, can be followed closely with serial CT scans. In patients in whom the severity of the clinical deficits exceeds expectations, magnetic resonance (MR) imaging can be used to assess for possible causes, such as diffuse axonal injury (DAI).

MECHANISMS OF HEAD TRAUMA

Blunt trauma results in mechanical injury to the brain, primarily as a result of shear-strain deformation. This type of injury is characterized by a change in the shape of the brain without an associated change in its volume.[3] Although various other mechanisms play a small role, superficial brain injury is a primarily a consequence of skull deformation, often with associated fracture, as a result of direct impact. Deeper intraaxial lesions arise in the setting of shear strain related to rotational acceleration.[3] Cerebral contusions and DAI are addressed in more detail in separate sections.

Penetrating trauma to the head can be subclassified as superficial (object remains trapped in

[a] Section of Neuroradiology, Department of Radiology, Feinberg School of Medicine of Northwestern University, 676 North Saint Clair Street, Suite 1400, Chicago, IL 60611, USA
[b] Department of Radiology, Harvard Medical School, 55 Fruit Street, FND-210, Boston, MA 02114, USA
* Corresponding author.
E-mail address: thijaz@nmff.org

Radiol Clin N Am 49 (2011) 81–103
doi:10.1016/j.rcl.2010.07.012

extracranial soft tissues), tangential (object traverses and exits extracranial soft tissues), penetrating (object penetrates calvarium and remains within it), and perforating (object penetrates and exits calvarium) (**Fig. 1**A, B). These injuries can also be characterized as projectile (missile) or nonprojectile (nonmissile). The former usually involves a gunshot injury, whereas the latter may be caused by stabbing or impalement. Projectile injuries can be further characterized as either low or high velocity.[4]

Nonprojectile injuries in which the brain is injured are not common given the degree of protection afforded by the calvarium. When objects do penetrate into the brain, the resulting damage is usually restricted to the area immediately along the path of travel (**Fig. 2**A, B). In contrast, in projectile injuries, the damage is often more extensive. Initial imaging is performed with CT, and the scout image usually obviates separate skull radiographs.

Projectile trauma, which results in serious brain injury more commonly than nonprojectile trauma, is different in the military and civilian settings. Most injuries in the military setting are high velocity and involve jacketed bullets, which tend not to fragment. In contrast, civilian injuries are usually low velocity and involve nonjacketed bullets, which can fragment on impact (**Fig. 3**). This fragmentation can result in additional tissue damage and can preclude removal of all of the bullet fragments, potentially increasing the chance of subsequent infection.[4]

Projectile injuries can result in permanent cavitation as a result of crushing of tissue. The high pressure in the immediate vicinity of the projectile forms the tissue cavity, which often contains bullet and bone fragments as well as additional foreign material. The size of the cavity is increased if the projectile yaws, pitches, or tumbles along its trajectory. Temporary cavitation, which is also accentuated by eccentricity in the movement of the projectile, occurs when the force of the projectile results in a temporary cavity that oscillates in size. The centrifugal movement of the tissue leads to blunt trauma and shearing injuries.[4]

The unequivocal study of choice for penetrating head trauma is CT because the images can be acquired rapidly, and the risks associated with metallic foreign bodies in the setting of MR imaging are avoided. Furthermore, CT offers excellent delineation of the extent of both soft tissue and osseous injuries, and multidetector acquisition of a volume dataset allows postprocessing, including three-dimensional (3D) volume-rendered images, which can assist in presurgical planning. When the penetrating object is metallic, evaluation of the surrounding tissues on CT can be limited because of streak artifact. Some have advocated the use of cone beam CT to minimize this artifact.[5] Cone beam CT has been available in the United States only for the past few years. Rather than using a fan-shaped x-ray beam and one or more rows of detectors as in conventional CT, cone beam CT acquires a volume dataset using a cone-shaped x-ray beam and a two-dimensional detector array.

Penetrating injuries can result in damage to major vascular structures, including dissection, thrombosis, occlusion, and pseudoaneurysm

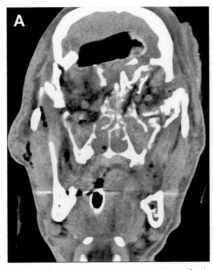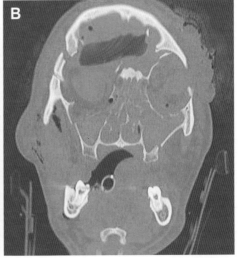

Fig. 1. (*A*) Coronal reformatted CT image in soft-tissue window and level settings showing penetrating injury secondary to a wooden plank. (*B*) Coronal reformatted CT image in bone window and level settings better showing the grain in the wooden plank.

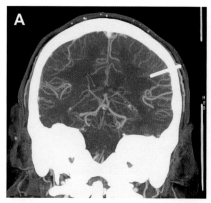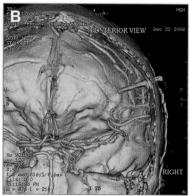

Fig. 2. (A) Coronal maximum-intensity projection (MIP) CTA image revealing a penetrating injury from a nail. (B) Coronal three-dimensional reformatted CTA image of penetrating injury from a nail.

formation. Once the study of choice for evaluating such injuries, digital subtraction angiography (DSA) has been supplanted by CT angiography (CTA). This modality offers the advantages of being noninvasive and simultaneously allowing assessment of the brain, calvarium, and extracalvarial soft tissues. CTA remains limited by streak artifact in the setting of metallic foreign bodies, and DSA still has a role in some cases, particularly for complications such as arteriovenous fistulae (AVFs).[4]

Infections are a known complication of penetrating head trauma, although there is conflicting information in the literature regarding the factors

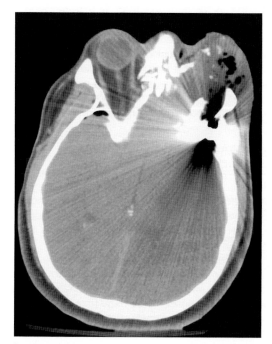

Fig. 3. Axial CT image showing fractures and soft tissue injuries caused by a bullet. Note the accompanying streak artifact.

that most predispose to infections and how best to treat and prevent them. Most cases of infection develop within 3 to 5 weeks of the initial trauma, and the overall incidence is 5% to 7%.[4] Aarabi and colleagues[6] reviewed 964 patients who had sustained military penetrating head trauma and found that 105 (11%) developed infections in the form of abscesses, cerebritis, and meningitis. The infections were most often caused by gram-negative bacteria, in particular *Klebsiella pneumoniae*, although gram-positive organisms, usually *Staphylococcus aureus*, were also seen. The investigators also found that the presence of cerebrospinal fluid (CSF) fistulae, transventricular injury, or paranasal sinus injury all increased the risk of infection. The presence of retained bullet or bone fragments was found to be a less important predisposing factor for infection.

Other complications of penetrating head trauma include delayed hemorrhage, migration/embolization of bullet fragments, hydrocephalus, and CSF leaks. The latter complication can present as CSF otorrhea or rhinorrhea and can be diagnosed with nuclear or CT cisternography.[4]

CALVARIAL FRACTURES

Calvarial fractures, as in fractures elsewhere in the body, can be classified by several features, including location, size, comminution (fragmentation into multiple parts), diastasis (widening of sutures or joints), and, most importantly, the presence of any associated depression. Depression of fracture fragments can be associated with underlying cerebral contusions or dural tears, which can predispose to CSF leaks or infection (Fig. 4A, B). Furthermore, if not corrected, they can result in permanent cosmetic deformity. Pediatric fractures and facial fractures are complex subjects in their own right, and they

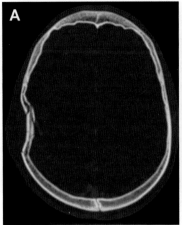 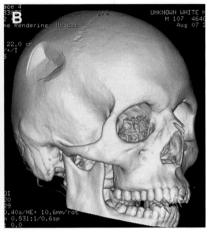

Fig. 4. (*A*) Axial CT image showing a comminuted, depressed calvarial fracture. (*B*) Surface shaded 3D volume-rendered CT image of a comminuted, depressed calvarial fracture.

are addressed in separate articles by Avery and colleagues and Patrick Barnes elsewhere in this issue.

The recognition of calvarial fractures, particularly those that are nondisplaced, is facilitated by a comprehensive knowledge of the location and appearance of normal cranial sutures and synchondroses. As a last resort, the presence or absence of symmetry can be an important diagnostic clue. Variant appearances, including a persistent metopic suture, which runs in the sagittal plane and bisects the frontal bones, can occur. The calvarium can also vary in shape, sometimes as a consequence of different forms of craniosynostosis, or premature sutural closure. For example, premature closure of the sagittal suture results in scaphocephaly (dolichocephaly), which is elongation of the anteroposterior dimension of the calvarium.

The immediate consequences of calvarial fractures include lacerations of the dural sinuses and cortical veins as well as arterial injuries, classically involving the middle meningeal artery. Almost without exception, such vascular injuries are accompanied by extraaxial hemorrhage, usually some combination of its epidural, subdural, and subarachnoid forms. Another potential result of vascular injury is thrombosis, often venous, which can be accompanied by infarction. Vascular injuries are addressed in more detail in a separate subsection.

Other immediate consequences of calvarial fractures include dural tears (with or without accompanying arachnoid tears) and cerebral contusions. The former may close spontaneously, although surgical intervention in the form of a dura-plasty may be required. The latter may or may not

be accompanied by intraaxial hemorrhage. Arachnoid tears can result in subdural hygroma formation. These fluid collections are often nearly isodense and isointense to CSF on CT and MR imaging, respectively, particularly if they do not contain any proteinaceous or hemorrhagic material. If both the arachnoid and dura are compromised, CSF and/or hemorrhage can accumulate in the epidural space. Furthermore, dural tears can result in CSF leakage, which may manifest clinically as CSF rhinorrhea or otorrhea, depending on the location of the tear. A tear resulting in a separation of the dura-arachnoid interface can result in the formation of a subdural hygroma.[7] Whereas radionuclide scintigraphy can confirm the presence of a leak, CT cisternography, using iodinated contrast introduced via a lumbar puncture, is sometimes required for more accurate presurgical localization (**Fig. 5A, B**).[8]

EXTRAAXIAL HEMORRHAGE
Subarachnoid Hemorrhage

Overall, trauma is the most common cause of subarachnoid hemorrhage (SAH). Others include aneurysm rupture and dural AVFs.[9] The incidence of SAH associated with head trauma has been reported to range from 33% to 60%.[10]

Sources of SAH in trauma include tearing of pial vessels, extraaxial extension of a hemorrhagic contusion, and redistribution of intraventricular hemorrhage caused by damage to subependymal veins. Often the highest concentration of SAH occurs contralateral to the side of direct impact.[8] Traumatic SAH most often occurs in superficial cerebral sulci near calvarial fractures and/or cerebral contusions (**Fig. 6**). In particularly severe

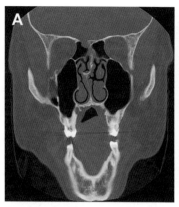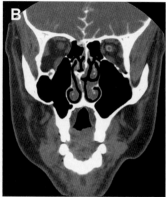

Fig. 5. (*A*) Coronal CT image showing skullbase fractures. (*B*) Coronal CT cisternogram image showing a small encephalocele with an accompanying CSF leak.

traumas, injury to one or more of the arteries in the vertebrobasilar circulation can result in massive SAH at the base of the brain.[11]

SAH has a characteristic appearance. In the acute and subacute phases, CT shows hyperattenuation in the sulci and basal cisterns and occasionally also in portions of the ventricular system. SAH is commonly seen in the interpenduncular and ambient cisterns, Sylvian fissures, and occipital horns of the lateral ventricles. Occasionally, hemorrhage in the region of the ambient cistern represents the most pronounced area of hemorrhage. It has been suggested that this may occur as a consequence of impaction of a vein along the edge of the tentorial incisura.[11] Differentiation of SAH from subdural hemorrhage (SDH) can be

difficult in certain locations, particularly along the tentorium cerebelli. A useful hint for recognizing SAH is extension of the blood into the cerebral sulci.[8]

On MR imaging, hyperintense signal may be seen in the locations mentioned earlier on fluid-attenuated inversion recovery (FLAIR) imaging (**Fig. 7**). Postcontrast FLAIR images have been shown to be even more sensitive for the detection of SAH. Flow artifacts limit the usefulness of FLAIR images for detection of SAH in the posterior fossa.

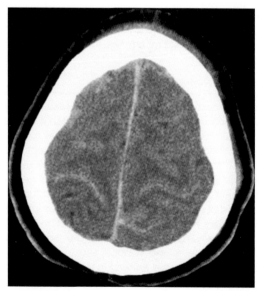

Fig. 6. Axial CT image showing acute traumatic SAH in several bilateral cerebral sulci.

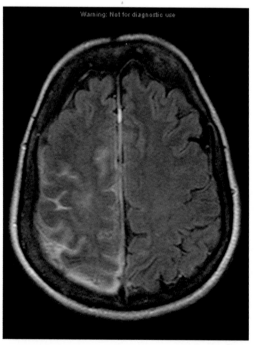

Fig. 7. Axial FLAIR image showing hyperintense signal within several right frontal lobe sulci consistent with SAH.

On gradient-recalled echo (GRE) T2 imaging, susceptibility effects may result in hypointense signal associated with SAH (**Fig. 8**). T1 images may show subacute hemorrhage as hyperintense signal (**Fig. 9**). Overall, MR imaging is not particularly practical as the primary modality for detection of SAH for several reasons, including cost, limited availability of scanners, long scan times, and motion and flow artifacts.

SAH can result in communicating hydrocephalus, presumably as a result of interference with reabsorption of CSF at the level of the arachnoid villi. Less frequently, obstructive hydrocephalus can result from impairment of CSF flow at the level of the cerebral aqueduct.

Another sequela of SAH is arterial vasospasm, although this complication is more common in the setting of aneurysmal rather than traumatic SAH. If severe enough, vasospasm can result in cerebral infarction corresponding to the vascular territories of the affected arteries. As with infarction as a result of other causes, CT shows hypoattenuation and loss of gray-white differentiation, and MR imaging reveals restricted diffusion. Vasospasm may be suspected if there is a change in the patient's clinical examination or if increased arterial velocities are detected on transcranial Doppler ultrasonography.

CTA and MR angiography (MRA) have become useful noninvasive techniques for detecting

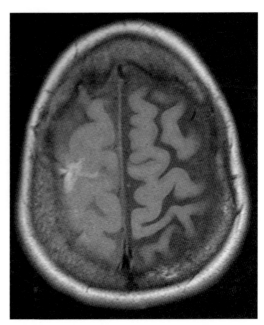

Fig. 9. Axial T1 image T1 shortening within several right frontal lobe sulci consistent with SAH.

vasospasm, and comparison with previous cross-sectional vascular imaging studies is particularly useful for detecting decreases in arterial caliber, either focal or diffuse. CT and MR perfusion can also be useful adjuncts. Rather than showing the vasospasm itself, these studies reveal the resulting ischemia or frank infarction. If there is high suspicion for vasospasm, DSA may be performed, and treatment options include infusion of calcium channel blockers such as verapamil or nimodipine and angioplasty, usually of the supraclinoid internal carotid arteries and M1 segments of the middle cerebral arteries.

Epidural Hemorrhage

Arterial epidural hemorrhage (EDH) results from laceration of arteries along the inner table of the calvarium. These hemorrhages often have a lentiform, biconvex appearance and do not cross the tough attachments of the dura at the cranial sutures (**Fig. 10A–C**). An exception to this rule is that arterial EDH can cross the sagittal suture at the vertex because the periosteal layer of the dura is less tightly attached in this location.[8]

Classically, direct trauma to the squamous portion of the temporal bone causes tearing of the middle meningeal artery. Up to 90% of arterial EDH is associated with a calvarial fracture.[9] Large arterial EDHs may require emergent surgical intervention because arterial pressure can result in

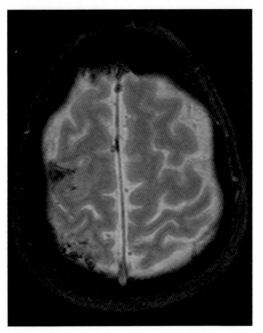

Fig. 8. Axial T2* GRE image gradient susceptibility within several right frontal lobe sulci consistent with SAH.

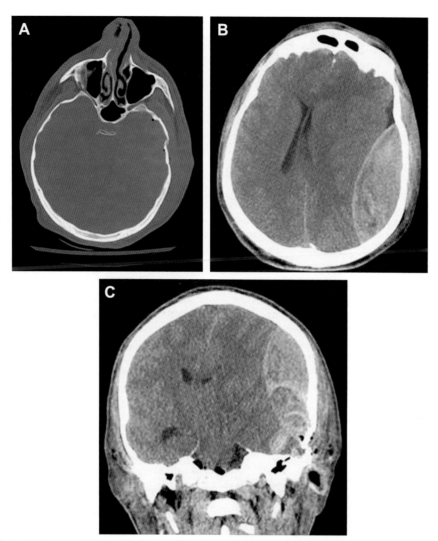

Fig. 10. (A) Axial CT image in bone window and level settings showing a fracture of the squamous portion of the left temporal bone. (B) Axial CT image showing a large epidural hematoma with a typical biconvex shape and resulting midline shift. (C) Coronal reformatted CT image showing a large epidural hematoma and left temporal lobe hemorrhagic contusions.

brain herniation because of the rapid accumulation of a large amount of extraaxial hemorrhage (Fig. 11A, B). In contrast, small arterial EDHs are often managed conservatively and followed with serial CT imaging. Mixed high- and low-attenuation regions within an arterial EDH suggest active hemorrhage and rapid enlargement of the hematoma.[8] A similar appearance can be seen as a result of poor clotting in anticoagulated patients, which is addressed in more detail at the end of the section on extraaxial hemorrhage (Fig. 12).

In contrast to arterial EDH, venous EDH can cross cranial sutures because these hemorrhages result from laceration of the dural sinuses, most commonly the transverse or superior sagittal sinuses or region of the torcular herophili (Fig. 13A, B).[10] Venous EDH can manifest as delayed neurologic decline related to the slow accumulation of blood under venous pressure.[9] Venous EDH is more easily diagnosed with MR imaging than CT because of the multiplanar capability of the former.[8]

SDH

SDH has a crescentic appearance with a concave margin abutting the brain (Fig. 14A, B). These hematomas can be either supra- or infratentorial, and the hemorrhage can extend along the

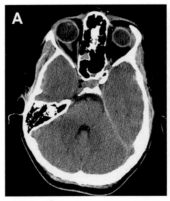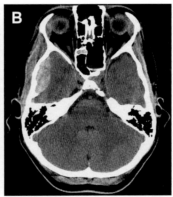

Fig. 11. (*A*) Initial axial CT image showing minimal EDH in the right middle cranial fossa. (*B*) Axial CT image obtained a few hours later showing a marked increase in the size of the epidural hematoma.

surfaces of the falx cerebri and tentorium cerebelli, although they do not violate the margins of these structures. Subdural hematomas can cross the cranial sutures, and if large enough, they may completely surround a cerebral hemisphere. SDH results from tearing of bridging veins, and they often occur on the opposite side of a direct blow to the head in a contrecoup fashion.[9] Other sources of SDH include injury to arachnoid granulations and pial vessels.[8]

Brain atrophy, whether caused by aging, chronic alcoholism, or other causes, increases the size of the extraaxial CSF spaces and exposes

the bridging veins to a higher degree of stretching and torsion than in patients without atrophy. This situation renders patients with atrophy more susceptible to SDH.[8] In such patients, even seemingly minor trauma can result in hemorrhage. Overly rapid or aggressive shunting in the setting of hydrocephalus can also result in SDH because there is a lag between retraction of the cortical surface because of decompression of the hydrocephalus and reexpansion of the substance of the brain.[8]

Surgical drainage of the hematoma may be required to preclude impending brain herniation. Hematocrit levels, formed by the gravity-induced settling of cellular elements to the dependent portions of the collection, often occur in SDH.[9] Occasionally, recurrent bleeding or coagulopathy can also result in this appearance.[8]

Delayed SDH, if unrecognized, is a potentially devastating sequela of trauma, and there are at least 6 published cases in the literature (**Fig. 15**A, B). Most recently, Matsuda and colleagues[12] reported a case in which a subdural hematoma developed approximately 1 week after the patient's initial mild head trauma, which was sustained during a football game. Although the patient had a persistent headache, a head CT performed 4 days after the injury had revealed no evidence of intracranial hemorrhage, and the patient had no underlying intracranial tumor, vascular malformation, or coagulopathy. The patient returned a few days later after the onset of a more severe headache, which was temporally related to his straining to tighten a bolt, and it was theorized that the Valsalva maneuver may have resulted in the hemorrhage by causing venous congestion in vessels with increased permeability as a result of local hypoxia and inflammation. The investigators also conceded that there may have been minimal hemorrhage on the initial CT

Fig. 12. Axial CT image showing an acute, low-attenuation epidural fluid collection. This appearance can be seen in anemic patients or when CSF comprises most of the fluid collection.

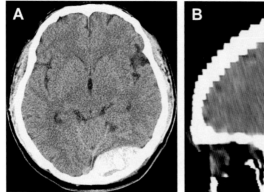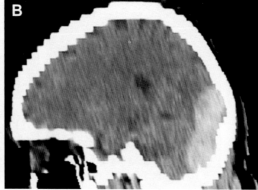

Fig. 13. (*A*) Axial CT image showing an acute epidural hematoma. (*B*) Coronal reformatted CT image revealing that the epidural hematoma extends both above and below the tentorium cerebelli, suggesting that the hematoma may be caused by venous hemorrhage from laceration of the transverse sinus.

that was not detected. Delayed intracerebral and EDHs have also been documented in the literature.[12]

Subacute, isodense subdural hematomas may be difficult to recognize, although this is less of a diagnostic dilemma than in the past given the quality of the images from most modern CT scanners. Secondary signs suggesting the presence of an isodense subdural hematoma include buckling of the gray-white matter junction and effacement of the cerebral sulci (**Fig. 16**A–C).[8]

Chronic subdural hematomas can have a complex appearance, and differentiating a chronic subdural hematoma from cerebral atrophy can be problematic on occasion. Contrast-enhanced imaging can help by revealing displacement of the cortical veins and/or a surrounding enhancing membrane.[8] Enhancing septa may also be seen within a chronic subdural hematoma.

Chronic SDH also can be difficult to distinguish from a subdural hygroma, which forms as a result of small rents in the arachnoid membrane (**Fig. 17**). Although they occasionally form acutely following trauma, hygromas tend to form several weeks later, which can sometimes help to differentiate them from chronic SDH, which appears contemporaneously with the trauma and then evolves in attenuation and signal characteristics. Chronic SDH is also more common adjacent to the frontal lobes because of the rough surface of the inner table of the calvarium in the anterior cranial fossa (**Fig. 18**A–C).[9]

Generally, intra- and extraaxial hemorrhage on CT has a typical initial appearance and pattern of evolution. Usually, acute to subacute hemorrhage is hyperattenuating and gradually becomes iso- and ultimately hypointense to the brain in days and weeks. In anemic patients, initial hemorrhage may be lower in attenuation than expected. Also, in anticoagulated or actively extravasating patients, hemorrhage may initially manifest as areas of mixed high and low attenuation.

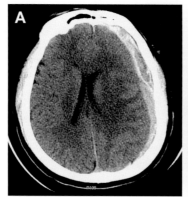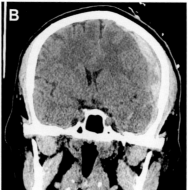

Fig. 14. (*A*) Axial CT image showing an acute SDH caused by penetrating injury with a knife. Note the typical crescentic configuration. (*B*) Coronal reformatted CT image showing an acute SDH with midline shift.

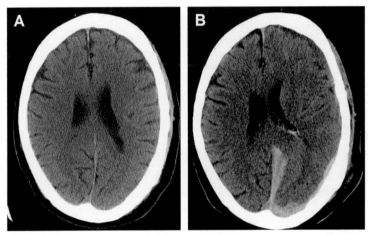

Fig. 15. (A) Axial CT image following blunt head trauma in a patient on Coumadin therapy showing no intracranial hemorrhage. (B) Axial CT image obtained several hours later showing delayed development of subdural and intraventricular hemorrhage.

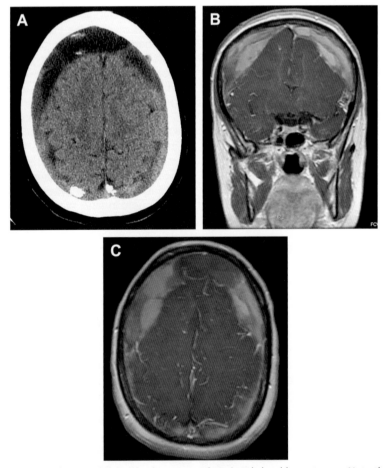

Fig. 16. (A) Axial CT image showing bilateral subacute on chronic subdural hematomas. Note the septations and the varying densities within both collections. (B) Coronal T1 postcontrast image showing bilateral subacute on chronic subdural hematomas. (C) Axial T1 postcontrast image showing bilateral subacute on chronic subdural hematomas.

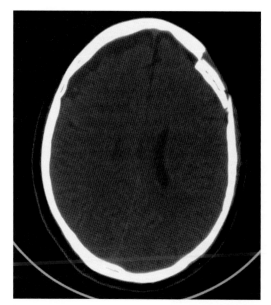

Fig. 17. Axial CT image showing a depressed calvarial fracture and bilateral subdural hygromas, right larger than left.

Radiologists are also familiar with a pattern of changing MR signal characteristics of hemorrhage as it evolves through the following stages: oxyhemoglobin, deoxyhemoglobin, intra- and extracellular methemoglobin, and ultimately, ferritin and hemosiderin. Typically, the signal changes (T1 and T2, respectively) follow a characteristic progression: hyperacute (isointense/hyperintense), acute (isointense/hypointense), early subacute (hyperintense/hypointense), late subacute (hyperintense/hyperintense), and chronic (hypointense/hypointense).[13]

Although the evolution of the signal characteristics of intraaxial hemorrhage is fairly predictable, extrapolation of this pattern of signal changes to extraaxial hemorrhage, including SDH, should be made cautiously. The appearance of hemorrhage on MR imaging is contingent on multiple factors, including red cell packing, hemoglobin level, sequence parameters, and field strength. Furthermore, the signal characteristics of extraaxial hemorrhage may evolve at a slower rate than in the setting of intraaxial hemorrhage because of the higher extraaxial oxygen tension.[14]

Before leaving extraaxial hemorrhage and before addressing cerebral contusions and associated intraparenchymal hemorrhage, anticoagulation is addressed briefly. As the US population ages, the number of patients on anticoagulation for various indications increases. In patients on anticoagulation, a minor trauma may elicit intracranial hemorrhage. Overall, anticoagulation increases the risk of intracranial hemorrhage by a factor of 7 to 10. Almost 70% of these hemorrhages are intraparenchymal, and most of the remaining hemorrhages are subdural.[15]

The risk of hemorrhage is increased regardless of the intensity of anticoagulation. For example, even patients on warfarin therapy who are within the preferred international normalized ratio range can experience intracranial hemorrhage. Regardless of the dose, aspirin increases the risk of intracranial hemorrhage by a factor of 2, and there are data suggesting that combined aspirin and warfarin therapy increases the risk even more.[15]

Hemorrhages in many patients on anticoagulation can continue for several hours, and short-term serial imaging can be critical in tracking the amount of hemorrhage and its effects on the surrounding brain. In patients who are not anticoagulated, the bleeding usually occurs over a short period and is self-limited.[15]

CEREBRAL CONTUSIONS

The most common locations for brain contusions, which result from injury to capillaries and associated edema, are the anterior and inferior surfaces of the frontal lobes as well as the temporal and occipital poles (Fig. 19). The differential acceleration of the brain relative to the calvarium in the setting of trauma results in abrasion and impaction of the brain along the inner table. Both coup injuries, which are at the site of direct impact, and contrecoup injuries, which occur on the opposite surface of the brain, may or may not be associated with frank intraaxial hemorrhage (Figs. 20A, B and Fig. 21A–C).[3]

In 2004, Drew and Drew[16] set out to explain the observation that contrecoup injuries are often more severe than coup injuries. Using the hypothesis that in blunt trauma, denser CSF shifts toward the site of impact whereas the less dense brain moves away, these investigators devised a model in which a balloon filled with pure water was immersed in salt water with a slightly higher density. The model confirmed that in blunt trauma, the less dense brain initially moves away from the point of impact and strikes the contrecoup location on the inner surface of the calvarium.

In a study of 40 patients, Gentry and colleagues[3] found cortical contusions to be most common in the temporal lobes (45.9%) followed by the frontal lobes (31.1%). Contusions tend to increase in size on subsequent imaging studies because of an increase in the amount of hemorrhage within the contusion or in the amount of edema surrounding it. Follow-up imaging often also reveals new areas

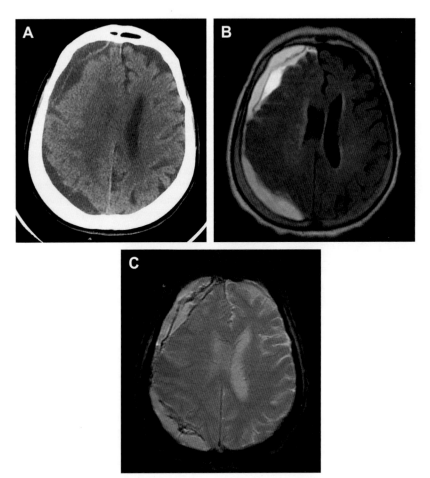

Fig. 18. (*A*) Axial CT image showing a chronic subdural hematoma. Note the septations and that although the collection is relatively hypodense, it remains mildly hyperdense to CSF. (*B*) Axial FLAIR image showing a chronic subdural hematoma. (*C*) Axial T2*GRE image showing a chronic subdural hematoma with septations. Note that the signal from the fluid within the hematoma does not suppress and that different portions of the hematoma have different signal characteristics.

of hemorrhagic contusion not present on initial imaging.[17]

Studies have shown a higher incidence of hemorrhage in cerebral contusions (51.9%) than in DAI (18.8%), and it has been proposed that this is because of the higher vascularity of gray matter than white matter.[3] Even contusions that show no detectable hemorrhage on imaging, almost without exception, are associated with hemorrhage on a microscopic level.[9]

GRE T2* images can improve detection of hemorrhagic brain contusions by revealing signal loss and blooming (**Fig. 22**A–C). Occasionally, this effect can also aid in the detection of extraaxial hemorrhage. This sequence is less helpful when hemorrhage lies close to the calvarium because susceptibility effects from the bone can obscure areas of interest. The same limitation applies when the area of interest is close to the paranasal

sinuses because of the susceptibility characteristics of air.[8]

In 2004, Wintermark and colleagues[18] published an article that showed the usefulness of perfusion CT for detection of brain contusions and found it to be more sensitive than conventional CT for this purpose. These investigators conducted a prospective study of 130 trauma patients, and all of the patients underwent perfusion CT imaging on admission. Clinical and imaging data at 3 months were reviewed. The data revealed that normal or increased perfusion, reported as cerebral blood flow (CBF) and volume (CBV), on admission was associated with a favorable clinical outcome, whereas decreased perfusion was associated with a poor clinical course. Furthermore, the investigators found that the more arterial territories with decreased CBV were revealed by the perfusion CT, the worse the prognosis.

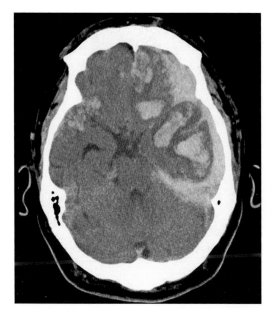

Fig. 19. Axial CT image showing typical bilateral frontal and temporal lobe hemorrhagic contusions with subdural and SAH.

CT perfusion has also been used to evaluate the tissue surrounding cerebral contusions. In a study published in 2002, von Oettingen and colleagues[19] evaluated CBF in 17 patients with brain contusions using xenon-enhanced CT, and they found, as had previous investigators, that the contusions themselves represented areas of irreversible ischemia. These investigators also revealed that, in a fashion similar to ischemic infarcts, there was a surrounding zone of relative hypoperfusion. It has been suggested that ischemia in the setting

of contusions is due to a combination of shearing of the microvasculature and compression by edema and the hemorrhage itself. The investigators proposed that increasing edema and mass effect associated with cerebral contusions may further decrease CBF in the already hypoperfused zone surrounding the hemorrhage, resulting in secondary ischemic injuries. Furthermore, this risk may be higher with larger contusions, which may compromise cerebral perfusion pressure by increasing intracranial pressure.

Delayed hemorrhage in brain contusions may occur, and this usually reflects a severe injury. The burst lobe phenomenon occurs when a severe brain contusion ruptures into the subdural compartment. This entity carries a poor prognosis.[9]

Alahmadi and colleagues[17] performed a retrospective review of 98 patients with brain contusions and found that radiographic progression, defined as a 30% or greater increase in volume, of the contusions occurred more commonly in larger contusions. The initial volume of the contusion and the presence of associated SDH, which might be caused by the burst lobe phenomenon, were found to predict radiographic progression. Furthermore, the investigators found that patients with large contusions and low Glasgow Coma Scale (GCS) scores were at risk for delayed clinical deterioration.

Other investigators have shown the usefulness of CTA in helping to predict hematoma expansion, which is a predictor of increased morbidity and mortality. In 2007, Wada and colleagues[20] found that the presence of a spot sign on CTA independently predicted cerebral hematoma

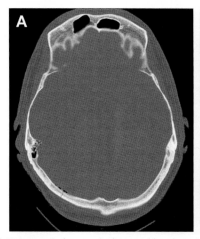
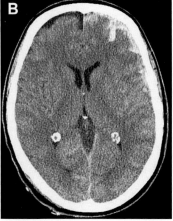

Fig. 20. (A) Axial CT image in bone window and level settings showing a fracture in the right side of the occipital bone indicating the location of direct impact. (B) Axial CT image in brain window and level settings showing a contrecoup hemorrhagic contusion in the left frontal lobe with associated extraaxial hemorrhage.

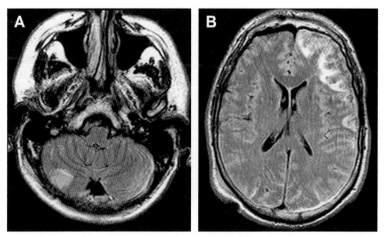

Fig. 21. (*A*) Axial FLAIR image showing a coup contusion in the right cerebellar hemisphere. (*B*) Axial FLAIR image showing a contrecoup contusion in the left frontal lobe.

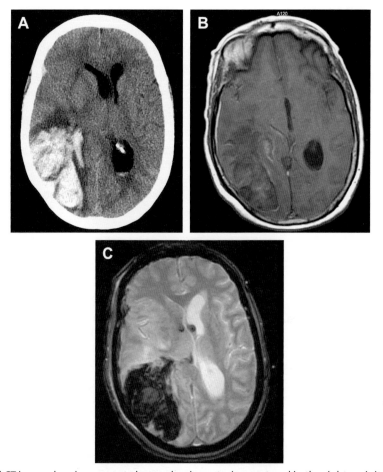

Fig. 22. (*A*) Axial CT image showing an acute hemorrhagic contusion centered in the right occipital lobe. (*B*) Axial T1 image showing mild intrinsic T1 shortening within the hemorrhagic contusion. (*C*) Axial T2*GRE image showing increased conspicuity of the hemorrhage as a result of gradient susceptibility blooming.

expansion. A spot sign was defined in the study as one or more small enhancing foci within a cerebral hematoma, regardless of whether contrast extravasation could be clearly identified. The patients in the study by Wada and his colleagues presented with spontaneous hemorrhages; however, there is no reason that the presence of a spot sign associated with a traumatic cerebral hematoma does not also predict subsequent expansion of the hemorrhage.

DAI

DAI is sustained as a result of shearing of axons related to the differential acceleration of tissues of different densities, most often in the setting of trauma involving rapid, high-magnitude acceleration or deceleration. It can occur with or without a direct blow to the head.[9] Estimates suggest that DAI occurs in more than 50% of all severe head trauma and in more than 85% of the subset related to motor vehicle collisions.[21]

The most common locations for this type of injury are at the gray-white matter junction, in the corpus callosum, and in the brainstem (**Fig. 23**A, B). Most DAI lesions occur at the gray-white matter junction, and they are most common in the frontal and temporal lobes. Lesions can occur elsewhere in the cerebral hemispheres and in the cerebellum.[3] Callosal injuries, the second most common location, are most often sustained in the region of the splenium, presumably because this portion of the corpus callosum is relatively mobile in relation to the falx cerebri. In their series of 25 patients, Huisman and colleagues[21] found that most of the DAI lesions occurred at the gray-white matter junction (43%) and in deep white matter (24%). Smaller

numbers of lesions were located in the corpus callosum (8%) and brainstem (7%). Gentry and colleagues[3] found a high association between callosal DAI and intraventricular hemorrhage.

DAI is graded by its anatomic location. Grade I injuries are isolated to the gray-white matter junction, whereas the presence of lesions in the corpus callosum or brainstem increase the grade to II or III, respectively.[8] Overall, the presence of DAI worsens a patient's prognosis, and the higher the grade, the more dire the prognosis. DAI is believed to be a contributing factor explaining persistent neurologic problems, including memory and attention deficits and headaches, which occasionally plague even patients who suffered mild head trauma.[22]

CT is relatively insensitive for the detection of DAI, particularly if the lesions are nonhemorrhagic. A prospective study of 40 patients by Gentry and colleagues[3] found that only about 19% of the DAI lesions showed associated hemorrhage. Hemorrhagic lesions appear as punctate hyperattenuating foci in typical locations.

Blood-sensitive MR sequences, such as GRE T2* sequences, detect more lesions than CT and consequently may change the grade of injury (**Fig. 24**).[8] DAI can also be detected using diffusion-weighted imaging (DWI), and a typical lesion shows restricted diffusion, characterized by high-signal intensity on the b1000 sequence and corresponding dark spot on the adjusted diffusion coefficient (ADC) map. Huisman and colleagues[21] retrospectively evaluated 25 patients imaged within 48 hours of their sustaining head trauma and reported that DWI detected more DAI lesions than T2/FLAIR or T2* GRE, although T2* GRE images were more sensitive than DWI for detection of hemorrhagic DAI.

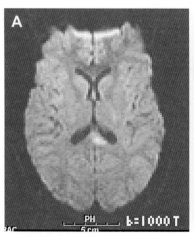
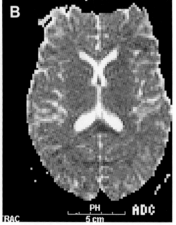

Fig. 23. (*A*) B1000 image showing DAI in the splenium of the corpus callosum. (*B*) ADC map image showing DAI in the splenium of the corpus callosum.

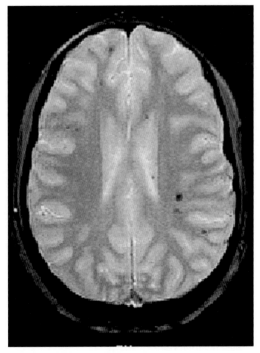

Fig. 24. Axial T2* GRE image showing hemorrhagic DAI at the gray-white matter junction.

More recently, the advent of susceptibility-weighted imaging (SWI), essentially a super-charged GRE sequence, has further increased the sensitivity of MR imaging for detection of DAI (**Figs. 25** and **26**). There is evidence that important clinical information can be gleaned from an assessment of the number of DAI lesions. In 2004, Tong and colleagues[23] published a study in which they found that both greater numbers and larger volumes of DAI lesions in children with traumatic brain injury correlated with lower GCS scores and prolonged coma. Another study found correlations between lesion volume and number and various cognitive indices, such as motor function, intelligence, memory, and language skills.[24] The results of these and other studies suggest that the increased sensitivity of SWI over conventional GRE T2* for detection of DAI lesions may have significant clinical usefulness.

Diffusion-tensor imaging (DTI) and tractography also have shown promise in the evaluation of DAI. DTI not only measures average ADC, but it reveals the direction of water diffusion in 3 dimensions.[25] This technique shows preferential diffusion of water parallel to intact white-matter tracts, a phenomenon known as diffusion anisotropy. When white-matter tracts are damaged or disrupted, this anisotropy is reduced. Fiber tractography is a 3D visual representation of white-matter tracts generated from DTI data. Le and colleagues[25] published a case report in which they used DTI and 3D fiber tractography to image shearing injuries in the splenium of the corpus callosum. These injuries resulted in left hemialexia arising from disconnection of the right visual cortex from the left hemispheric language centers, and the clinical and imaging findings correlated with one another.

VASCULAR INJURY

Arterial injuries caused by head trauma can result from rotational or stretching forces on vessels, or they may be a result of laceration by penetrating foreign bodies or bone fragments. Complete tearing of a vessel results in active extravasation,

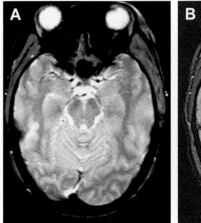
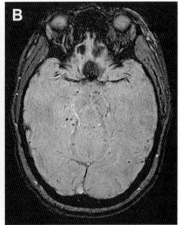

Fig. 25. (A) Axial T2* GRE image showing foci of gradient susceptibility, consistent with hemorrhagic DAI. (B) Axial SWI image showing increased conspicuity and number of foci of hemorrhagic DAI.

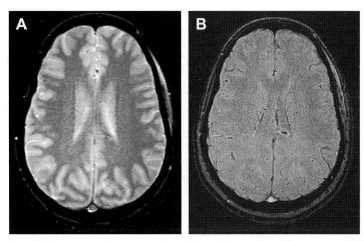

Fig. 26. (*A*) Axial T2* GRE image showing an equivocal, faint focus of gradient susceptibility in the posterior portion of the corpus callosum. (*B*) Axial SWI image showing increased conspicuity of a focus of hemorrhagic DAI in the posterior portion of the corpus callosum.

the extent of which depends on the surrounding tissues, which if durable enough eventually tampo-nades the hemorrhage. More commonly, head trauma leads to arterial dissections.

Because this article deals exclusively with head trauma, dissections of the major cervical arteries are not addressed, although the basic principles are essentially the same. The two major subtypes of dissection are subintimal and subadventitial. In their intracranial forms, the former results in nar-rowing of the true lumen of the vessel, often leading to downstream ischemia, whereas the latter causes pseudoaneurysm formation and, if intradural, SAH. When subintimal dissections extend through the intima into the lumen, frag-ments of coagulated blood can break off and lead to embolic infarcts.[26]

CTA is commonly used as a first-line modality for detection of vascular injury. Intuitively, the larger the vessel, the easier it is to detect an abnor-mality. Frank vascular occlusions or complete tears are usually readily identifiable. In larger vessels, dissection flaps (linear filling defects within the vessel) or pseudoaneurysm formation (focal outpouchings of the vessel wall) are also easily seen (**Fig. 27**). In dissections of smaller vessels, one may see only irregularity of the vessel contour with no discernible flap, and pseudo-aneurysms of small vessels may also be subtle. Intraluminal thrombus appears as an irregularly shaped filling defect.

A subtype of pseudoaneurysm sometimes seen in head trauma involves the superficial temporal artery (STA). These pseudoaneurysms are a conse-quence of trauma to the side of the head, whether or not it results in fractures. Clinically, STA

pseudoaneurysms often present as a pulsatile preauricular mass after head trauma. Although most pseudoaneuryms arise within 2 to 6 weeks after the initial injury, up to 20% may present as late as 3 years afterwards. Occasionally, STA pseudoaneurysms may be initially confused with STA AVFs, which can also result from trauma. In this entity, there is arteriovenous shunting at the level of a previous injury to the STA. CTA has

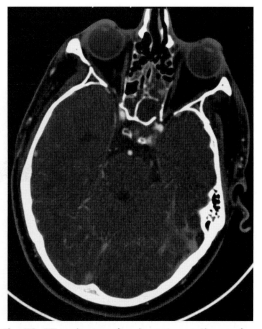

Fig. 27. CT angiogram showing a traumatic pseudoa-neurysm of the left ICA with an associated fracture of the sphenoid sinus wall.

been shown to be an effective, noninvasive modality for the accurate depiction of the anatomy of injuries to the STA.[27]

MRA can also be used for initial evaluation of vascular injuries, although it may be impractical for a variety of reasons including limited scanner availability, longer scan time than CTA, and image degradation caused by patient motion (**Fig. 28**A, B). The findings are the same as in CTA, although MRA has a few additional features. Fat-saturated T1-weighted images can show the presence of T1 hyperintense mural thrombus. The diagnostic usefulness of this technique diminishes with the size of the vessel being evaluated. Often this finding is seen in conjunction with narrowing of the vascular flow void or abnormally hyperintense signal within the vessel lumen on T2-weighted images.[8]

If CTA or MRA fail to provide adequate diagnostic information or if endovascular therapy, such as stenting or embolization, is required, DSA may be performed. DSA is no longer commonly performed as a first-line study for the diagnosis of traumatic arterial injuries.

In addition to dissections, with or without vessel occlusion, and complete tears of arteries, head trauma can lead to the formation of AVFs. AVFs sometimes are associated with sphenoid bone fractures and may manifest as carotid-cavernous shunting. A direct carotid-cavernous fistula can result from laceration of the internal carotid artery (ICA), and this injury can occur either in the setting of blunt or penetrating trauma. The usual ancillary findings, including proptosis, chemosis, and enlargement of the cavernous sinus and superior ophthalmic vein often accompany this injury. The

fistula may not manifest until weeks after the trauma.[8] Delayed presentations are even more common with peripheral AVFs, such as those at the cerebral convexities. These fistulae may be revealed by hemorrhaging several years after the initial trauma.[9]

Both CTA and MRA can detect traumatic AVFs, but detection of subtler cases has traditionally required DSA. Although low when performed by an experienced angiographer, the risks associated with DSA are real, and such an invasive procedure should be avoided whenever possible. Time-resolved MRA provides a noninvasive alternative for detection of AVFs. A study published in 2009 by Nishimura and colleagues[28] compared time-resolved (four-dimensional) contrast-enhanced MRA with DSA for detection of intracranial dural AVFs. These investigators found good to excellent agreement between the 2 modalities with respect to localization of the fistulae and identification of the venous drainage. These results suggest that time-resolved MRA should be considered as a first-line choice for detection of intracranial AVFs, regardless of their underlying cause.

A study published in 2005 by York and colleagues[29] examined how often fractures of the carotid canal and other CT findings, including sphenoid air-fluid levels, brain contusions, SAH, SDH, and basilar skull fractures, are associated with ICA injuries. The investigators identified a total of 21 fractures of the carotid canal in 17 patients and 11 injuries to the ICA in 10 patients, and evaluated for vascular injury using DSA. They determined that carotid canal fractures had a sensitivity of 60% and a specificity of 67% for associated ICA injury. Similar values were

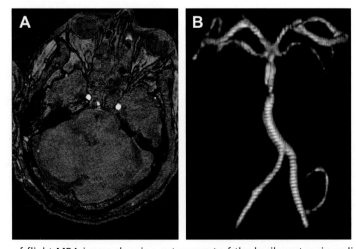

Fig. 28. (*A*) 3D time-of-flight MRA image showing entrapment of the basilar artery in a clival fracture. (*B*) MIP image from 3D time-of-flight MRA showing narrowing of the basilar artery as a result of entrapment in a clival fracture.

obtained for the other CT findings listed earlier, suggesting that the presence of carotid canal fractures, although raising the level of suspicion for ICA injury, are only moderately predictive. The presence of a sphenoid sinus air-fluid level had a higher sensitivity (90%) for associated ICA injury than did the presence of a carotid canal fracture. Nevertheless, the investigators found that the rate of ICA injury was twice as high (35%) in patients who had carotid canal fractures when compared with those who did not.[29] Consequently, further evaluation with CTA or DSA is warranted.

RELATIVE ADVANTAGES OF CT AND MR IMAGING

In current practice, CT is used as the initial imaging modality of choice in trauma because of its availability, speed, and ability to readily detect osseous injury, foreign bodies, and intracranial hemorrhage.[8] Modern CT scanners also have the capability to perform CTA and CT perfusion imaging, adding useful diagnostic information on vascular injuries, cerebral contusions, and infarctions. In general, CT is more readily available than MR imaging at most hospitals because of the greater number of scanners and because CT scanners are often staffed 24 hours a day. Despite its usefulness, correlation with pathologic conditions has revealed that various forms of traumatic brain injury, including DAI, nonhemorrhagic brain contusion, and primary brainstem injury, are underestimated by noncontrast CT.[3]

MR imaging tends to be used when the patient's neurologic symptoms cannot be explained adequately by the findings on CT, often in the setting of DAI. It is also useful when evaluating delayed sequelae of trauma, including encephalomalacia and brain atrophy.[8] In addition to standard sequences, MR imaging also offers other diagnostic techniques, such as DTI, spectroscopy, and volumetric imaging, providing information that correlates with a patient's clinical status and prognosis.

Acute epidural and subdural hematomas can be detected almost equally well by CT and MR imaging, but MR imaging has superior sensitivity for detection of nonhemorrhagic contusions, brainstem injuries, and small amounts of SAH.[8] Overall, the unequivocal choice for first-line imaging of SAH is CT, mostly because of its sensitivity and speed. SAH can be detected on MR imaging, usually using FLAIR images to show hyperintensity in the sulci and/or cisterns, but detection of SAH in the posterior fossa is problematic given CSF flow artifacts. Furthermore, in intubated patients receiving a high inspired-oxygen fraction, FLAIR images often show artifactual signal hyperintensity in the subarachnoid space. Subacute SAH may be isodense to CSF on CT, thus presenting a diagnostic challenge. In this special case, MR imaging, in particular the FLAIR sequence, is more sensitive for detection of subacute SAH.[8]

SECONDARY OR DELAYED INJURIES AND LONG-TERM SEQUELAE

According to the CDC, in the United States at least 5.3 million victims of traumatic brain injury require long-term or lifelong assistance performing activities of daily living.[30] Traumatic brain injury can result in difficulties with memory and cognition and emotional disturbances, including anxiety, depression, aggression, and personality changes. Language impairment and alterations of various senses, such as olfaction, vision, and touch may also manifest.[31]

Although a single, severe trauma often results in varying degrees of cognitive and neurologic impairment, milder injuries are not innocuous. When several mild traumatic brain injuries are clustered within a short period (hours to weeks), serious deficits or even death can result. Even when distributed over months or years, mild injuries can have a cumulative detrimental effect.[32]

Much of the literature on head trauma divides injuries into primary forms, which are immediately manifest, and secondary forms, which occur at some point in time after the trauma. The significance of secondary injuries is that in some cases, actions can be taken to prevent them.[8] An example of a secondary injury is diffuse cerebral edema. Disruption of cerebrovascular autoregulation is implicated as the cause of vasogenic edema and hyperemia, whereas cytotoxic edema can also result from direct tissue injury. Generalized edema is recognized by effacement of the cerebral sulci, and, if severe enough, the basal cisterns.[8]

Ischemic changes and frank brain infarction are other secondary injuries occurring in head trauma. These injuries may be the result of compression of arteries by brain herniation, as in the anterior cerebral arteries under the falx cerebri and the posterior cerebral arteries along the tentorium cerebelli. Ischemia can also follow diffuse cerebral edema or local mass effect, sometimes as a result of extraaxial hemorrhage.[8] Often, an initial noncontrast CT does not reveal trauma-related ischemic changes, and for this reason, radiologists must be vigilant when looking for signs of ischemia on serial follow-up CT scans, particularly if the patient has developed herniation.

Another important secondary injury is brain herniation, which can occur secondary to other sequelae of trauma, such as space-occupying extraaxial hemorrhages (**Fig. 29**A, B). The most easily recognized of these forms is subfalcine herniation, in which the cingulate gyrus on one side crosses the midline. In uncal herniation, the mesial temporal lobe narrows the ipsilateral side of the suprasellar cistern. Transtentorial herniation, which has upward and downward forms, can be more difficult to recognize if one is not vigilant. In the former, the contents of the posterior fossa are displaced cephalad via the tentorial incisura, resulting in effacement of the CSF spaces at this level. In the latter, the cerebellar tonsils efface the CSF spaces at the level of the foramen magnum, and downward displacement of the supratentorial contents effaces the suprasellar and perimesencephalic cisterns.[8] The various forms of herniation may be present on an initial head CT, and even if not initially present, they can develop rapidly.

Cerebral venous thrombosis can occur secondary to trauma (**Fig. 30**). This entity was first described specifically as a sequela of trauma in 1915, although it had been reported in the medical literature as early as 1825. The cause of thrombosis in this setting has not been fully elucidated, although hypotheses include direct injury to venous sinuses by fracture fragments, dissection of the sinuses, and alterations in blood flow caused by distortion of the contours of the sinuses.[33] Clinical symptoms and signs are

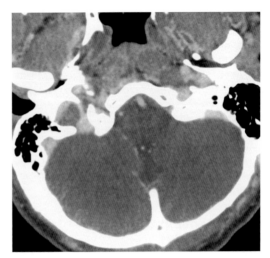

Fig. 30. Axial CT image showing thrombus in the right internal jugular bulb related to a right temporal bone fracture.

nonspecific and include headaches, nausea, vomiting, and papilledema.

As in cerebral venous thrombosis resulting from other causes, infarction and hemorrhage can result. The diagnosis is often made using CT or MR venography or DSA, although noncontrast CT and MR imaging of the brain can suggest the diagnosis. On noncontrast CT, one may see hyperdensity in the venous structures reflecting the presence of thrombus. MR imaging may show abnormal signal in the dural sinuses on multiple sequences. T1-weighted images can be particularly helpful and often reveal T1 shortening in the thrombosed sinus.

More delayed sequelae of calvarial fractures include infection as well as the formation of leptomeningeal cysts and epidermoid cysts. Although leptomeningeal cysts are most often associated with pediatric skull fractures, there are documented cases in adults.[34] Typically, radiographs or CT show scalloping and erosion along the margins of a prior skull fracture, and there may be progressive diastasis of the fracture fragments.[35] The presumed mechanism for formation of a leptomeningeal cyst involves herniation of the arachnoid membrane via a tear in the dura at the site of a fracture, and fractures with associated diastasis of 4 mm or greater have a greater propensity for the development of cysts. The dura adheres to the edges of herniated arachnoid, and a one-way valve mechanism results in an enlarging arachnoid cyst because of the transmission of CSF pulsations via the dural defect.[35] CT cisternography, the introduction of iodinated contrast into the subarachnoid space surrounding

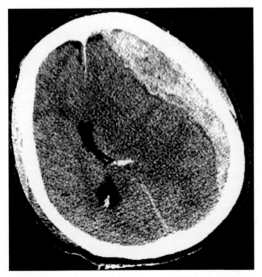

Fig. 29. Axial CT image showing subfalcine herniation and partial effacement of the suprasellar cistern caused by a subdural hematoma.

the brain via lumbar puncture, may help to confirm the diagnosis. Features that help to distinguish an epidermoid cyst from a leptomeningeal cyst include displacement of the inner table of the calvarium toward the brain and the presence of bone debris within the lesion.[35]

Another delayed consequence of head trauma is encephalomalacia, which develops at the sites of previous brain contusions (**Fig. 31**A, B). The location and size of these areas of encephalomalacia dictate the nature of any associated symptoms. For example, posttraumatic encephalomalacia in the frontal lobes may result in frontal lobe syndrome, which can include disinhibition and inappropriate behavior, whereas encephalomalacia at the occipital poles may result in cortical blindness.

Patients with posttraumatic encephalomalacia, which by definition includes damage to the cerebral cortex, may also suffer from seizures. Furthermore, data suggest that suffering traumatic brain injury can increase one's chances of developing neurodegenerative disorders, including Alzheimer disease and Parkinson disease.[31]

Although encephalomalacia represents local volume loss, repeat imaging of patients who have sustained severe head trauma often shows progressive generalized cerebral volume loss. In many patients, initial imaging was either normal or may have shown a few focal lesions. Presumably, this progressive atrophy results at least in part from extensive DAI, and even MR imaging likely underestimates the extent of shearing injury, particularly because many of the lesions are microscopic.[21]

As noted earlier, the long-term sequelae of head trauma can be life altering for the patient, and various more advanced imaging modalities are helping to better define associated anatomic changes and predict clinical outcomes. An example is MR spectroscopy, which has been used to evaluate patients with head trauma. There is a correlation between a reduced N-acetyl aspartate to creatine ratio and a poor clinical prognosis in the setting of head trauma. Poor clinical outcomes have also been associated with reduced magnetization transfer ratios, a metric reflecting the "structural integrity of tissue."[8]

Other advanced imaging techniques, in particular DTI with tractography, hold promise for further increased sensitivity for detection of DAI and an improved understanding of its long-term sequelae. Arfanakis and colleagues,[22] in a study of 5 patients with traumatic brain injury and 10 controls, found reduced diffusion anisotropy in the brains of the trauma patients imaged within 24 hours of their injury. Diffusion anisotropy refers to the preferential diffusion of water molecules along intact white-matter tracts in particular directions. When white-matter tracts are injured, diffusion anisotropy is reduced. Arfanakis and his colleagues noted that the reduced diffusion anisotropy observed in the trauma patients was less evident when they were reimaged approximately 1 month later.

The importance of DAI in long-term outcome has been suggested by multiple studies.

Huisman and colleagues[21] noted that calculated ADC maps allowed the separation of DAI lesions into those with increased and those with decreased diffusion, with the latter representing the larger subgroup (65%). Although these researchers acknowledged that current understanding of changes in ADC in the setting of trauma is

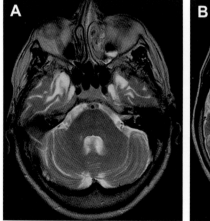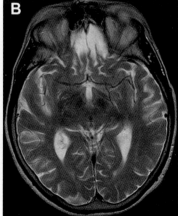

Fig. 31. (*A*) Axial T2 image showing encephalomalacia in the anterior inferior temporal lobes. (*B*) Axial T2 image showing encephalomalacia in the inferior paramedian frontal lobes.

incomplete, decreased ADC may be an independent determinant of long-term prognosis. Furthermore, increased ADC may reflect vasogenic edema related to less severe injury.

SUMMARY

This article reviews the essential concepts related to the imaging of head trauma. However, it is only a starting point, because there is a large and continually expanding body of literature on the subject. Furthermore, imaging technologies and techniques continue to evolve at an ever-accelerating rate. It is incumbent on each of us to try to stay abreast of these developments so that we can provide the best possible care to our patients and so that as radiologists, we remain collectively at the cutting edge of imaging. Continued advances in CT and MR imaging technology, including progressively faster image acquisition and postprocessing, higher image resolution, and increased safety through various radiation dose-limiting measures, help radiologists to continue to play an integral part in the assessment and care of patients with head trauma in the years to come. By keeping ourselves informed of these developments, we may even make ourselves more indispensable.

ACKNOWLEDGMENTS

I would like to thank the following individuals for contributing images for this article: Eric Russell, MD, Steve Futterer, MD, Alyssa Volk, MD, Jim Gehl, MD, Mike Lin, MD, Corey Bregman, MD, Enzo Cento, MD, Jeet Minocha, MD, Nicholas Kolanko, MD, Rick Yeh, MD, Jimmy Wang, MD, Kush Desai, MD, Tom Rhee, MD. I would also like to thank Mari Fitzgibbons (fourth-year medical student at the Feinberg School of Medicine of Northwestern University) for her assistance in compiling and organizing many of the images for this article.

REFERENCES

1. Langlois JA, Rutland-Brown W, Thomas KE. Traumatic brain injury in the United States: emergency department visits, hospitalizations, and deaths. Atlanta (GA): Centers for Disease Control and Prevention, National Center for Injury Prevention and Control; 2004. Available at: http://www.cdc.gov/ncipc/pub-res/TBI_in_US_04/TBI_ED.htm. Accessed December 13, 2009.

2. Finkelstein E, Corso P, Miller T, et al. The incidence and economic burden of injuries in the United States. New York: Oxford University Press; 2006.

3. Gentry LR, Godersky JC, Thompson B. MR imaging of head trauma: review of the distribution and radiopathologic features of traumatic lesions. Am J Roentgenol 1988;150(3):663–72.

4. Offiah C, Twigg S. Imaging assessment of penetrating craniocerebral and spinal trauma. Clin Radiol 2009;64(12):1146–57.

5. Stuehmer C, Blum KS, Kokemueller H, et al. Influence of different types of guns, projectiles, and propellants on patterns of injury to the viscerocranium. J Oral Maxillofac Surg 2009;67(4):775–81.

6. Aarabi B, Taghipur M, Alibaii E, et al. Central nervous system infections after military missile head wounds. Neurosurgery 1998;42(3):500–9.

7. Lee KS. The pathogenesis and clinical significance of traumatic subdural hygroma. Brain Inj 1998;12(7):595–603.

8. Le TH, Gean AD. Neuroimaging of traumatic brain injury. Mt Sinai J Med 2009;76(2):145–62.

9. Klufas RA, Hsu L, Patel MR, et al. Unusual manifestations of head trauma. Am J Roentgenol 1996;166(3):675–81.

10. Armin SS, Colohan ART, Zhang JH. Traumatic subarachnoid hemorrhage: our current understanding and its evolution over the past half century. Neurol Res 2006;28(4):445–52.

11. Rinkel GJ, van Gijn J, Wijdicks EF. Subarachnoid hemorrhage without detectable aneurysm: a review of the causes. Stroke 1993;24(9):1403–9.

12. Matsuda W, Sugimoto K, Naoaki S, et al. Delayed onset of posttraumatic acute subdural hematoma after mild head injury with normal computed tomography: a case report and brief review. J Trauma 2008;65(2):461–3.

13. Gomori JM, Grossman RI. Mechanisms responsible for the MR appearance and evolution of intracranial hemorrhage. Radiographics 1988;8(3):427–40.

14. Kleinman PK. Diagnostic imaging of child abuse. 2nd edition. St. Louis (MO): Mosby; 1998.

15. Hart RG, Boop BS, Anderson DC. Oral anticoagulants and intracranial hemorrhage: facts and hypotheses. Stroke 1995;26(8):1471–7.

16. Drew LB, Drew WE. The contrecoup-coup phenomenon: a new understanding. Neurocrit Care 2004;1(3):385–90.

17. Alahmadi H, Vachhrajani S, Cusimano MD. The natural history of brain contusion: an analysis of radiological and clinical progression. J Neurosurg 2010;112:1139–45.

18. Wintermark M, van Melle G, Schnyder P, et al. Admission perfusion CT: prognostic value in patients with severe head trauma. Radiology 2004;232(1):211–20.

19. von Oettingen G, Bergholt B, Gyldenstad C, et al. Blood flow and ischemia with traumatic cerebral contusions. Neurosurgery 2002;50(4):781–9.

20. Wada R, Aviv RI, Fox AJ, et al. CT angiography "spot sign" predicts hematoma expansion in acute intra-cerebral hemorrhage. Stroke 2007;38:1257–62.

21. Huisman TA, Sorensen AG, Hergan K, et al. Diffusion-weighted imaging for the evaluation of diffuse axonal injury in closed head injury. J Comput Assist Tomogr 2003;27(1):5–11.

22. Arfanakis K, Haughton VM, Carew JD, et al. Diffusion tensor MR imaging in diffuse axonal injury. AJNR Am J Neuroradiol 2002;23:794–802.

23. Tong KA, Ashwal S, Holshouser BA, et al. Diffuse axonal injury in children: clinical correlation with hemorrhagic lesions. Ann Neurol 2004;56:36–50.

24. Babikian T, Freier MC, Tong KA, et al. Susceptibility-weighted imaging: neuropsychological outcome and pediatric head injury. Pediatr Neurol 2005;33: 179–89.

25. Le TH, Mukherjee P, Henry RG, et al. Diffusion tensor imaging with three-dimensional fiber tractography of traumatic axonal shearing injury: an imaging correlate for the posterior callosal "disconnection" syndrome: case report. Neurosurgery 2005;56(1):189.

26. Caplan LR. Dissections of brain-supplying arteries. Nat Clin Pract Neurol 2008;4(1):34–42.

27. Walker MT, Liu BP, Salehi SA, et al. Superficial temporal artery pseudoaneurysm: diagnosis and preoperative planning with CT angiography. AJNR Am J Neuroradiol 2003;24:147–50.

28. Nishimura S, Hirai T, Sasao A, et al. Evaluation of dural arteriovenous fistulas with 4D contrast-enhanced MR angiography at 3T. AJNR Am J Neuroradiol 2010; 31(1):80–5.

29. York G, Barboriak D, Petrella J, et al. Association of internal carotid artery injury with carotid canal fractures in patients with head trauma. Am J Roentgenol 2005;184:1672–8.

30. Thurman D, Alverson C, Dunn K, et al. Traumatic brain injury in the United States: a public health perspective. J Head Trauma Rehabil 1999;14(6):602–15.

31. National Institute of Neurological Disorders and Stroke. Traumatic brain injury: hope through research. Bethesda (MD): National Institutes of Health; 2002. NIH publication no. 02–158. Available at: http://www.ninds.nih.gov/disorders/tbi/detail_tbi.htm. Accessed November 17, 2009.

32. Centers for Disease Control and Prevention (CDC). Sports-related recurrent brain injuries-United States. MMWR Morb Mortal Wkly Rep 1997;46(10):224–7. Available at: http://www.cdc.gov/mmwr/preview/mmwrhtml/00046702.htm. Accessed November 20, 2009.

33. D'Alise MD, Fichtel F, Horowitz M. Sagittal sinus thrombosis following minor head injury treated with continuous urokinase infusion. Surg Neurol 1998;49(4):430–5.

34. Britz GW, Kim DK, Mayberg MR. Traumatic lepto-meningeal cyst in an adult: a case report and review of the literature. Surg Neurol 1998;50(5): 465–9.

35. Gruber F. Post-traumatic leptomeningeal cysts. Am J Roentgenol 1969;105:305–7.

Spine Infection/ Inflammation

Jeffrey DeSanto, MD*, Jeffrey S. Ross, MD

KEYWORDS

• Spine • Infection • Inflammation • MR imaging

This article discusses the imaging of infectious and other inflammatory conditions that affect the spinal cord, spinal column, intradural spinal nerve roots, and spinal meninges with emphasis on magnetic resonance (MR) imaging. Inflammatory lesions of the spine are often indistinguishable on imaging and even on pathologic examination. However, infectious causes are treatable so it is important for the radiologist to make the diagnosis. The most common inflammatory and infectious conditions affecting the anatomic compartments of the spine are described, following an external to internal anatomic approach. Subsequently, several infectious pathogenic agents are discussed individually as they affect the spinal column and its contents.

INFECTIOUS SPONDYLODISCITIS

Infectious spondylitis can be caused by bacterial, fungal, or parasitic organisms. Vertebral bodies and intervertebral discs are most frequently affected with primary or secondary involvement of the epidural space, posterior elements, and paraspinal soft tissues.

PHYSIOPATHOLOGY OF SPINAL INFECTIONS

The vasculature of the vertebral bodies and intervertebral discs changes significantly with age.[1] In adults there are secondary periosteal arteries arising from the segmental arteries, which ramify on the surface of the bone and give rise to a large number of peripheral intraosseous arteries supplying the outer third of the vertebral body. Anastomoses between intraosseous arteries are widespread in infants and small children but become less prominent by age 7 years and regress by age 15 years, when the adult configuration peripheral periosteal arteries develop. Intraosseous anastomoses have completely involuted in adult life.[2–4] The vascular supply of the discs also changes significantly with age. The intervertebral discs of infants and children have a much more profuse vascular supply than adults. The capillary network at the vertebral margins adjacent to the discs is denser in infants and children than in adults. Several vessels penetrate deeply into the discs of infants, whereas in most adolescents and in all adults no such vessels are present. In contrast to the vertebral margins, the free margins of the discs are almost equally richly vascularized in children and adults.[5]

The most accepted hypothesis is that vertebral osteomyelitis results from hematogenous spread from an infected microembolus in the arterial system becoming lodged in one of the metaphyseal arteries resulting in infarction and subsequent infection.[6] Osteomyelitis is most frequent at the end plates because of the greater number of arteries in this location.[4] The mere presence of bacteria in the bone is insufficient to result in osteomyelitis.[7,8] Subsequent infarct is also a necessary precondition for the pathogenesis of osteomyelitis.

A septic embolus in a metaphyseal artery of a child causes only a small infarct because of the rich intraosseous anastomoses. In adults, however, the intraosseous metaphyseal artery is an end artery, and a septic embolus causes a septic infarct of a wedge-shaped subdiscal area of bone. Infection can then extend to the opposite vertebral end plate through primary periosteal arteries or to the adjacent end plate, across the interspace through the intermetaphyseal

Neuroradiology Department, Barrow Neurological Institute, St Joseph's Hospital and Medical Center, 350 West Thomas Road, Phoenix, AZ 85013, USA
* Corresponding author.
E-mail address: jeffrey_desanto@yahoo.com

Radiol Clin N Am 49 (2011) 105–127
doi:10.1016/j.rcl.2010.07.018
0033-8389/11/$ — see front matter © 2011 Elsevier Inc. All rights reserved.

arteries without necessarily affecting the central part of the vertebral body. In both children and adults the disc is involved early by infection from the metaphysis. Because the adult disc is an almost avascular structure there are no immediate blood-borne immune defense mechanisms and infection can readily become established and quickly progress. Primary involvement of the disc by blood-borne pathogens occurs only in the pediatric age groups because of persistent blood supply to the disc.[9,10]

PYOGENIC SPONDYLITIS

Pyogenic spondylitis is most frequently caused by hematogenous spread from infectious foci elsewhere in the body, but it can occur also by direct extension from instrumentation or surgery or by contiguous spread from neighboring infected organs such as the oropharynx, pleural space of the lung, and thoracic or abdominal wall.[11,12] The most common sources of septic emboli are, in decreasing order of frequency, infections from the genitourinary tract, skin, and upper respiratory tract.[13] *Staphylococcus aureus* is the most common organism identified (up to 60%), followed by Enterobacteriaceae (up to 30%). Other organism commonly isolated include *Staphylococcus epidermidis*, *Haemophilus influenzae*, and different groups of *Streptococcus*.[14] *Escherichia coli* is the most common source of the gram-negative bacilli. *Salmonella* infection is more common in patients with sickle-cell disease. *Pseudomonas* species are the most common causative agents in intravenous drug abusers.[15] Elderly diabetic patients, 60 to 70 years old, are more frequently affected. Men used to be affected more frequently than women, but this trend is changing, and recent series show similar incidence in both sexes.[16] Intravenous drug use, immunosuppression, and chronic medical disease (renal failure, cirrhosis, cancer) also predispose to vertebral osteomyelitis. The number of pyogenic spinal infections has increased in recent decades because of the larger proportion of the elderly population and prolongation of the life of patients suffering from chronic and debilitating diseases. In addition, the number of iatrogenic spinal infections related to spinal instrumentation has been increasing. The lumbar spine is most frequently involved (48%) followed by the thoracic (35%) and cervical spine (6.5%).[17]

The clinical presentation of vertebral osteomyelitis and discitis can be variable but the cardinal signs are focal back pain and muscle spasm, which are present in more than 90% of cases.[18] Fever and leukocytosis are present in only 40%

to 50%. The erythrocyte sedimentation rate (ESR) is almost always increased.[19] C-reactive protein may be a superior laboratory marker to monitor response to therapy as a result of quicker normalization with effective therapy.[20] Percutaneous needle biopsy sampling of the infected vertebral body or disc can be performed under fluoroscopic or computed tomography (CT) guidance to isolate the causative organism and may be diagnostic in 68% to 86% of cases.[21–23] In cases in which percutaneous biopsy sampling fails, is nondiagnostic, or cannot be performed, an open surgical biopsy procedure can be performed. Diagnosis can be established without direct biopsy sampling in patients with positive blood cultures, but bacterial growth on blood cultures occurs in less than 25% of cases.[18] Cultures of biopsied specimens may be falsely negative in up to 40% to 65% of cases of osteomyelitis.[24–27] Treatment of the neurologically intact patient primarily involves immobilization and antibiotics.[17] In most cases surgical intervention is not required, however, destruction of the vertebral body and intervertebral disc may lead to spinal deformity and instability placing the spinal cord at risk, thereby requiring stabilizing surgical fusion.[18]

The earliest plain radiograph findings of vertebral osteomyelitis and discitis are usually not evident until 2 to 8 weeks after onset of symptoms. Radiographs may show demineralization, loss of definition of end-plate margins, narrowing of intervertebral space, associated soft tissue swelling, and eventually destructive changes of the vertebral end plate and the vertebral body. CT has played a minor role in cases with bony or soft tissue components and is not considered a mainstay for the diagnosis of disk space infection.[28,29] Noncontrast CT findings of osteolytic and osteosclerotic changes of the end-plate cortex and spinal deformity best seen on coronal and sagittal reformations are evident earlier than with plain film radiographs. Prominent isodense to hypodense paraspinal soft tissue with or without soft tissue gas may also be seen in the setting of paraspinal abscess.

Radionuclides most commonly used for detecting inflammatory changes of the spine are technetium 99m (^{99m}Tc) phosphate complexes, gallium 67 (^{67}Ga) citrate, and indium 111 (^{111}In)-labeled white blood cells. A 3-phase technetium Tc-99m diphosphonate scan shows increased activity in all phases. Although scintigraphy with ^{99m}Tc and ^{67}Ga compounds is sensitive to infection, it is also nonspecific. Healing fractures, sterile inflammatory reactions, tumors, and loosened prosthetic devices can show increased uptake.[1–3] ^{111}In has several advantages compared with other radionuclides, including higher target-to-background ratios, better image quality (compared with gallium), and more intense uptake by abscesses. Its main disadvantage is its accumulation within any inflammatory lesion, whether infectious or not.[30] The radionuclide study also takes time to perform (hours to days).

Modic and colleagues[31,32] showed that MR was as accurate as and more sensitive than radionuclide scanning in the characterization of osteomyelitis. Despite being the most sensitive tool to detect early osteomyelitis, MR findings may still lag behind the clinical symptoms. When the diagnosis is uncertain, a follow-up MR in 1 week may be helpful to show the evolution of the early changes. It is imperative to obtain both T1-weighted and T2-weighted images in the sagittal plane to optimize sensitivity of the examination. The T1-weighted spin echo (SE) image allows detection of the increased water content or marrow fluid seen with inflammatory exudates or edema. The sagittal T1-weighted sequence typically shows ill-defined hypointense vertebral marrow in the adjacent vertebral bodies and involved intervertebral disc space with loss of end-plate definition on both sides of the disc. Loss of disc space height is a characteristic but late finding. T2-weighted images show increased signal intensity of the vertebral bodies adjacent to the involved disk, and an abnormal morphology and increased signal intensity from the disk itself, with the absence of the normal intranuclear cleft. Postcontrast sequences show enhancement of the disc and adjacent end plates. These MR findings are much more typical of pyogenic than of tuberculous or fungal spondylitis (**Fig. 1**).[33]

Dagirmanjian and colleagues[34] showed 95% of disk space infection levels had typical T1-weighted vertebral body changes, and 90% had increased nonanatomic signal of the disc on T2-weighted images. However, only 54% of the abnormal levels showed increased signal of the vertebral bodies on T2-weighted images. Thus, although 84% of patients showed the typical T1 vertebral body, and T1 and T2 disc changes, only 49% of cases showed both the typical T1- and T2-weighted vertebral body and disc findings as originally described. T1-weighted vertebral body, disc and end-plate changes, and T2-weighted imaging disc changes are the most reliable findings of disk space infection and vertebral osteomyelitis. Thus, when confronted with the typical T1-weighted vertebral body and disc changes and T2-weighted disc signal intensity changes of discitis, one should not be dissuaded from the MR diagnosis of discitis with associated vertebral osteomyelitis by the absence of increased vertebral body signal on the T2-weighted images. Seventy-one percent of patients with decreased or isointense signal of the body on T2-weighted images had sclerosis on plain films, in contrast with 45% of patients with high signal of the body on T2-weoghted images. T2 signal intensity of the vertebral body on MR imaging reflects the marrow space, whereas the sclerosis seen on plain films reflects the bony trabecula. Trabecular sclerosis may increase to such an extent that it obliterates the marrow space with associated decreased signal intensity on T2-weighted images.

Just as the MR findings lag behind the early signs of disc space infection, they also lag behind in the healing phase of vertebral osteomyelitis. Radiographic and MR findings may be very slow or inconsistent in resolution of infection-related abnormalities.[35] Kowalski and colleagues[36] reported no specific associations between follow-up MR imaging findings and clinical status in their cohort of patients with spine infections. Gillams and colleagues[37] found that diminished soft tissue inflammation in 8 of 14 patients (57%) was one of the first signs of improvement. The finding of high signal intensity on T1-weighted images from a previously infected vertebra reflects replacement of cellular marrow by fat, indicating healing.[14] The efficacy of conservative care may be estimated in individual cases by diminution of pain, resolution of fever and leukocytosis, and decreasing ESR. A decreasing ESR during the first month of nonsurgical treatment is a good prognostic sign, however, success of conservative treatment is seen in 40% of cases with persistently high or increasing ESR.[38]

DIFFERENTIAL DIAGNOSIS OF SPONDYLODISCITIS DEGENERATIVE CHANGES

The 3 patterns of end-plate changes in degenerative lumbar disc disease are well known.[39] The type I degenerative changes with low T1 and high T2 signal in the end plates can potentially mimic spondylodiscitis. Distinction between this inflammatory stage of osteoarthritis and disc space infection can be made by the lack of abnormal disc signal or by hypointensity of the disc on T2-weighted images. Tuberculosis and brucellosis, however, may involve adjacent vertebral bodies without affecting the intervening disc.[40] Although a degenerated disc can enhance in its central portion or at the periphery, it usually does not occur at the same intensity that is observed in spondylodiscitis. The end plates can

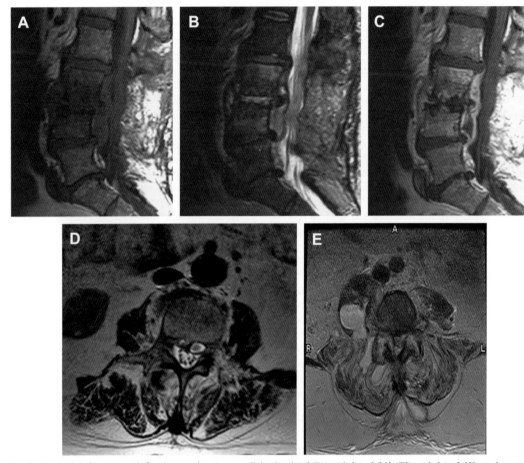

Fig. 1. Bacterial disc space infection and osteomyelitis. Sagittal T1-weighted (*A*), T2-weighted (*B*) and postcontrast T1-weighted (*C*) images show the typical findings of disc space infection with abnormal low T1 signal, disc T2 hyperintensity, and irregular end plate and disc enhancement. There is a large ventral epidural abscess at the L4 level. Axial T2-weighted images from a different patient (*D*) shows characteristic appearance of abscess in the anterior epidural space bounded by midline septum and lateral membranes with posterior displacement of the posterior longitudinal ligament. There is prominent inflammatory changes in the paraspinous soft tissues with abscess formation (*E*).

enhance with either the inflammatory stage of degenerative changes or with infection. An early follow-up study can be of benefit in making this distinction as it will demonstrate no changes in the degenerated disc or alteration in end-plate marrow signal in the setting of degenerative disc disease.

An atypical-appearing disk space infection can also be present if it complicates a degenerated disk with an associated type II marrow change (ie, increased signal from the end plates on T1-weighted images). In these cases the T1-weighted images may continue to show increased signal, in effect masking the usual characteristically confluent decreased intensity. The key observation to make in these cases is the abnormal disk signal hyperintensity on T2-weighted images, a finding that does not occur

in uncomplicated type II marrow change. Very early on in vertebral osteomyelitis, there may be decreased signal involving the end plates without an appreciable increase in signal from the bodies or disk on T2-weighted images.

POSTOPERATIVE SPONDYLODISCITIS

Postoperative spondylodiscitis is an infrequent complication of lumbar disc surgery. The most probable cause is intraoperative contamination rather than hematogenous spread,[41,42] although either may occur. The typical clinical presentation is recurrent pain after initial postoperative relief, muscle spasm, fever, and positive straight leg-raising test. The ESR is almost always increased, however this is nonspecific because it may be increased postoperatively in the absence of infection. A more reliable screening test for post-operative spondylodiscitis is C-reactive protein,[43] especially if it was known to be negative before surgery. The roentgenographic findings appear several weeks after the initial symptoms. MR may be helpful earlier, but it is usually not possible to reliably diagnose infection until 3 weeks after surgery. Contrast enhancement and signal changes in the intervertebral disc or the vertebral end plates can be seen both in the setting of disci-tis and in normal postoperative asymptomatic patients. However, absence of signal changes in the vertebral end plates, contrast enhancement of the disc, or enhancing paravertebral soft tissues does help rule out spondylodiscitis.[44] MR imaging may therefore be more useful for the exclusion rather than the confirmation of postoperative spondylodiscitis. CT or fluoroscopically guided needle biopsy and aspiration frequently allows isolation of a causative pathogen. Conservative management based on bed rest, immobilization, and antibiotics remains the treatment of choice. Early surgical treatment may be indicated in some cases.

Distinguishing early MR postoperative discitis from normal postoperative changes in the disc space can be challenging. The postoperative disc may change as a result of the intervention with related aseptic inflammatory changes that may mask early infectious alterations.[44] Boden and colleagues[45] suggested that in the postopera-tive spine the triad of intervertebral disk space enhancement, annular enhancement, and verte-bral body enhancement lead to the diagnosis of disk space infection when found in conjunction with appropriate laboratory findings such as an increased ESR. However, there is a group of normal postoperative patients with annulus enhancement (at the surgical curette site), inter-vertebral disk enhancement, and vertebral end-plate enhancement without evidence of disk space infection. In these cases, the intervertebral disk enhancement is typically seen as thin bands paral-leling the adjacent end plates, and the vertebral body enhancement is enhancement associated with type I degenerative end-plate changes. This pattern should be distinguished from the amor-phous enhancement present within the interverte-bral disk with disk space infection.

Other differential considerations for pyogenic spondylodiscitis include dialysis-related spondy-loarthropathy, pseudoarthrosis and neuropathic spine, granulomatous spondylitis, neoplasm, and idiopathic and autoimmune inflammatory processes.[46] These processes can usually be reli-ably distinguished based on the combination of imaging findings and clinical presentation.

Granulomatous infectious and inflammatory processes are discussed separately.

SPINAL EPIDURAL ABSCESS

Early diagnosis of spinal epidural abscess (SEA) remains difficult and treatment is often delayed.[47] The morbidity of SEA is high with mortality ranging from 18% to 31% in modern series.[48–50] Its prev-alence is apparently increasing.[51,52] The risk factors of SEA are similar for those of spondylodis-citis including diabetes mellitus, intravenous drug use, chronic renal failure, alcohol abuse, and immunodeficiency.[51,52] Human immunodeficiency virus (HIV) infection does not seem to play a role in the overall increasing incidence of the disease. Prompt diagnosis and treatment are critical because SEA can rapidly progress to paraplegia, quadriplegia, and death if untreated or if treatment is delayed. The clinical features include acute or subacute back pain, tenderness, progressive rad-iculopathy or myelopathy, and fever. Fever may be absent in the subacute and chronic cases.[52] Leukocytosis is present in approximately 60% of patients, and ESR is usually increased. A meta-analysis of 915 patients with SEA showed 71% of patients had back pain as the initial symptom and 66% had fever. The second stage of radicular irritation was followed by the third stage of begin-ning neurologic deficit including muscle weakness and sphincter incontinence as well as sensory deficits. The fourth stage of paralysis affected only 34% of the patients. Functional compromise of the spinal cord usually results in mechanical compression, but clinical deterioration can occur without significant mechanical compression and may be secondary to ischemia.[15] Treatment includes emergent surgical drainage and decom-pression. Wide spectrum antibiotics can be used until the causative pathogen is isolated.

S aureus is the causative agent in 62% to 67% of cases,[47,52,53] and in 15% of infections these organisms are methicillin resistant.[47] *Mycobacte-rium tuberculosis* is the next most frequent cause accounting for approximately 25% of reported cases. SEA may be encountered in all segments of the spinal canal. SEA occurs most commonly in the lower thoracic and lumbar spine, followed by the cervical and upper thoracic spine. SEA can be classified as diffuse when it involves 6 or more vertebral segments and as focal when it involves 5 or fewer vertebral segments as defined by Numaguchi and colleagues[50] The most common concomitant infections are spondylodis-citis, facet infection, posterior paraspinal abscess, and retroperitoneal abscess. Most cases are ante-rior to the dural sac or involve it circumferentially and are associated with spondylodiscitis.[52] When abscess involves the ventral epidural space, it tends to conform to a pattern anatomically dictated by the posterior longitudinal ligament/central septum complex and lateral membranes (see **Fig. 1**).[54] MR is the most effective diagnostic technique for SEA, its sensitivity varying between 91%[52] and 100%.[47]

The primary diagnostic modality in the evaluation of epidural abscess is MR. MR is as sensitive as CT myelography for epidural infection, but it also allows the exclusion of other diagnostic choices such as herniation, syrinx, tumor and cord infarction.[55] MR imaging of epidural abscess shows a soft tissue mass in the epidural space with tapered edges and an associated mass effect on the thecal sac and cord (**Fig. 2**). The epidural masses are usually isointense to the cord on T1-weighted images and of increased signal on T2-weighted images. Post and colleagues[56,57] recommended that in these ambiguous cases either CT myelography or perhaps Gd-diethylene triamine pentaacetic acid (DTPA) enhancement is necessary for full elucidation of the abscess. The patterns of Gd-DTPA enhancement of epidural abscess include (1) diffuse and homogeneous, (2) heterogeneous, and (3) thin peripheral. Post and colleagues[57] found that Gd-DTPA enhancement was a useful adjunct for identifying the extent of a lesion when the plain MR scan was equivocal,

for demonstrating activity of an infection, and for directing needle biopsy and follow-up treatment. Successful therapy should cause a progressive decrease in enhancement of the paraspinal soft tissues, disk, and vertebral bodies. Differential diagnostic considerations for SEA include extra-dural metastases, epidural hematoma, extruded or migrated disc fragment, and epidural lipomatosis. There is a case report of tophaceous gout mimicking an epidural abscess.[58]

INTRAMEDULLARY ABSCESSES

Intramedullary abscesses are uncommon with only approximately 70 cases reported in the literature. The symptoms of intramedullary abscess are indistinguishable from those of epidural abscess.[59] They can occur secondary to hematogenous spread, continuous spread from adjacent infection, implantation secondary to trauma or surgery, or from congenital dermal sinus or other congenital conditions with open dural defects. S aureus and Streptococcus are the most common pathogens. Medical therapy alone can be attempted but laminectomy and surgical debridement may be necessary if neurologic symptoms progress. Because it is an uncommon entity there is a relative paucity of accumulated experience and thus no consensus criteria have been established for appropriate surgical intervention.[60] Murphy and colleagues[59] reported a preferential location in the distal thoracic spinal cord and conus medullaris. Fever may be present, and the ESR tends to be increased. Cerebrospinal fluid (CSF) cultures are usually sterile.[61]

The MR findings of 1 case of staphylococcal myelitis and of 6 cases with proven intramedullary spinal cord abscesses have been described.[62] According to the imaging patterns observed, the cord involvement begins as an ill-defined myelitis and gradually evolves to a localized abscess. The initial imaging studies may show areas of intramedullary high signal on T2-weighted images. Enhanced T1-weighted images show ill-defined low signal in an expanded cord. Postcontrast T1-weighted sequences show an irregular ring-enhancing lesion with cord expansion. This abnormal enhancement tends to be more localized than the diffuse and extensive T2 high-signal abnormality (**Fig. 3**). Differential diagnostic considerations include cord ischemia, Guillain-Barré syndrome (GBS), acute transverse myelitis, multiple sclerosis, hemangioblastoma, and other cavitary neoplasm. An infected syrinx can also appear as an intramedullary abscess. Diffusion-weighted imaging may show restricted diffusion although the absence of restricted diffusion does not exclude abscess.

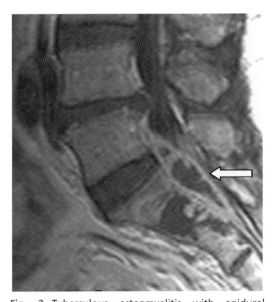

Fig. 2. Tuberculous osteomyelitis with epidural abscess. Sagittal T1-weighted image following contrast shows irregular decreased enhancement involving the S1 and S2 bodies, and a large ventral epidural abscess with peripheral enhancement (*arrow*).

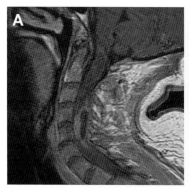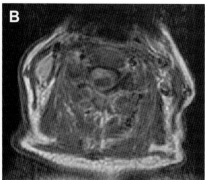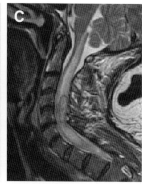

Fig. 3. Intramedullary abscess. Sagittal and axial T1-weighted images (*A, B*) show irregular ring-enhancing lesion with cord expansion. Sagittal T2 image (*C*) shows more extensive intramedullary signal hyperintensity.

MULTIPLE SCLEROSIS

The spinal cord is the site of much motor disability in patients with multiple sclerosis (MS), yet imaging of the spinal cord has always been subordinate to brain imaging in clinical investigations in MS. None of the recent, large, therapeutic trials on patients with MS include assessment of cord disease, even though brain MR findings may be the primary objective determinant of disease activity. The reasons for the omission include a lack of established relationships between cord disease and disability in MS, the complexity and duration of MR examinations when obtaining both brain and cord data, and technical difficulties in cord imaging because of the small size of the spinal cord, its orientation, and the presence of artifacts from pulsatile CSF flow, as well as cardiac, respiratory, and oropharyngeal motion. Because some of the clinical disease activity in MS is related to the spinal cord, it is important to investigate cord disease activity to gain further insights into the nature of disability in these patients and to determine if any objective imaging improvements in brain and cord lesion burden observed in a therapeutic trial are associated with correlative changes in clinical disability scoring.

PATTERNS OF CORD MS

Tartaglino and colleagues[63,64] described in detail the MR appearances of MS in the spinal cord. They found that most focal plaques were less than 2 vertebral body lengths in size, occupied less than half the cross-sectional diameter of the cord, and were characteristically peripherally located with respect to a transverse cross-sectional reference (**Fig. 4**). Approximately 60% to 75% of the MS lesions in the spinal cord are present in the cervical region, and more than half of the patients with MS with cord plaques had multiple plaques. Of the patients with cord plaques, 90% had intracranial MS plaques. Most plaques did not significantly alter cord morphology. However, more than half of the cord plaques longer than 2 vertebral segments were accompanied by cord atrophy, or conversely, cord swelling. Cord swelling occurred only in patients with relapsing-remitting MS and in patients with Devic syndrome of optic neuritis and myelitis. Characteristic imaging findings described for Devic syndrome (neuromyelitis optica [NMO]) include cord lesions involving a long segment (up to 9 vertebral body lengths), holocord signal abnormality with cord swelling and mild, patchy gadolinium enhancement. Wiebe and colleagues[65] found approximately 14% of cord plaques enhanced following gadolinium administration.

CORD MS ACTIVITY AND CLINICAL IMPAIRMENT

A study by Kidd and colleagues[66] with current MR coil and sequence technologies reveal spinal cord lesions in nearly 75% of patients with clinically definite MS, and cord lesions are seen in every clinical subtype of MS. Approximately 10% to 15% of patients with spinal cord plaques have no intracranial disease. The cord lesion burden did not correlate with the brain lesion load. Cord atrophy, defined as a cross-sectional diameter less than 2 SD less than normal for the specific cord level, was present in 40% of patients with MS, most frequently at the C5 level. There was a tendency for focal cord lesions to be more prevalent in normal-sized cords. Those patients with atrophy had a mean Expanded Disability Status Scale (EDSS) that was significantly worse than those without atrophy. Losseff and colleagues[67] also found a statistically significant difference in

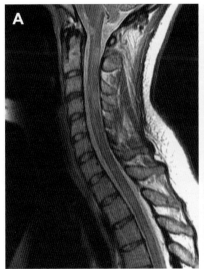
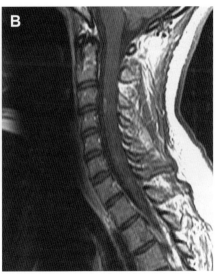

Fig. 4. Multiple sclerosis. Sagittal short time inversion recovery image shows multiple focal areas of T2 hyperintensity involving the cervical cord (A). After contrast (B), the sagittal T1-weighted image shows several foci of cord enhancement consistent with areas of active demyelination.

cord cross-sectional area between patients with MS and normal volunteers, and did find a significant correlation between the presence of cord atrophy and clinical disability. Wiebe and colleagues[65] found 12 of 25 newly detected cord plaques were not associated with any new clinical signs. Thus, a similar lack of precise clinical and MR correlation of anatomic localization of disease activity exists for spinal cord as well as brain MS. Lycklama a Nijeholt and colleagues[68] found that diffuse cord abnormalities were correlated with primary or secondary progressive clinical MS subtypes, and diffuse disease was associated with cord atrophy, and had a weak but significant correlation with clinical disability. Another study by Kidd and colleagues[69] in patients with primary progressive and secondary progressive MS showed no correlation between brain or spinal cord activity over 12 months and change in clinical disability in a patient cohort in which 80% showed a change in EDSS of 1 or greater during the study period. They summarized by suggesting that serial imaging of the cord to detect new activity would not make a useful contribution to clinical therapeutic trials in patients with progressive MS.

NMO (DEVIC SYNDROME)

NMO is an uncommon autoimmune, inflammatory, demyelinating disorder involving myelin of the neurons of optic nerves and spinal cord with limited brain parenchymal involvement.[70–73] The disease is characterized clinically by optic neuritis

and transverse myelopathy. The interval between optic neuritis and transverse myelitis is usually days or weeks, but sometimes it may take as long as several years. The course of NMO is unpredictable and may have a mono- or multiphasic course.[74] This disease has a clinical pattern distinct from MS in that it almost exclusively affects women, typically in the fourth decade, and leads to a more severe neurologic impairment. A previous infectious-inflammatory event may be involved in the pathogenesis of the disease, which probably triggers an autoimmune mechanism. An association of NMO with anti-DNA antibodies, systemic lupus erythematosus (SLE), Sjogren syndrome, and autoimmune thyroiditis has been shown. Pathologically, there are areas of necrosis of gray and white matter, cavitation, vascular hyalinization, and fibrosis, as well as lack of inflammatory infiltration.[75] The classic imaging pattern is the presence of lesions with longitudinally extensive (>3 vertebral segments) T2 hyperintensity within the spinal cord and enhancement of the optic nerves (85% of cases) (Fig. 5). There may be swelling and enhancement in approximately 25% of cases.[70] Some cases result in spinal cord atrophy.

NMO was formerly believed to be a severe variant of MS because both can cause attacks of optic neuritis and myelitis. It is now believed that they are different diseases. Recently, a new serum autoantibody called NMO-IgG has been discovered that apparently distinguishes between NMO and MS.[76–78] This laboratory test has a 58% to

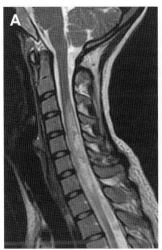
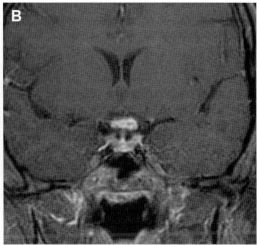

Fig. 5. NMO. A 28-year-old female with optic neuritis and myelopathy. Sagittal T2-weighted image (A) shows a longitudinal extensive segment of T2 hyperintensity throughout the cervical cord. Coronal T1-weighted image through the optic nerves (B) shows diffuse enhancement of the optic chiasm.

73% sensitivity and more than 90% specificity for detecting NMO. The proposed target for this antibody is a protein designated Aquaporin-4 (AQP4), which is the most abundant protein water channel expressed in the central nervous system (CNS), highly concentrated in astrocytic foot processes.[79] Aquaporins are a family of transmembrane channel proteins that are highly selective for the transport of water. These proteins function as bidirectional channels that facilitate the transport of water by diffusion along osmotic and hydrostatic gradients. AQP4 is the predominant water channel expressed in the brain, and is primarily an astroglial membrane protein with highly polarized expression localized to astrocytic foot processes surrounding the cerebral capillary endothelium.

Revised NMO diagnostic criteria require optic neuritis, acute myelitis, and 2 of the following 3 characteristics: disease-onset brain MR imaging that is nondiagnostic for MS, contiguous spinal cord MR imaging lesion extending more than 3 or more vertebral segments, and NMO-IgG seropositive status. Symptoms referable to CNS regions other than the optic nerve and spinal cord do not necessarily exclude the diagnosis of NMO.[76] This does not necessarily imply that white-matter lesions in the brain need to be absent to diagnose NMO. Pittock and colleagues[80] found that asymptomatic brain lesions are common in NMO, and symptomatic brain lesions do not exclude the diagnosis of NMO.

ACUTE DISSEMINATED ENCEPHALOMYELITIS

Acute disseminated encephalomyelitis (ADEM) is an uncommon inflammatory disorder of the CNS characterized by widespread demyelination predominantly affecting the white matter of the brain and spinal cord. The peripheral nerves can also be involved. ADEM can occur at any age but is more common in children and young adults. The pathogenesis is believed to be immune mediated following a predisposing viral infection with a subsequent cross-reaction with a viral protein resulting in a cell-mediated immune response against myelin basic protein. Symptoms usually develop within 3 weeks following a prodromal phase of fever, myalgia, and malaise. Tanembaum and colleagues[81] showed that in a cohort of 84 pediatric patients 70% reported a clinically evident antecedent infection or vaccination during the previous few weeks. However, in a study of ADEM in adults, such an antecedent infection or vaccination occurred in less than 35% of cases.[82] The symptoms and signs of ADEM include a rapid onset of encephalopathy associated with seizures and/or a combination of multiple neurologic deficits. A prodromal phase with nonspecific symptoms is followed rapidly by meningeal signs and drowsiness. The clinical course is rapidly progressive and the nadir is reached within days. Peripheral nervous system syndromes such as acute polyradiculoneuropathy may occur in ADEM in adult patients but are rare in children.[83] The diagnosis of ADEM is based on clinical and radiologic features. Although ADEM usually has a monophasic course in contrast to MS, recurrent or multiphasic forms have been reported, leading to difficulties in distinguishing these cases from MS.[84] Although infrequent in children, up to 35% of cases of ADEM in adults develop definite MS on follow-up.[82]

ADEM is characterized pathologically by a perivascular lymphocytic infiltrate within the brain and spinal cord white matter with a corresponding zone of demyelination. There may be small perivascular hemorrhages. Although loss of myelin predominates, there may be some axonal destruction. There are often inflammatory cells in the leptomeninges. Subpial inflammation and demyelination may occur in the brainstem and spinal cord.[84] The basis of the inflammatory response and subsequent demyelination is believed to be an autoimmune phenomenon. When severe hemorrhagic necrosis is identified as a major component, the disease is referred to as acute hemorrhagic leukoencephalopathy or acute hemorrhagic encephalomyelitis. A rapid progression to a fatal outcome is usual in these cases.

Spinal cord involvement in ADEM has been described in 11% to 28% of patients,[81] although it is probably under diagnosed. Lesions are more common in the brain, which is almost always involved. Lesions can occur anywhere in the cord but are more common in the thoracic region followed by the cervical cord. There are reported cases in which the spinal involvement predominates more than the brain component.[85]

Imaging of spinal ADEM is characterized by multifocal flame-shaped white-matter lesions with slight cord swelling and showing variable enhancement. Lesions occur most frequently in the thoracic region.[84] ADEM is usually clinically differentiated from MS by its clinically monophasic course, in contrast to MS, which classically has periods of exacerbation and remission. Myelopathy in MS is frequently partial,[86] but in ADEM it is often complete and associated with areflexia. Up to 90% of patients with ADEM have a good or complete recovery; however, the outcome of the disease in the acute phase may be fatal.

ACUTE TRANSVERSE MYELOPATHY

Acute transverse myelopathy (ATM) is a monophasic, acute inflammatory process involving both halves of the spinal cord, producing paraplegia, a sensory impairment level, and sphincter dysfunction.[87] The clinical course of ATM is highly variable. Longitudinal case series of ATM reveal that approximately one-third of patients recover with little or no sequelae, one-third are left with a moderate degree of permanent disability, and one-third with severe disabilities.[88]

ATM and acute transverse myelitis have often been used interchangeably in the literature, creating considerable confusion. ATM has inflammatory and noninflammatory causes such as MS, viral infections, postviral and postvaccinal processes such as acute disseminated encephalomyelitis, collagen vascular disorders such as systemic lupus erythematosis, vascular disorders, paraneoplastic syndromes, and idiopathic.[89–92] There was a time when the term acute transverse myelitis was reserved for idiopathic cases, but currently the term acute transverse myelopathy is used to encompass the general clinical syndrome, whether or not the cause is known.

The MR imaging appearance is quite variable, with a large range in size of T2 hyperintense regions in the cord, although most commonly the lesions extend for 3 or 4 spinal segments. Lesions occur most frequently in the thoracic cord. Unlike typical MS plaques, the area of high signal generally occupies more than two-thirds of the cross-sectional area of the cord on transverse images (**Fig. 6**). There is variable enlargement of the cord, and variable enhancement patterns following gadolinium administration, including diffuse, patchy, and peripheral patterns.[93] Occasionally, the lesions of ATM mimic spinal cord tumors, and if the patient's clinical history is unrevealing, biopsy may be needed for diagnosis. Up to 40% to 50% of cases of ATM have no findings on MR imaging. Follow-up MR imaging in these patients may show resolution of the abnormal signal and return of the cord to a normal caliber or evolution to cord atrophy.

There is considerable interest in ATM as a clinically isolated syndrome in patients who do not yet fulfill diagnostic criteria for MS. MR scanning of the brain is a useful additional study. It reveals typical white-matter changes of MS in approximately one-third of patients with ATM; these patients have a high likelihood of developing clinically definite MS.[89,91] Campi and colleagues[89] showed that patients with small, ovoid, enhancing spinal cord lesions without cord swelling had a high likelihood of developing clinically definite MS. Those with long segments of cord swelling, with inhomogeneous gadolinium enhancement, had no evolution to MS.

Inclusion criteria for acute transverse myelitis include[94] (1) development of sensory, motor, or autonomic dysfunction attributable to the spinal cord; (2) bilateral signs and/or symptoms; (3) clearly defined sensory level; (4) exclusion of extraaxial compressive cause by neuroimaging; (5) inflammation within the spinal cord demonstrated by CSF pleocytosis or increased IgG index or gadolinium enhancement; and (6) progression to nadir between 4 hours and 21 days after the onset of symptoms. For the myelitis diagnosis, there are notable exclusion criteria including evidence of connective tissue diseases, CNS manifestations of syphilis, Lyme disease, HIV,

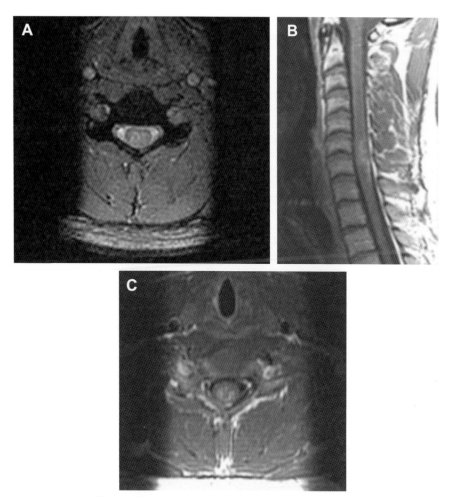

Fig. 6. Acute transverse myelitis. A 30-year-old with monophasic episode of myelopathy. Axial gradient echo image (*A*) shows abnormal hyperintensity within the cervical cord. Enhanced T1-weighted sagittal (*B*) and axial (*C*) images show expansion and focal enhancement within the cervical cord at C6 and C7.

human T-lymphotrophic virus type 1 (HTLV-1), *Mycoplasma*, and other viral infections.

SLE-RELATED MYELOPATHY

Transverse myelopathy is an uncommon but well-recognized complication of SLE.[95–99] Women are much more commonly affected than men with a ratio of 8:1. Transverse myelopathy secondary to SLE is clinically characterized by back pain, par-aparesis or tetraparesis, and sensory loss caudad to the lesion, and tends to be recurrent. Most patients with SLE who present with transverse myelopathy[100–103] test positive for the presence of antiphospholipid antibodies although the precise causative pathophysiologic mecha-nism has not been established. Recurrent myelitis

associated with SLE is a subset of a broader group of conditions associated with antiphospholipid antibody syndrome (APS), which includes the anti-cardiolipin antibody and the lupus anticoagulant antiphospholipid syndromes. CNS involvement in SLE is most often seen in the setting of APS with IgG type of anticardiolipin antibodies. Sequelae of APS include cerebrovascular diseases, migraine, epilepsy, chorea, dementia, depression, deep brain reversible encephalopathy, and myelitis.[104,105]

The MR imaging pattern of spinal cord involve-ment is the same as that described earlier for ATM of other causes, usually demonstrating a cen-trally located increased signal intensity on T2-weighted images, occupying more than two-thirds of the cross-sectional area of the cord, and extending more than 3 to 4 vertebral segments in length. Enhancement by paramagnetic agents is variable.[101,102]

AIDS

Spinal cord disease in AIDS is frequently overshadowed by other manifestations of the disease, however the incidence of spinal cord disease at autopsy is high.[106] There are several major categories of spinal cord disease in AIDS: those caused by direct HIV infection (HIV myelitis); those caused by opportunistic diseases or lymphoma; those associated with HIV, although the cause is unclear; and those related to vascular or metabolic disorders. HIV myelitis, which occurs in 5% to 8% of patients with AIDS, is caused by primary infection of the spinal cord, and is most often seen when the cerebral involvement is severe. Inflammation with typical microglial nodules and multinucleated giant cells is seen, predominately in the central gray region. Imaging findings on MR imaging for HIV myelitis include spinal cord T2 hyperintensity, which may show patchy enhancement, more common in the thoracic than cervical cord. There tends to be increased rostral involvement as the disease progresses. Opportunistic infections of the spinal cord in AIDS include cytomegalovirus, fungal, toxoplasmosis, herpes simplex virus (HSV), varicella zoster virus (VZV), tuberculosis, syphilis, and PML.

Vacuolar myelopathy refers to a spongy degeneration in the spinal cord, predominately involving the posterior and lateral columns.[106–108] Vacuolar myelopathy is by far the most common spinal cord disease in AIDS, approaching an incidence of 50% in autopsy studies. It is a frequent cause of progressive ataxia and paraparesis in patients with AIDS. The disease is most prominent in the mid to lower thoracic cord, and is usually fairly symmetric in distribution over the cross-section of the cord. It is frequently most severe in the fasciculus gracilis. Histopathologically, there is prominent vacuolation of spinal white matter, with swelling within the myelin sheaths and splitting of lamellae. Axons may be normal, atrophic, or show secondary Wallerian degeneration. There is little active demyelination or inflammation, and there are some similarities to the changes seen in subacute combined degeneration. Many patients with AIDS are deficient in vitamin B_{12} and this has resulted in speculation about possible causative links between the disorders, but this has not been confirmed. MR findings include cord atrophy and symmetric hyperintensity in the dorsal columns on T2-weighted MR images that can be traced over several spinal segments. Involvement

of the lateral columns is less common. There is no cord swelling or deformity, and characteristically, in contrast to HIV myelitis, there is no gadolinium enhancement. The MR findings of vacuolar myelopathy are generally distinctive, such that it can be differentiated from other spinal tract pathologies in AIDS such as viral myelitis caused by VZV, or cytomegalovirus radiculomyelitis, as discussed in the next section.

VIRAL DISEASES

VZV infection in the CNS is rare in healthy populations, and it is also an infrequent opportunistic infection in patients with AIDS. Clinical recognition of the disease is difficult, because only one-third of patients present with characteristic skin eruptions of shingles. A neuropathologic study by Gray and colleagues[109] proposed 5 different patterns of CNS involvement in patients with AIDS: multifocal leukoencephalitis, ventriculitis, acute meningomyeloradiculitis, focal necrotizing myelitis, and necrotizing angiitis involving leptomeningeal arteries with cerebral infarction. The multiple patterns of disease in the CNS from VZV suggest that multiple routes of spread to the CNS exist, including direct transneuronal and hematogenous routes, via CSF seeding, as well as the classically described reactivation of latent virus in the dorsal root ganglia that produces cutaneous shingles. This latter method is likely in VZV myelitis because it typically involves the posterior horn regions and spreads along axonal pathways primarily in the posterior columns. Pathologic changes of inflammation, demyelination, and hemorrhagic necrosis are seen. Thoracic cord involvement is most common, as a result of the high frequency of thoracic-level dermatomal involvement in shingles. MR imaging reveals a swollen cord with patchy gadolinium enhancement, usually more posteriorly (**Fig. 7**).[109,110] When VZV myelitis develops associated with cutaneous shingles, it typically is in the region of the cord corresponding to the involved dermatome, and focal enhancement of the corresponding dorsal root ganglia, nerve roots, and root entry zone may be seen. Myelitis may occur in conjunction with other CNS manifestations of VZV infection such as leukoencephalitis.

Cytomegalovirus infection in the spinal cord produces a polyradiculomyelitis that frequently involves the conus and nerve roots of the cauda equina.[107,111] AIDS and other immune-compromised patients as well as immune-competent individuals may be affected. Typically patients develop a flaccid paraparesis, saddle dysesthesia, and urinary retention. The paraparesis may be ascending and

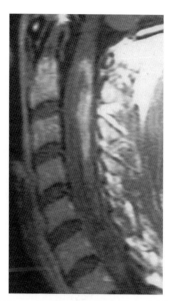

Fig. 7. Herpes myelitis. Sagittal T1-weighted image after contrast administration shows enlargement and diffuse enhancement of the cervical cord.

a Guillian-Barré—like syndrome may be observed, which is frequently associated with leg and/or back pain. CSF analysis reveals a polymorphonuclear pleocytosis. MR imaging reveals abnormal thickening, clumping, and enhancement of the nerve roots of the cauda equina consistent with an inflammatory arachnoiditis. There is frequently abnormal peripheral pial and leptomeningeal enhancement over the spinal cord. The MR imaging pattern suggests a differential diagnosis including carcinomatous or lymphomatous meningitis.

Poliomyelitis infection involves the anterior horn cells (lower motor neurons) in the ventral horns of the spinal cord. It classically produces an asymmetric flaccid paralysis. Although poliomyelitis caused by the natural virus has been virtually eradicated in Western countries, there are still several cases a year in the United States of vaccine-associated paralytic poliomyelitis, estimated to occur at a rate of approximately 1 per 2.5 million doses administered. In the acute infection there is active inflammation, gliosis, and destruction of anterior horn cells, and the characteristic MR appearance described is that of local enlargement and abnormal signal in the ventral horns.[112] Chronically, the spinal cord of polio patients shows loss of anterior horn cells, severe reactive gliosis, and persistent inflammation. There are rare poliolike paralytic syndromes associated with other viruses such as coxsackie virus, echovirus, and enterovirus. A striking case of an acute paralytic syndrome secondary to Epstein-Barr virus

encephalomyelitis was reported by Donovan and colleagues,[113] with striking inflammation and edema confined to the central gray matter of the cervical cord, as well as involvement of the cerebral gray matter structures in the basal ganglia and insula.

HTLV-1 infection can produce a slowly progressive myelopathy associated with spastic paraparesis.[114] The virus is highly endemic in Japan, Melanesia, the Caribbean, and in some parts of Africa. The 2 disorders, HTLV-1 associated myelopathy (HAM), and tropical spastic paraparesis (TSP), are clinically, epidemiologically, and pathologically identical. Patients usually have a slowly progressive course over several years, at which time MR examinations of the spinal cord reveal diffuse atrophy and abnormal signal intensity most frequently involving the anterior and lateral columns. Rarely, patients have periods of rather acute progression of myelopathy, at which time mild cord swelling may be seen. Typically there is peripheral gadolinium enhancement. Pathologically, there is loss of myelin and axons with perivascular and parenchymal infiltration of inflammatory cells in white and gray matter tracts of the cord. HTLV-1 and HIV are both human retroviruses that produce myelopathies, however, the clinico-pathologic and MR imaging changes in HAM/TSP are quite different from those of vacuolar myelopathy in AIDS.

BACTERIAL DISEASES

Bacterial spinal cord abscesses are relatively rare but can occur in septicemia, after spinal surgery, penetrating trauma, complicated meningitis, and associated with dysraphisms and dermal sinus tracts. The most common causative organisms are staphylococcal and streptococcus species. Cord swelling and edema are present with a local, rim-enhancing collection in well-formed spinal cord abscesses. Unlike cerebral abscesses, whose temporal course of development is well documented, the natural history of spinal cord abscesses is not well described. Murphy and colleagues[59] described the evolutionary changes in the cord as infection progressing from myelitis to abscess formation. Patients may develop neurologic dysfunction before the development of a well-formed abscess, and thus the gadolinium enhancement characteristics may be variable depending on the stage of evolution at the time of imaging.[115]

Listeria monocytogenes may produce a primary meningoencephalomyelitis in healthy and immune-compromised patients.[116] *Listeria* produces abscesses in the brainstem and upper cervical cord as well as in the cerebral hemispheres. CSF analysis demonstrates a lymphocytic pleocytosis, but the organism is rarely discovered or cultured from CSF. Blood cultures may yield the gram-positive bacillus. *Listeria* meningoencephalomyelitis is a difficult clinical diagnosis, and fatal infections in patients with no predisposing factors have occurred.

GRANULOMATOUS DISEASES

Infectious granulomatous diseases such as tuberculosis, brucellosis, and syphilis produce similar pathologic and MR imaging findings to sarcoidosis, the major noninfectious granulomatous disease. All of these entities can produce any combination of granulomatous meningitis, myelitis, or radiculitis. Patients with tuberculous myelitis usually have evidence of primary or secondary tuberculous infection in the lungs, brain, or spine. Intramedullary tuberculomas may be solitary or multiple, and generally are well-defined, circumscribed lesions demonstrating avid gadolinium enhancement in a nodular or rim-enhancing fashion.[90,117,118] There is prominent cord edema and swelling, which may be related to cord ischemia secondary to vasculopathic changes. Myelitis is a rare presentation of syphilis, and the granulomatous process has a predilection for the meninges, pial vessels, and subpial portions of the cord.[119] Imaging findings include a swollen cord with patchy or nodular gadolinium enhancement, especially in the cord periphery. Pathologic changes in the cord are believed to be caused by a combination of granulomatous myelitis, and simultaneous cord ischemia caused by granulomatous vasculitic changes.

TUBERCULOUS SPONDYLODISCITIS

Tuberculosis is caused by *Mycobacterium tuberculosis*. The prevalence of tuberculosis has continued to decline in the United States. However, the smallest annual decrease in the past 10 years occurred in 2003 with some states actually showing a slight increase.[120] There has also been in increase in global prevalence, particularly in immunosuppressed populations. Tuberculosis usually affects the respiratory system, however any organ system can be involved. The clinical syndromes of tuberculosis are related to the host's defenses because tubercle bacilli do not elaborate classic endotoxins or exotoxins, and the inflammatory illness and tissue destruction are immune mediated.[121] Skeletal involvement in tuberculosis occurs mainly by hematologic dissemination. The clinical presentation of tuberculosis is insidious, with onset of

symptoms ranging from months to 2 to 3 years.[86,122–124] By comparison, pyogenic infections tend to have onset of symptoms ranging from days to months.[125] Spinal tuberculosis usually starts in the anteroinferior portion of the vertebral body.[126] Spread of infection can occur beneath the anterior longitudinal ligament involving the adjacent vertebral bodies. Narrowing of disc space occurs secondarily and is not as prominent as in pyogenic infection. A lack of proteolytic enzymes in *Mycobacterium* compared with pyogenic infection has been proposed as the cause of relative preservation of the intervertebral disc.[127] The disc may not show increased T2 signal in contradistinction to pyogenic infections.[14,31,128] Cortical definition of affected vertebrae is invariably lost, in contrast to pyogenic spondylitis. T1-weighted images usually show decreased marrow signal in the affected vertebrae. T2 signal hyperintensity is usually present in the affected vertebrae, discs, and soft tissues. Involvement of the posterior elements is more common in tuberculous than pyogenic infection,[129] which can make differentiation of infection from tumor difficult, particularly when there is relative preservation of the disc space. Tuberculous infection commonly spreads to the adjacent ligaments and soft issues, varying in the literature from 55% to 96%.[122–130] This extension usually occurs anterolaterally. Postachini and Montanaro[131] reported a case of tuberculoma mimicking a disc herniation. Paravertebral phelgmon is characterized by a thick, irregular enhancement on CT and MR imaging.[130] Rim enhancement around intraosseous and paraspinal soft tissue abscess is more common than in other spinal infections (see **Fig. 2**). The paraspinal masses are generally larger in tuberculosis than in pyogenic infections.[125] Collapse of partially destroyed vertebral bodies with resultant gibbous deformity is characteristic. The vertebral column is affected in approximately 25% to 60% of cases of skeletal tuberculosis.[132] The thoracolumbar junction is the most frequent spinal segment affected. Involvement of the cervical and sacral segments of the spine is relatively infrequent. Intramedullary involvement of the spinal cord is rare and typically affects young adults.[133] Intramedullary tuberculomas are seen in 0.002% of cases and in 0.2% cases of CNS tuberculosis.[134] Lesions are usually solitary, although additional lesions may be present in the brain or spinal cord.[135] A nuclear medicine gallium scan can show increased radionuclide uptake in affected vertebrae and paraspinal soft tissues and is considered highly sensitive and specific for vertebral osteomyelitis.[136]

Sarcoidosis is a multisystem, idiopathic granulomatous disease that involves the CNS in approximately 5% of patients. Generally, patients with CNS sarcoidosis have evidence of pulmonary disease. Spinal sarcoidosis includes vertebral, disc space, intramedullary, intradural extramedullary, and extradural lesions. Bone involvement is reported in 1% to 13% of cases,[137] is usually late, and is commonly associated with cutaneous lesions. The tubular bones of the hands and feet are most often involved. Sarcoidosis of the vertebral bodies is rare, and there is a predilection for involvement of the thoracolumbar spine. Spinal sarcoidosis may involve the intradural nerve roots. Typically, plain radiographs reveal lytic lesions with or without regions of surrounding sclerosis, mixed lytic and sclerotic lesions, and, infrequently, predominantly sclerotic lesions involving single or multiple bones.[137–139] Only a few cases of MR of vertebral sarcoidosis have been described.[140,141] An associated paraspinal mass may be present, and disc space involvement is rare. The acutely involved spinal cord is swollen, with variable patterns of enhancement following gadolinium administration, including uniform diffuse, multifocal patchy, nodular, or linear leptomeningeal enhancement.[142] The lesions of sarcoidosis have a nonspecific appearance with low T1 and variably increased T2 signal. The differential diagnosis is therefore broad and includes metastatic disease, myeloma, lymphoma, and tuberculous infection. However, the diagnosis of sarcoidosis should be considered in any patient with known sarcoidosis if lytic lesions are seen on CT or if MR imaging shows multiple or single lesions.[141]

PARASITIC DISEASES

Schistosomal infections are a common parasitic infection worldwide, with endemic regions in Asia, the Caribbean, South America, and in portions of Africa and Arabia. Immigration has brought patients with schistosomal infections to North America, and therefore it is important that this disease is considered. Schistosomes are parasitic worms. The life cycle includes an asexual stage in an intermediate snail host, and an adult sexual stage in vertebrate definitive hosts. Schistosomal larvae penetrate the skin of hosts while swimming in infested water. The larvae enter lymphatic and venous systems and migrate to lung and liver, where they mature and take final residence in the mesenteric veins and vesical venous plexus. There are 3 schistosomes of clinical importance: *Schistosoma mansoni*, *Schistosoma haematobium*, and *Schistosoma japonicum*. Schistosomal myelitis is a relatively rare clinical manifestation of the disease, and *Schistosoma mansoni* is responsible for most cases. The organisms are believed to reach the spinal axis by migrating from pelvic and rectal veins into the paravertebral venous plexus, and finally to perimedullary veins. Schistosomal myelitis characteristically involves the conus, lower thoracic spinal cord, and cauda equina. Several basic patterns of spinal cord disease are seen, most commonly an intramedullary granulomatous mass, or an intradural, extramedullary granulomatous mass with compression of the conus.[143] Other forms include an acute transverse myelitis,[144] which may be hemorrhagic and necrotizing,[145] and an acute, anterior spinal artery syndrome. MR imaging reveals enlargement of the conus, occasionally somewhat irregular, nodular, or asymmetric, with increased signal intensity and patchy or nodular gadolinium enhancement. The appearance most frequently mimics a cord neoplasm. Schistosomal infection can be diagnosed by blood or CSF serology and the ova may be recovered from the patient's stool. It is therefore important to elicit a clinical history of travel from endemic areas. This should prompt appropriate laboratory studies, enabling the diagnosis to be made without biopsy. Treatment with antiparasitic agents is usually curative although occasionally laminectomy, myelotomy, and resection of the granulomatous mass are needed.

The parasitic disease toxoplasmosis is a common CNS pathogen in immunocompromised patients, but it rarely involves the spinal cord.[107] In patients with AIDS, toxoplasmosis spinal abscesses usually present as enhancing intramedullary mass lesions with extensive associated edema. Frequently, the presence of coexisting acute cerebral toxoplasma abscesses assists in making the diagnosis of the spinal disease.

SPINAL CYSTICERCOSIS

Cysticercosis is the most common parasitic infection of the CNS.[146] Neurocysticercosis can involve the entire craniospinal axis, with cystic lesions in the brain, cord, and subarachnoid spaces (see **Fig. 7**).[147,148] It is a worldwide disease that affects 50 million people, with a prevalence of 3% to 6% of the population in endemic areas such as Central and South America, Eastern Europe, Africa, and some regions of Asia.[149] The disease has increased in frequency in the United States with the growing number of immigrants from these countries. A population study in a Hispanic community in California found the prevalence of *Taenia solium* cysticercosis to be 2.8% in adult Latinos, similar to the prevalence data from some endemic regions in Latin America.[150] Seizures occur in more than 90% of patients. Cysticercosis is the most common cause of seizures in Latin America. Encephalopathic symptoms are also common. Treatment is with anticysticercus drugs such as praziquantel and albendazole. The organism responsible for the disease is the larva form of the pork tapeworm *Taenia solium*. Humans can become the incidental host of its larval form by ingestion. When the eggs reach the stomach they are lysed by gastric juice and the embryos are released, crossing the walls of the bowel to reach the arterial system. Subsequently, they lodge preferentially in neural and subcutaneous tissues, as well as in skeletal muscles and ocular globes, where they finally develop into the larvae form of *Cysticercus cellulosae* or *Cysticercus racemosae*.[151] The most frequent form is *Cysticercus cellulosae*, which has a characteristic scolex and results in brain intraparenchymal lesions or, rarely, spinal intramedullary lesions. In most cases it remains small, approximately 1 cm in diameter, and eventually dies. After its death it is surrounded by a collagenous capsule that elicits a variable-intensity inflammatory reaction. *Cysticercus racemosae*, which lacks a scolex, grows in grapelike clusters of thin-walled cysts and shows a tendency to predominate in the subarachnoid space.[152–154]

Although the CNS is involved in 60% to 90% of cases, spinal cord involvement is rare and varies from 0.7% to 5.85%.[155,156] Leptomeningeal cysts are much more common than intramedullary cysts. The extradural form is rare with only a few cases reported.[157,158] Neurologic symptoms and signs might arise from an inflammatory reaction caused by the metabolites of the parasite or the degenerated larva, mass effect from intramedullary or extramedullary cysts, or from leptomeningitis or vascular insufficiency.[154] MR imaging is useful in the evaluation of neurocysticercosis. The intensity of the cystic fluid, whether in the spinal cord or in the subarachnoid space, is usually similar to that of the CSF on both T1- and T2-weighted images. MR findings include mass effect from the cysts, enhancement of the cyst rim, and lack of a CSF flow void adjacent to these cysts.[159] Myelography may demonstrate cysts in the spinal subarachnoid space (**Fig. 8**).

FUNGAL INFECTIONS

The incidence of fungal infections has increased in the last decade as the population of immunocompromised patients has increased.[160] *Candida* and *Aspergillus* are the most common causes of human opportunistic mycotic infections.[9] Manifestations of fungal infection in the spine include osteomyelitis, discitis, and meningitis. These

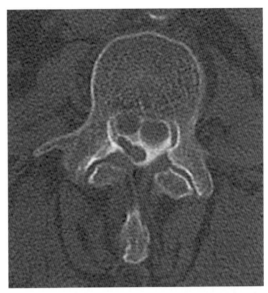

Fig. 8. Neurocysticercosis. Axial CT through the lumbar spine after intrathecal contrast administration shows several rounded filling defects within the lumbar subarachnoid space.

pathogens can result in the formation of abscesses and granulomas. Vascular invasion can result in thrombosis and subsequent cord infarction. Infection can occur by direct implantation, invasion, or hematogenous spread from elsewhere in the body.[128,160,161] The diagnosis is achieved by the isolation of the fungus or by the presence of characteristic histopathologic changes. Imaging findings with fungal osteomyelitis can vary from those classically described in association with pyogenic infection, particularly in the immunocompromised host. Although the usual findings of low T1 signal intensity in the end plates and discs tends to be present, there is often less T2 signal changes in the vertebral bodies and relative sparing of the disc with preservation of the intranuclear cleft.[160] These alterations in appearance compared with classic pyogenic infection may reflect the blunted immune response of the immunocompromised host. As in the case of tuberculosis there tends to be greater involvement of the posterior elements and a prominent paraspinous soft tissue inflammatory component.

Coccidioidomycosis is a systemic infection caused by *Coccidioides immitis* and is endemic in the southwestern United States, as well as in parts of Central and South America. Approximately two-thirds of infections are asymptomatic. Symptomatic patients usually present with a mild pulmonary syndrome. Some patients develop complications or progressive forms of infection that display a broad variety of manifestations affecting the skin, bones, meninges, and other viscera. Disseminated coccidioidomycosis usually stems from a primary lung infection in an immunosuppressed patient. Osseous manifestations occur in 10% to 50% of patients with disseminated disease.[162] Involvement of the spine, ribs, and pelvis predominates, although any bone may be affected.[163] The spine is the most common site of bone infection in the setting of disseminated coccidioidomycosis.[164] Vertebral osteomyelitis can involve 1 or more vertebral bodies, paraspinal masses, and contiguous ribs. The intervertebral discs are relatively spared, and vertebral collapse and fistulous tracts are uncommon late manifestations. Unlike tuberculosis, gibbous deformity in coccidioidomycosis spondylitis is unusual but has been reported.[162,164] Plain films and CT may demonstrate lucent lesions with or without endosteal new bone formation leading to sclerosis.[162,163] The MR findings are nonspecific and diagnosis is made by biopsy in a patient from an endemic area. Meningitis occurs in one-third to one-half of patients with disseminated coccidioidomycosis but intraparenchymal abscesses are rare.

GBS

GBS is an acute inflammatory demyelinating polyneuropathy characterized clinically by weakness or paralysis affecting more than 1 limb, usually symmetrically, associated with loss of tendon reflexes with little or no sensory loss and increased levels of protein in the CSF without pleocytosis. The incidence of GBS is 1 to 3 per 100,000 inhabitants, making GBS the most common cause of acute flaccid paralysis in the United States.[165] It is also the most frequent cause of acute flaccid paralysis worldwide. The proposed mechanism for GBS is that an antecedent infection evokes an immune response that results in a cross-reaction with peripheral nerve components. Most patients report an infectious process in the weeks preceding the onset of GBS. The pathophysiologic mechanism of an antecedent illness and of GBS is typified by *Campylobacter jejuni* infections. There are specific antigens in the capsule of *Campylobacter jejuni* that are shared with peripheral nerves. Immune responses directed against the capsular components produce antibodies that cross-react with myelin to cause demyelination. Ganglioside GM1 seems to cross-react with *Campylobacter jejuni* lipopolysaccharide antigens, resulting in the immunologic damage to the peripheral nervous system via a process that has been termed molecular mimicry.[166,167] Indicators of poor outcome are advanced age, need for mechanical ventilation, shorter latency to nadir, particular antecedent infections (especially *Campylobacter jejuni* or cytomegalovirus), and evidence of axonal degeneration.[168]

Two forms of GBS have been defined based on electrophysiologic and pathologic findings[169]: acute inflammatory demyelinating polyneuropathy (AIDP) and acute motor axonal neuropathy (AMAN). AMAN is characterized by pure motor axial degeneration or dysfunction, presumably mediated by antiganglioside antibodies that may be induced by particular infectious agents such as *Campylobacter jejuni*.[166,170] In contrast, AIDP is associated with demyelination of motor and sensory nerves.[170] The initial symptoms are often tingling and paresthesias in the feet, sometimes accompanied by lumbar back pain. Weakness occurs within hours or a few days after onset of symptoms. Weakness may progress for up to 4 weeks, is usually symmetric, and involves the lower extremities before spreading to the upper extremities and face. Involvement of cranial nerves and autonomic dysfunction are common. Swallowing difficulty and respiratory insufficiency may occur. Treatment involves medical management with plasma exchange or intravenous gamma globulin. No definite benefit has been shown from use of corticosteroids.[171,172]

The diagnosis of GBS is determined mainly from clinical findings and CSF analysis. The role of imaging studies is primarily to exclude other causes. Imaging findings seen in GBS include enhancement and thickening of cauda equina nerve roots (more commonly in the anterior nerve roots) and slight precontrast intrinsic T1 signal hyperintensity within the nerve roots without corresponding T2 signal abnormality **(Fig. 9)**.[173] Enhancement and thickening of the spinal nerve roots decreased on follow-up MR imaging, commensurate with improvement in clinical and electrophysiologic findings. The differential diagnosis for enhancement and thickening of the nerve roots includes Miller-Fisher syndrome (considered by many to be a variant of GBS), chronic polyneuropathies (subacute inflammatory demyelinating polyradiculoneuropathy, chronic inflammatory demyelinating polyradiculoneuropathy), hereditary polyneuropathies (Charcot-Marie-Tooth, Dejerine-Sottas), vasculitic neuropathies, carcinomatous meningitis, lymphoma, and arachnoiditis. Although enhancement of spinal roots is a nonspecific finding that can be seen in neoplastic or other inflammatory processes, enhancement of only the anterior nerve roots may be suggestive of GBS.

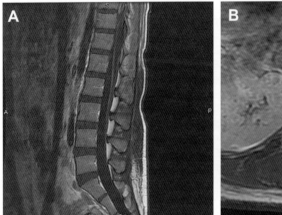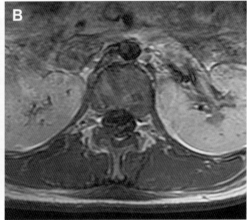

Fig. 9. GBS. Sagittal (*A*) and axial (*B*) T1-weighted images show enhancement and thickening of the cauda equina nerve roots.

METABOLIC/TOXIC DISEASES

Subacute combined degeneration (SCD) is a complication of vitamin B_{12} deficiency, as may occur in pernicious anemia or with prolonged insufficient dietary intake. The pathologic changes of demyelination, axonal loss and gliosis are seen in a roughly symmetric fashion involving the dorsal and lateral columns of the thoracic and lower cervical cords. MR scans may reveal increased signal intensity in the dorsal columns on T2-weighted scans.[174] MR has been less able to reveal the lateral column changes, even when present clinically. Improvement in the MR appearance has been described corresponding to improvement in clinical function following vitamin B_{12} supplementation. Nitrous oxide is a gaseous anesthetic agent used as a propellant in the food industry; it is also abused as a recreational drug. Nitrous oxide toxicity can result in the same pathophysiologic process as SCD, because nitrous oxide inactivates cobalamin (B_{12}), which is essential in the metabolic processes that form and maintain myelin.[175] The myelopathy typically develops several weeks after exposure. Myelopathy has been described in patients with normal B_{12} levels and high nitrous oxide exposure, as well as in patients with borderline B_{12} levels undergoing surgical procedures using nitrous oxide as an anesthetic agent. MR imaging again shows abnormal signal intensity in the dorsal columns.[175]

Cases of myelopathy have been reported as a result of intravenous use of heroin and probably other intravenous recreational drugs.[176] Ischemic myelopathy and cord infarction have been reported in association with cocaine abuse.[177]

RADIATION MYELOPATHY

Radiation myelopathy is a complication of radiation therapy, most commonly seen in the cervical spinal cord of patients treated for head and neck malignancies with doses of 50 to 70 Gy.[178,179] Radiation myelopathy is generally a subacute to chronic progressive myelopathy, with a variable latent period, generally several months to years after treatment. With the onset of clinical symptomatology, MR imaging reveals cord swelling, edema, and gadolinium enhancement, lasting for up to 8 months. During this phase, histopathologic changes of edema, necrosis, demyelination, gliosis, and fibrinoid necrosis of small blood vessels are seen. In patients with nasopharyngeal malignancies, the development of radiation myelopathy in the high cervical cord and medulla may be lethal. After approximately 8 months, the swelling gradually subsides, and progressive cord atrophy develops and eventually stabilizes over a few years in survivors. The pathologic gadolinium enhancement may persist even after the cord has become atrophic, but it has been shown to diminish over approximately 24 months. The cord damage frequently extends beyond the spatial distribution of the radiation exposure, although the main focus is always within the primary field.

REFERENCES

1. Daroviche RO, Hamill RJ, Greenberg SB, et al. Bacterial spinal epidural abscess. Review of 43 cases and literature survey. Medicine 1992;71: 369–85.

2. Rattcliffe JF. Microarteriography of the cadaveric human lumbar spine. Evaluation of a new technique of injection in the anastomotic arterial system. Acta Radiol Diagn 1978;19:656.

3. Rattcliffe JF. The arterial anatomy of the adult human vertebral body. J Anat 1980;131:57.

4. Rattcliffe JF. The arterial anatomy of the developing human dorsal and lumbar vertebral body. A microarteriographic study. J Anat 1981;133:625.

5. Hassler O. The human intervertebral disc. Acta Orthop Scand 1969;40:765–72.

6. Wiley AM, Trueta J. The vascular anatomy of the spine and its relationship to pyogenic vertebral osteomyelitis. J Bone Joint Surg Br 1959;41:796.

7. Norden CW. Experimental osteomyelitis. A description of the model. J Infect Dis 1970;122:410.

8. Wilensky AO. The mechanism and pathogenesis of acute osteomyelitis. Am J Surg 1927;3:281.

9. Bertino RE, Porter BA, Stimac GK, et al. Imaging spinal osteomyelitis and epidural abscess with short TI inversion recovery (STIR). AJNR Am J Neuroradiol 1988;9:563–4.

10. Fischer GW, Popich GA, Sullivan DE, et al. Diskitis: a prospective diagnosis analysis. Pediatrics 1978; 62:543–8.

11. Resnick D, Niwayama G. Osteomyelitis, septic arthritis, and soft tissue infection: axial skeleton. In: Resnick D, Niwayama G, editors. Diagnosis of bone and joint disorders, vol. 4. 3rd edition. Philadelphia: WB Saunders; 1995. p. 2419–47.

12. Sharif HS, Clark DC, Aabed MY, et al. MR imaging of thoracic and abdominal wall infections: comparison with other imaging procedures. AJR Am J Roentgenol 1990;154:989–95.

13. Waldvogel FA, Vasey H. Osteomyelitis: the past decade. N Engl J Med 1980;303:360–70.

14. Sharif HS. Role of MR imaging in management of spinal infections. AJR Am J Roentgenol 1992;158: 1333–45.

15. Reihsaus E, Waldbaur H, Seeling W. Spinal epidural abscess: a meta-analysis of 915 patients. Neurosurg Rev 2000;23(4):175–204.

16. Butler JS, Shelly MJ, Timlin M, et al. Nontuberculous pyogenic spinal infections in adults. A 12 year experience from a tertiary referral center. Spine 2003;31(23):2695–700.

17. Quinones-Hinojosa A, et al. General principles in the medical and surgical management of spinal infections: a multidisciplinary approach. Neurosurg Focus 2004;17(6):E1.

18. Hsieh PC, et al. Pyogenic vertebral osteomyelitis: report of 9 cases and review of the literature. Rev Infect Dis 1979;1:754–76.

19. Leal FS, de Tella OI Jr, Bonatelli Ade PL, et al. [Septic spondylodiscitis: diagnosis and treatment]. Arq Neuropsiquiatr 2003;61(3-B):829–35 [in Portuguese].

20. Przybylski GJ, Sharan AD. Single-state autogenous bone grafting and internal fixation in the surgical management of pyogenic discitis and vertebral osteomyelitis. J Neurosurg (Spine) 2001;94:1–7.

21. Eismont FJ, Bohlman HH, Soni PL, et al. Pyogenic and fungal vertebral osteomyelitis with paralysis. J Bone Joint Surg Am 1983;65:19–29.

22. Garcia A Jr, Grantham SA. Hematogenous pyogenic vertebral osteomyelitis. Am J Orthop 1960;42: 429–36.

23. Sapico FL, Montgomerie JZ. Vertebral osteomyelitis. Infect Dis Clin North Am 1990;4:539–50.

24. Armstrong P, Chalmers AH. Needle aspiration/biopsy of the spine in suspected disc space infection. Br J Radiol 1978;51:333–7.

25. Carrasco CH, Wallace S, Richli WR. Percutaneous skeletal biopsy. Cardiovasc Intervent Radiol 1991; 14:69–72.

26. Rawlings CE, Wilkins RH, Gallis HA, et al. Postoperative intervertebral disc space infection. Neurosurgery 1983;13:371–5.

27. Tehranzadeh J, Freiberger RH, Ghelman B. Closed skeletal biopsy: review of 120 cases. AJR Am J Roentgenol 1983;140:113–5.

28. Golimbu C, Firooznia H, Rafii M. CT of osteomyelitis of the spine. AJR Am J Roentgenol 1984;142: 159–63.

29. Jeffrey RB, Callen PW, Federle MP. Computed tomography of psoas abscesses. J Comput Assist Tomogr 1980;4:639–41.

30. McAfee JG, Samin A. In-111 labeled leukocytes: a review of problems in image interpretation. Radiology 1985;155:221–9.

31. Modic MT, Feiglin DH, Piraino DW, et al. Vertebral osteomyelitis: assessment using MR. Radiology 1985;157:157–66.

32. Modic MT, Weinstein MA, Pavlicek W, et al. Nuclear magnetic resonance imaging of the spine. Radiology 1983;148:757–62.

33. deRoos A, Van Meerten EL, Bloem JL, et al. MRI of tuberculosis spondylitis. AJR Am J Roentgenol 1986;146:79–82.

34. Dagirmanjian A, Schils J, Modic MT. Vertebral osteomyelitis revisited. Radiology 1993;189(Suppl P):193.

35. Carragee E. The clinical use of magnetic resonance imaging in a pyogenic vertebral osteomyelitis. Spine 1997;22:780–5.

36. Kowalski TJ, Layton KF, Berbari EF, et al. Follow-up MR imaging in patients with pyogenic spine infections: lack of correlation with clinical features. AJNR Am J Neuroradiol 2007;28:693–9.

37. Gillams AR, Chaddha B, Carter AP. MR appearances of the temporal evolution and resolution of infectious spondylitis. AJR Am J Roentgenol 1996;166:903–7.

38. Carragee EJ, Kim D, van der Vlugt T, et al. The clinical use of erythrocyte sedimentation rate in

pyogenic vertebral osteomyelitis. Spine 1997;22: 2089–93.

39. Ross JS, Masaryk TJ, Modic MT, et al. MR imaging of lumbar arachnoiditis. AJNR Am J Neuroradiol 1987;8:885–92.

40. Ergan M, Macro M, Benhamou CL. Septic arthritis of lumbar facet joints: a review of six cases. Rev Rhum Engl Ed 1997;64:386–95.

41. Grane P, Josephsson A, Seferlis A, et al. Septic and aseptic postoperative discitis in the lumbar spine— evaluation by MRI. Acta Radiol 1998;39:108–15.

42. Peruzzi P, Rosseaux P, Sherpereel B, et al. Spondylodiscitis after surgery of lumbar disc hernia. Neurochirurgie 1988;34:394–400.

43. Meyer B, Schaller K, Rohde V, et al. The C-reactive protein for detection of early infections after lumbar microdiscectomy. Acta Neurochir 1995;136: 145–50.

44. Van Goethem JW, Parizel PM, van den Haywe L, et al. The value of MRI in the diagnosis of postoperative spondylodiscitis. Neuroradiology 2000;42: 580–5.

45. Boden SD, Davis DO, Dina TS, et al. Postoperative diskitis: distinguishing early MR imaging findings from normal postoperative disk space changes. Radiology 1992;184(3):765–71.

46. Resnick D, Niwayama G. Osteomyelitis, septic arthritis, and soft tissue infection: organisms. In: Resnick D, Niwayama G, editiors. Diagnosis of bone and joint disorders vol. 4. 3rd edition. Philadelphia: WB Saunders; 1995. p.2448–558.

47. Rigamonti D, Liem L, Sampath P, et al. Spinal epidural abscess: contemporary trends in etiology, evaluation and management. Surg Neurol 1999;52: 189–96 [discussion: 197].

48. Baker AS, Osemann RG, Swartz MN, et al. Spinal epidural abscess. N Engl J Med 1975;293:463–8.

49. Kaufman DM, Kaplan JG, Litman N. Infectious agents in spinal epidural abscesses. Neurology 1980;30:844–52.

50. Numaguchi Y, Rigamonti D, Rothman MI, et al. Spinal epidural abscess: evaluation with gadolinium enhanced MR imaging. Radiographics 1993;13:545.

51. Danner RL, Hartman BJ. Update of spinal epidural abscess: 35 cases and review of the literature. Rev Infect Dis 1987;9:265–74.

52. Hlavin ML, Kaminski HJ, Ross JS, et al. Spinal epidural abscess: a ten year perspective. Neurosurgery 1990;27:177–84.

53. Endress C, Guyot DR, Fata J, et al. Cervical osteomyelitis due to IV heroin use. Radiologic findings in 14 patients. AJR Am J Roentgenol 1990;155: 333–5.

54. Schellinger D. Patterns of anterior spinal canal involvement by neoplasms and infections. AJNR Am J Neuroradiol 1996;17:953–9.

55. Angtuaco EJC, McConnell JR, Chadduck WM, et al. MR imaging of spinal epidural sepsis. AJNR Am J Neuroradiol 1987;8:879–83.

56. Post MJD, Quencer RM, Montalvo BM, et al. Spinal infection: evaluation with MR imaging and intraoperative US. Radiology 1988;169:765–71.

57. Post MJ, Sze G, Quencer RM, et al. Gadoliniumenhanced MR in spinal infection. J Comput Assist Tomogr 1990;14(5):721–9.

58. Bonaldi VM, Duong H, Starr MR, et al. Tophaceous gout of the lumbar spine mimicking an epidural abscess: MR features. AJNR Am J Neuroradiol 1996;17:1949–52.

59. Murphy KJ, Brunberg JA, Quint DJ, et al. Spinal cord infection: myelitis and abscess formation. AJNR Am J Neuroradiol 1998;19:341–8.

60. Ditullio MV. Intramedullary spinal abscess: case report with a review of 53 previously described cases. Surg Neurol 1977;7:351–3.

61. Candon E, Frerebeau P. [Bacterial abscesses of the spinal cord: review of the literature (73 cases)]. Rev Neurol (Paris) 1994;150:370–6 [in French].

62. Fries HM, Wasenko JJ. MR of staphylococcal myelitis of the cervical spinal cord. AJNR Am J Neuroradiol 1997;18:455–8.

63. Tartaglino LM, Friedman DP, Flanders AE, et al. Multiple sclerosis in the spinal cord: MR appearance and correlation with clinical parameters. Radiology 1995;195:725–32.

64. Tartaglino LM, Flanders AE, Rapoport RJ. Intramedullary causes of myelopathy. Semin Ultrasound CT MR 1994;15:158–88.

65. Wiebe S, Lee DH, Karlik SJ, et al. Serial cranial and spinal cord magnetic resonance imaging in multiple sclerosis. Ann Neurol 1992;32:643–50.

66. Kidd D, Thorpe JW, Thompson AJ, et al. Spinal cord MRI using multi-array coils and fast spin echo. Findings in multiple sclerosis. Neurology 1993;43:2632–7.

67. Losseff NA, Webb SL, O'Riordan J, et al. Spinal cord atrophy and disability in multiple sclerosis. Brain 1996;119:701–8.

68. Lycklama a Nijeholt GJ, Barkof F, Scheltens P, et al. MR of the spinal cord in multiple sclerosis: relation to clinical subtype and disability. AJNR AM J Neuroradiol 1997;18:1041–8.

69. Kidd D, Thorpe JW, Kendall BE, et al. MRI dynamics of brain and spinal cord in progressive multiple sclerosis. J Neurol Neurosurg Psychiatry 1996;60:15–9.

70. Ghezzi A, Bergamaschi R, Martinelli V, et al. Clinical characteristics, course and prognosis of relapsing Devic's Neuromyelitis Optica. J Neurol 2004;251:47–52.

71. Wingerchuk DM, Lennon VA, Pittock SJ, et al. Revised diagnostic criteria for neuromyelitis optica. Neurology 2006;66:1485–9.

72. Weinshenker BG, Wingerchuk DM, Vukusic S, et al. Neuromyelitis optica IgG predicts relapse after longitudinally extensive transverse myelitis. Ann Neurol 2006;59:566–9.

73. Wingerchuk DM. Weinshenker BG neuromyelitis optica: clinical predictors of a relapsing course and survival. Neurology 2003;60:848–53.

74. Filippi M, Rocca MA. MR imaging of Devic's neuromyelitis optica. Neurol Sci 2004;25: S371–3.

75. Mandler RN, Gambarelli D, Gayraud D, et al. Devic's neuromyelitis optica: a clinicopathological study of 8 patients. Ann Neurol 1993;34:162–8.

76. Wingerchuk DM. Diagnosis and treatment of neuromyelitis optica. Neurologist 2007;13(1):2–11.

77. Giovannoni G. Neuromyelitis optica and anti-aquaporin-4 antibodies: widening the clinical phenotype. J Neurol Neurosurg Psychiatry 2006; 77:1001–2.

78. Bloch O, Manley GT. The role of aquaporin-4 in cerebral water transport and edema. Neurosurg Focus 2007;22(5):E3.

79. Menge T, Hemmer B, Nessler S, et al. Acute disseminated encephalomyelitis. Arch Neurol 2005;62:1673–80.

80. Pittock SJ, Lennon VA, Krecke K, et al. Brain abnormalities in neuromyelitis optica. Arch Neurol 2006; 63:390–6.

81. Tanembaum S, Chamoles N, Fejerman N. Acute disseminated encephalomyelitis: a long-term follow-up study of 84 pediatric patients. Neurology 2002;59:1224–31.

82. Schwarz S, Mohr A, Knauth M, et al. Acute disseminated encephalomyelitis: a follow-up study of 40 adult patients. Neurology 2001;56:1313–8.

83. Amit R, Glick B, Itzchak Y, et al. Acute severe combined demyelination. Childs Nerv Syst 1992; 8:354–6.

84. Tanembaum S, Chitnis T, Ness J, et al. Acute disseminated encephalomyelitis. Neurology 2007; 68:23–36.

85. David P, Baleriaux D, Bank WO, et al. MRI of acute disseminated encephalomyelitis after coxsackie B infection. J Neuroradiol 1993;20:258–65.

86. Myller HG, Evans MJ. Prognosis in acute disseminated encephalomyelitis: with a note on neuromyelitis optica. Q J Med 1953;22:347–479.

87. Choi KH, Lee KS, Chung SO, et al. Idiopathic transverse myelitis: MR characteristics. AJNR Am J Neuroradiol 1996;17:1151–60.

88. De Seze J, Lanctin C, Lebrun C, et al. Idiopathic acute transverse myelitis: application of the recent diagnostic criteria. Neurology 2005;65:1950–3.

89. Campi A, Filippi M, Comi G, et al. Acute transverse myelopathy: spinal and cranial MR study with clinical follow-up. AJNR Am J Neuroradiol 1995;16: 115–23.

90. Gero B, Sze G, Sharif H. MR imaging of intradural inflammatory diseases of the spine. AJNR Am J Neuroradiol 1991;12:1009–19.

91. Holtas S, Basibuyuk N, Fredriksson K. MRI in acute transverse myelopathy. Neuroradiology 1993;35: 221–6.

92. Mascalchi M, Cosottini M, Cellerini M, et al. MR of spinal cord involvement in Bechet's disease: case report. Neuroradiology 1998;40:255–7.

93. Pardatscher K, Fiore DL, Lavano A. MR imaging of transverse myelitis using Gd-DTPA. J Neuroradiol 1992;19:63–7.

94. Transverse Myelitis Consortium Working Group. Proposed diagnostic criteria and nosology of acute transverse myelitis. Neurology 2002;59: 499–505.

95. Al-Husaini A, Jamal GA. Myelopathy as the main presenting feature of systemic lupus erythematosus. Eur Neurol 1985;24:94–106.

96. Johnson RT, Richardson EP. The neurological manifestation of systemic lupus erythematosus: a clinical-pathological study of 24 cases and review of the literature. Medicine 1968;47:337–69.

97. Granger DP. Transverse myelitis with recovery: the only manifestation of systemic lupus erythematosus. Neurology 1960;10:325–9.

98. Provenzale JM, Barboriak DP, Gaensler EH, et al. Lupus-related myelitis: serial MR findings. AJNR Am J Neuroradiol 1994;15:1911–7.

99. Warren RW, Kredich DW. Transverse myelitis and acute central nervous system manifestation of systemic lupus erythematosus. Arthritis Rheum 1984;27:1058–60.

100. Lavalle C, Pizarro S, Drenkard C, et al. Transverse myelitis: a manifestation of systemic lupus erythematosus strongly associated with antiphospholipid antibodies. J Rheumatol 1990;17:34–7.

101. Campi A, Fillipi M, Comi G, et al. Acute transverse myelopathy associated with anticardiolipin antibodies. AJNR Am J Neuroradiol 1998;19:781–6.

102. Krishnan AV, Gabor MH. Acute transverse myelitis in SLE. Neurology 2004;62:2087.

103. Lenhardt FG, Impekoven P, Rubbert A, et al. Recurrent longitudinal myelitis as primary manifestation of SLE. Neurology 2004;63:1976.

104. Sanna G, Bertolaccini ML, Cuadrado MJ, et al. Central nervous system involvement in the antiphospholipid (Hughes) syndrome. Rheumatology 2003;42:200–13.

105. Parikh T, Shifteh K, Lipton ML, et al. Deep brain reversible encephalopathy: association with secondary antiphospholipid syndrome. AJNR Am J Neuroradiol 2007;28:76–8.

106. Sartoretti-Schefer S, Blattler T, Wichmann W. Spinal MRI in patients with vacuolar myelopathy, and correlation with histopathological findings. Neuroradiology 1997;39:865–9.

107. Quencer RM, Post MJ. Spinal cord lesions in patients with AIDS. Neuroimaging Clin N Am 1997;7:359–73.

108. Santosh CG, Bell JE, Best JJ. Spinal tract pathology in AIDS: Postmortem MRI correlation with neuropathology. Neuroradiology 1995;37:134–8.

109. Gray F, Belec L, Lescs MC, et al. Varicella zoster virus infection of the central nervous system in the acquired immune deficiency syndrome. Brain 1994;117:987–99.

110. Hirai T, Korogi Y, Hamatake S, et al. Case report: Varicella zoster virus myelitis – serial MR findings. Br J Radiol 1996;69:1187–90.

111. Hansman Whiteman ML, Dandapani BK, Shebert RT, et al. MRI of AIDS-related polyradiculomyelitis. J Comput Assist Tomogr 1994;18:7–11.

112. Malzberg MS, Rogg JM, Tate CM, et al. Poliomyelitis: hyperintensity of the anterior horn cells on MR images of the spinal cord. AJR Am J Roentgenol 1993;161:863–5.

113. Donovan WD, Zimmerman RD. MRI findings of severe Epstein Barr virus encephalomyelitis. J Comput Assist Tomogr 1996;20:1027–9.

114. Shakudo M, Inoue Y, Tsutada T. HTLV-1 associated myelopathy: acute progression and atypical MR findings. AJNR Am J Neuroradiol 1999;20:1417–21.

115. Friess HM, Wasenko JJ. MR of staphylococcus myelitis of the cervical spinal cord. AJNR Am J Neuroradiol 1997;18:455–8.

116. King SJ, Jeffree MA. MRI of an abscess of the cervical spinal cord in a case of Listeria meningoencephalomyelitis. Neuroradiology 1993;35:495–6.

117. Sanchez Pernaute RS, Berciano J, Rebollo M, et al. Intramedullary tuberculoma of the spinal cord with syringomyelia. Neuroradiology 1996;38:s105–6.

118. Yunten N, Alper H, Zileli M, et al. Tuberculous radiculomyelitis as a complication of spondilodiscitis: MR demonstration. J Neuroradiol 1996;23:241–4.

119. Nabatame H, Nakamura K, Matuda M. MRI of syphilitic myelitis. Neuroradiology 1992;34:105–6.

120. Citow JS, Ammirati M. Intramedullary tuberculoma of the spinal cord: case report. Neurosurgery 1994;35:327–30.

121. Iseman MD. Tuberculosis. In: Bennett D, Plum F, editors. Cecil textbook of medicine. 20th edition. Philadelphia: WB Saunders; 1996. p. 1683–9.

122. LaBerge JM, Brant-Zawadzki M. Evaluation of Pott's disease with computer tomography. Neuroradiology 1984;26:429–34.

123. Shivaram U, Wollschlager C, Khan F, et al. Spinal tuberculosis revisited. South Med J 1985;78:681–4.

124. Weaver P, Lifeso RM. The radiological diagnosis of tuberculosis of the adult spine. Skeletal Radiol 1984;12:178–86.

125. Whelan MA, Schonfeld S, Post JD, et al. Computed tomography of nontuberculous spinal infection. J Comput Assist Tomogr 1985;9:280–7.

126. Westermark N, Frossman G. The roentgen diagnosis of tuberculous spondylitis. Acta Radiol 1938;19:207.

127. Chapman M, Murray RO, Stoker DJ. Tuberculosis of the bones and joints. Semin Roentgenol 1979;14:266–82.

128. Sharif HS, Clark DC, Aabed MY, et al. MR imaging of mycetoma: comparison with CT. Radiology 1991;178:865–70.

129. Bell D, Cockshot WP. Tuberculosis of the vertebral pedicles. Radiology 1971;99:43.

130. Whelan MA, Naidich DP, Post JD, et al. Computed tomography of spinal tuberculosis. J Comput Assist Tomogr 1983;7:25–30.

131. Postachini F, Montanaro A. Tuberculous spinal granuloma simulating a herniated lumbar disk: a report of a case. Clin Orthop 1980;148:182.

132. Hodgson AR. Infectious diseases of the spine. In: Rothman RH, Simeone FA, editors. The spine. Philadelphia: WB Saunders; 1975. p. 567.

133. Rhoton EL, Ballinger WE Jr, Wuisling R, et al. Intramedullary spineal tuberculoma. Neurosurgery 1988;22:773.

134. Alessi G, Lemmerling M, Nathoo N. Combined spinal subdural tuberculous empyema and intramedullary tuberculoma in an HIV-positive patient. Eur Radiol 2003;13:1899–901.

135. Kumar A, Montanera W, Willinsky R, et al. MR features of tubercular arachnoiditis. J Comput Assist Tomogr 1993;17:127–30.

136. Hadjipavlou AG, Cesani-Vazquez F, Villaneuva-Meyer J, et al. The effectiveness of gallium citrate Ga 67 radionuclide imaging in vertebral osteomyelitis revisited. Am J Orthop (Belle Mead NJ) 1998;27(3):179–83.

137. Sartoris DJ, Resnick D, Resnik C, et al. Musculoskeletal manifestation of sarcoidosis. Semin Roentgenol 1985;20:376–86.

138. Zener JC, Alpert M, Klainer LM. Vertebral sarcoidosis. Arch Intern Med 1963;111:696–702.

139. Brodey PA, Pripstein S, Strange G, et al. Vertebral sarcoidosis: a case report and review of the literature. AJR Am J Roentgenol 1976;126:900–2.

140. Fisher AJ, Guilula LA, Kyriakos M, et al. MRI changes of lumbar vertebral sarcoidosis. AJR Am J Roentgenol 1999;173:354–6.

141. Ginsberg LE, Stanton C, Williams DW III. MRI of vertebral sarcoidosis: clinical images. J Comput Assist Tomogr 1993;17:158–62.

142. Rieger J, Hosyen N. Spinal cord sarcoidosis. Neuroradiology 1994;36:627–8.

143. Bennett G, Provenzale JM. Schistosomal myelitis: findings at MR imaging. Eur J Radiol 1998;27:268–70.

144. Dupuis MJ, Atrouni S, Dooms GC, et al. MR imaging of schistosomal myelitis. AJNR Am J Neuroradiol 1990;11:782–3.

145. Silbergleit R. Schistosomal granuloma of the spinal cord: evaluation with MR imaging and intraoperative sonography. AJR Am J Roentgenol 1992;158: 1351–3.

146. Grisolia JS, Wiederholt WC. CNS cysticercosis. Arch Neurol 1982;39:540–4.

147. Leite CC, Jinkins JR, Escobar BE, et al. MR imaging of intramedullary and intradural-extramedullary spinal cysticercosis. AJR Am J Roentgenol 1997;169:1713–7.

148. Chang KH, Lee JH, Han MH, et al. The role of contrast-enhanced imaging in the diagnosis of neurocysticercosis. AJNR Am J Neuroradiol 1991; 12:509–12.

149. White AC. Neurocysticercosis update on epidemiology, pathogenesis, diagnosis and management. Annu Rev Med 2000;51:187–206.

150. DeGiorgio CM, Sorvillo F, Escueta SP. Neurocysticercose in the United States: review of an important emerging infection. Neurology 2005;64:1486 [correspondence].

151. Siqueira MG, Koury LS, Boer CA, et al. Cisticerco solitário intramedular: relato de caso e revisão da literatura. Arq Br Neurocirurg 1987;6:131–9.

152. Carbajal JR, Palacios E, Azar-Kia B, et al. Radiology of cysticercosis of the central nervous system including computed tomography. Radiology 1977;125:127–32.

153. Martinez-Lopez M, Quiroz y Ferrari F. Cisticercosis. J Clin Neuroophthalmol 1985;5:127–43.

154. Queiroz LD, Filho AP, Callegaro D, et al. Intramedullary cysticercosis: case report, literature review and comment on pathogenesis. J Neurol Sci 1975;26:61–70.

155. Torabi AM, Quiceno M, Mendeoshon DB, et al. Mutilevel intramedullary spinal neurocysticercosis with eosinophilic meningitis. Arch Neurol 2004;61:770–2.

156. Singh P, Sahai K. Intramedullary cysticercosis. Neurol India 2004;52:264–5.

157. Venkataraman VS, Roy AK, Dhamija RM, et al. Cysticercal meningoencephalitis: clinical presentation and autopsy findings. J Assoc Physicians India 1990;38:763–5.

158. Parmar H, Shah J, Patwardhan V, et al. MR imaging in intramedullary cysticercosis. Neuroradiology 2001;43:961–7.

159. Teitelbaum GP, Otto RJ, Lin M, et al. MR imaging of neurocysticercosis. AJR Am J Roentgenol 1989; 153:857–66.

160. Williams RL, Fukui MB, Meltzer CC, et al. Fungal spinal osteomyelitis in the immunocompromised patient: MR findings in three cases. AJNR Am J Neuroradiol 1999;20:381–5.

161. Scaravilli F. Parasitic and fungal infections of the nervous system. In: Hume Adams J, Corsellis JAN, Duchen LW, editors. Greenfield's neuropathology. 4th edition. New York: Wiley; 1984. p. 305–33.

162. McGahan JP, Graves DS, Palmer PE. Coccidioidal spondylosis; usual and unusual radiographic manifestations. Radiology 1980;136:5–9.

163. Eller JL, Siebert PE. Sclerotic vertebral bodies. An unusual manifestation of disseminated coccidioidomycosis. Radiology 1969;93:1099–100.

164. Dalinka CM, Greendyke CW. The spinal manifestations of coccidiomycosis. J Can Assoc Radiol 1971;22:93–9.

165. Winer JB. Guillain Barre syndrome. Mol Pathol 2001;54(6):381–5.

166. Jacobs BC, van Doorn PA, Schmitz PI, et al. Campylobacter jejuni infections and anti-GM1 antibodies in Guillain-Barré syndrome. Ann Neurol 1996;40(2):181–7.

167. Seneviratne U. Guillain-Barre syndrome. Postgrad Med J 2000;76(902):774–82.

168. Chiò A, Cocito D, Leone M, et al. Guillain-Barré syndrome: a prospective population-based incidence and outcome survey. Neurology 2003;60:1146–50.

169. Hiraga A, Mori M, Ogawara K, et al. Differences in patterns of progression in demyelinating and axonal Guillain-Barré syndromes. Neurology 2003; 61:471–4.

170. Ogawara K, Kuwabara S, Mori M, et al. Axonal Guillain-Barré syndrome: relation to anti-ganglioside antibodies and Campylobacter jejuni infection in Japan. Ann Neurol 2000;48:624–31.

171. Swick HM, McQuillen MP. The use of steroids in the treatment of idiopathic polyneuritis. Neurology 1976;26:205–12.

172. Van Koningsveld R, van der Meché FG, Schmitz PI, et al. Combined therapy of intravenous immunoglobulin and methylprednisolone in patients with Guillain-Barré syndrome: the results of a multicentre double blind placebo controlled clinical trial. J Peripher Nerv Syst 2001;6:186–7.

173. Byun WB, Park WK, Park BH, et al. Guillain-Barré syndrome: MRI findings of the spine in eight patients. Radiology 1998;208:137–41.

174. Timms SR, Cure JK, Kurent JE. Subacute combined degeneration of the spinal cord: MR findings. AJNR Am J Neuroradiol 1993;14:1224–7.

175. Pema PJ, Horak HA, Wyatt RH. Myelopathy caused by nitrous oxide toxicity. AJNR Am J Neuroradiol 1998;19:894–6.

176. Goodhart LC, Loizou LA, Anderson M. Heroin myelopathy. J Neurol Neurosurg Psychiatry 1982; 45(6):562–3.

177. Jumma O, Koulaouzidis A, Ferguson IT. Cocaine induced spinal cord infarction. Postgrad Med J 2008;84:391.

178. Wang PY, Shen WC, Jan JS. Serial MRI changes in radiation myelopathy. Neuroradiology 1995;37:374–7.

179. Wang PY, Shen WC, Jan JS. MR imaging in radiation myelopathy. AJNR Am J Neuroradiol 1992;13: 1049–55.

Spine Trauma

Seamus Looby, MD*, Adam Flanders, MD

KEYWORDS

• Spine • Trauma • Cervical • Thoracic • Lumbar

Spine trauma is a devastating event with a high morbidity and mortality and many additional medical, psychological, social, and financial consequences for patients, their families, and society. It is estimated that the annual incidence of spinal cord injury, not including those who die at the scene of the accident, is approximately 40 cases per million population in the United States or approximately 12,000 new cases each year. The number of people in the United States who were alive in 2008 with a spinal cord injury has been estimated to be approximately 259,000 persons (range of 229,000–306,000). The average age of the typical patient with spinal cord injury has increased to 40.2 years as of 2005, and approximately 80.9% of all spinal cord injuries occur in males.[1]

Motor vehicle accidents account for 42.1% of reported spinal cord injury cases. The next most common cause is falls (26.7%), followed by acts of violence (15.1%), and sporting activities (7.6%). The proportion of injuries that are due to sports has decreased over time whereas the proportion of injuries due to falls has increased. Violence caused 13.3% of spinal cord injuries before 1980, and peaked between 1990 and 1999 at 24.8%, before declining to 15.1% since 2005.[1,2]

The most frequent neurologic category at discharge of patients with spinal cord injury is incomplete tetraplegia (30.1%), followed by complete paraplegia (25.6%), complete tetraplegia (20.4%), and incomplete paraplegia (18.5%). More than half (57.5%) of patients with spinal cord injury are employed at the time of their injury. At postinjury year 1, 11.5% of persons with spinal cord injury are employed. By postinjury year 20, 35.4% are employed and a similar level of employment is observed 30 years after injury.[3] Today 87.8% of all persons with spinal cord injury who

are discharged alive from the system are sent to a private, noninstitutional residence (in most cases their homes before injury). Most patients with spinal cord injury (52.3%) are single when injured. The average hospital stay for a typical patient with spinal cord injury has declined from 24 days in 1973–1979 to 12 days in 2005–2008. The total cost of care for patients with spinal cord injury is dependent on the severity of injury; the first year cost of care for a tetraplegic patient costs an average of $801,161 and drops by an average of $143,507 a year thereafter.[1,4,5]

OVERVIEW OF SPINE TRAUMA

Spinal fractures represent 3% to 6% of all skeletal injuries.[6] A systematic review by Sekhon and Fehlings[7] found that 55% of all spinal injuries (including all types of spinal injuries) involve the cervical spine, 15% the thoracic spine, 15% the lumbar spine, and 15% the lumbosacral spine. The risk of damage to the spinal cord is greater in cervical spine injuries than in the thoracic and lumbar regions.[8] Many epidemiologic studies have shown that fractures of the thoracic and the lumbosacral spine are much more common than fractures of the cervical spine.[9,10]

Cervical spine injuries, including fractures and ligamentous injuries, primarily occur secondary to traumatic injuries to the head and neck. An individual with an unstable cervical fracture is at risk for cervical spinal cord injury unless the fracture is stabilized. The majority of cervical spine fractures occur at the upper or lower ends of the cervical spine. C1 vertebral fractures represent approximately 10%,[11] C2 vertebral fractures approximately 33%, fractures of the odontoid process of C2 approximately 15%, and C6 and C7 vertebral fractures approximately 50% of

Division of Neuroradiology, Department of Radiology, Thomas Jefferson University Hospital, 111 South 11th Street, Philadelphia, PA 19107, USA
* Corresponding author.
E-mail address: seamuslooby@hotmail.com

Radiol Clin N Am 49 (2011) 129–163
doi:10.1016/j.rcl.2010.07.019
0033-8389/11/$ — see front matter © 2011 Elsevier Inc. All rights reserved.

cervical spine fractures.[12] The overall incidence of cervical spine fracture without spinal cord injury is 3%.[13] There are many studies on the overall epidemiology of cervical spine injuries. A study by Grossman and colleagues[14] concluded that the overall incidence of all types of cervical spine injury in patients with trauma is 4.3%, cervical spinal injury without spinal cord injury 3%, spinal cord injury without fracture 0.7%, and delayed diagnosis of all types of cervical spine injury 0.01%.

The incidence, mechanism of injury, and type of cervical spinal injury in the elderly patient differs from those in younger patients because of osteopenia, degenerative changes, and low-velocity falls causing injury.[15] C2 fractures are much more common in the elderly.[16] The combination of osteopenia, degenerative changes, and difficulty in positioning the patient's head make imaging of the cervical spine difficult in the elderly. It is difficult to determine which patients require computed tomography (CT). In patients screened with plain radiography only, particular attention must be given to C2, with a low threshold for CT evaluation.[17]

Cervical spine fractures are uncommon in children.[18] The same criteria for imaging of the cervical spine cannot be applied to children because of the large radiation dose associated with CT.[19] Plain radiography is the imaging modality of choice, with CT reserved for cases where an abnormality is identified.[20]

Fractures of the thoracic and lumbar spine are more common than fractures of the cervical spine.[10] Major trauma is the most common cause of thoracolumbar fractures. In the United States, the incidence of spinal fractures from motor vehicle accidents is 5% to 6%.[21] However, the majority of thoracolumbar fractures occur in elderly patients as a consequence of minor injury in a patient with osteoporosis. In the United States, the incidence of vertebral fractures from osteoporosis requiring hospitalization is 150,000 per year.[22] The majority of thoracic spine fractures occur in the lower thoracic spine, with 60% to 70% of all thoracolumbar spine fractures occurring between T12 and L2. The majority of these fractures (75%–90%) occur without spinal cord injury.[23] Injury to the cord or the cauda equina occurs in approximately 10% to 38% of adult thoracolumbar fractures and in 50% to 60% of adult fracture-dislocations.[24]

CLEARING THE SPINE AND INDICATIONS FOR IMAGING

Cervical spine imaging is one of the most common imaging examinations performed in trauma centers in the United Stated and developed countries. The task of clearing the cervical spine for injury and the rationale for determining which patients require imaging can be challenging. There are additional challenges in special populations including the obtunded individual, the elderly individual, and children. Two large prospective multicenter trials have attempted to address the appropriate selection criteria for cervical spine imaging after blunt trauma.

In the multicenter National Emergency X-Radiography Use Study (NEXUS),[25] investigators identified the key clinical risk factors that had significant predictive value in determining if a cervical fracture was absent. From the analysis of clinical data and radiography of 34,069 blunt trauma patients with 818 confirmed cervical spine fractures (2.4%), the investigators concluded that no imaging was required in the *absence* of the following clinical features: no midline cervical spine tenderness, no focal neurologic deficit, normal level of alertness, no intoxication, and no painful distracting injury. The NEXUS group found that their clinical prediction rule could adequately identify subjects at risk for fracture with a sensitivity of 99.6%.

A similar trial was conducted by the Canadian Cervical Spine Group,[26] which identified the clinical criteria for which risk of cervical spine fracture is low after blunt trauma. The criteria included: (1) a fully alert patient with a Glasgow Coma Scale of 15; (2) absence of high-risk factors (e g. age >65 years, dangerous mechanism of injury such as a fall from greater than 3 m/5 stairs, axial load to head, high-speed vehicular crash, bicycle crash, or a motorcycle crash, or the presence of paresthesias in the extremities); (3) presence of low-risk factors (simple vehicular crash, sitting position in emergency department, ambulatory at any time, delayed onset of neck pain, and the absence of midline cervical tenderness), and (4) ability to actively rotate the neck 45° to the left and to the right. The Canadian group found that their clinical criteria had 100% sensitivity and 42.5% specificity for predicting absence of cervical injury. Although the recommendations of the 2 groups differ, no clear advantage of one clinical rule over the other has emerged. One problematic feature of both studies is that in practice it is rare to encounter a patient who fulfills either set of criteria, therefore in many instances some imaging is still required.

The advent of newer technologies (eg, CT, magnetic resonance [MR] imaging) has provided additional diagnostic imaging options for spinal clearance. For example, for cervical spine clearance, plain radiography consisting of the standard

3-view cervical spine radiographs (anteroposterior, lateral, odontoid/peg) was the primary radiological test in evaluating the bony structures of the cervical spine.[27] Although good-quality radiographs have provided excellent sensitivity for detection of cervical fractures, the method provides very little useful information on the integrity of the ligamentous or soft tissue injuries. Moreover, it has been shown that quality of radiography in the setting of multisystem trauma patients is often inadequate, requiring repeat imaging and delays in management.[28] One large series that assessed diagnostic sensitivity of cervical radiography in the trauma setting found that the standard 3 views failed to demonstrate 61% of all fractures and 36% of all subluxations and dislocations.[29]

Multidetector CT (MDCT) has replaced radiography as the primary modality for assessment of osseous injury in the adult in many major trauma centers. MDCT creates isotropic datasets, which permits reconstruction of data in any plane without loss of intrinsic resolution. The combination of MDCT, soft-copy review on PACS (picture archive and communication system) workstations, and retrospective reformatting capabilities has obviated the requirement to perform radiography in many instances. Moreover, the speed of acquisition and uniform image quality of MDCT makes it more cost effective to use in the emergency setting. For multisystem trauma, a single data acquisition can generate both a spine dataset and a visceral dataset.[30,31]

Flexion-extension radiography has been used in the past to assess for ligamentous stability. It is an aid in the diagnosis of unstable ligamentous cervical spinous injury or subtle fractures by demonstrating such radiographic signs as anterolisthesis or focal kyphosis. However, there are no reliable data regarding the appropriate use of flexion-extension radiography in the evaluation of acute cervical spinal trauma.[32] The few retrospective trials that have evaluated the value of this technique have demonstrated a very low diagnostic yield.[33] Moreover, isolated cervical ligamentous injury without fracture is relatively rare.[34]

MR imaging of the cervical spine is often difficult to perform in the acute setting, particularly in an obtunded patient. Moreover, there is currently little evidence in the medical literature to say it is superior to CT in the initial management of cervical spinal injury, as the majority of the findings (in patients with a normal CT) will require nonsurgical treatment.[35]

Plain radiography can be used to evaluate the thoracic and lumbar spine after trauma. However, with the ever increasing use of CT in multitrauma patients, reconstructions of the thoracic and lumbar spine from the raw data of a CT abdomen and pelvis study are used, obviating the need for plain radiographs. However, the radiologist needs to be aware that the quality of the data is less than that acquired from a dedicated CT of the spine, and equivocal findings may require a dedicated CT of the thoracolumbar spine.[36,37]

STABILITY VERSUS INSTABILITY

The concept of stable versus unstable spinal injuries is of critical importance in spinal imaging. Essentially, an unstable spinal injury is one in which the mechanically unstable spine moves and undergoes potentially deleterious deformation in response to physiologic loading and a normal range of movement. Many classification systems with regard to type and mechanism of injury have been proposed over the years. The most widely used of these systems is the 3-column theory of Denis,[38] which helps predict stability associated with the different patterns of injury to the spine.

The 3-column theory of Denis divides the spinal column into anterior, middle, and posterior columns. The anterior column consists of the anterior vertebral body, the anterior longitudinal ligament, and the anterior annulus fibrosis. The middle column consists of the posterior vertebral body, the posterior longitudinal ligament, and the posterior annulus. The posterior column consists of the posterior bony elements including the pedicles, the lamina, the facets, and the spinous processes, the ligaments including the ligamentum flavum, the interspinous, and supraspinous ligaments, and the facet joint capsule. When only one column is disrupted, the injury is considered mechanically stable. When 2 columns are disrupted, the injury is considered unstable. In general, this requires failure of the middle column with either the anterior or the posterior column.

It is important for the radiologist to be descriptive in terms of the spinal injury/fracture and its morphology, so as to be able to communicate accurately to the physician the type of spinal injury/fracture and its stability or instability. The radiological features of mechanical instability include displacement/translation greater than 2 mm indicating ligamentous disruption, widening of the interspinous space, the facet joints, and/or the interpediculate distance, disruption of the posterior vertebral body line, widening of the intervertebral canal, vertebral body height loss of greater than 50%, and kyphosis of greater than 20°.[39]

Awareness of the neurologic and mechanical stability allows the clinician to choose the appropriate treatment strategy, conservative or surgical.

CERVICAL SPINE INJURIES

Trauma to the cervical spine is frequently classified into injuries of the upper and lower cervical spine. The upper cervical spine injuries include injuries to the occipital condyles, the atlanto-occipital articulation, C1, C2, and the atlantoaxial joint. The lower cervical spine includes injuries to C3 to C7. However, more commonly cervical spine injuries are classified according to the underlying mechanism of injury. These mechanisms include hyperflexion, hyperflexion and rotation, hyperextension, hyperextension and rotation, vertical compression, lateral flexion, and indeterminate mechanisms that result in injuries.[40]

Upper Cervical Spine Injuries

Occipital condyle fractures are rare and are rarely, if ever, diagnosed with conventional radiography. The classification system most commonly used to describe them is the Anderson-Montesano system. Using this system, a type I occipital condyle fracture is a comminuted fracture that occurs due to axial loading (**Fig. 1**). Type II is a skull base fracture that propagates into one or both occipital condyles. Type III is an inferomedial avulsion fracture with medial displacement of the fracture fragment into the foramen magnum, and is considered unstable because of an avulsed alar ligament. Type III occipital condyle fractures are the commonest of the 3. High-resolution CT of the skull base provides the best evaluation of this type of injury, and the base of the skull should therefore be included on all CT cervical spine examinations.[41]

Atlanto-occipital dislocation results in disruption of the stabilizing ligaments between the occiput and C1, and this injury is more frequent in children due to the disproportionate size of the cranium. Atlanto-occipital dislocation has a high associated fatality rate because of stretching of the brainstem, which results in respiratory arrest. However, with improved on-scene and immediate management of patients with spinal cord injuries, this once uniformly fatal injury is now potentially survivable. No radiographic modality has 100% sensitivity for this injury, which is diagnosed on the basis of increased distance from the basion to the odontoid. Secondary radiographic signs include soft tissue swelling or subarachnoid/craniocervical junction/posterior cranial fossa hemorrhage. CT with coronal and sagittal reformats will demonstrate increased distance between the occipital condyles and the lateral masses of C1 (**Fig. 2**). MR imaging in the sagittal plain is the best modality for demonstrating ligamentous injury.[42]

Acute atlantoaxial dissociation (AAD) is a rare injury in which there is partial or complete derangement of the lateral atlantoaxial articulations directly related to trauma. AAD is characterized by excessive motion between C1 and C2 caused by either a bony or a ligamentous injury. AAD is associated with certain congenital conditions such as Down syndrome, osteogenesis imperfecta, neurofibromatosis, Morquio syndrome, spondyloepiphyseal dysplasia congenital, and chondrodysplasia punctata. The 3 mechanisms of AAD are flexion-extension, distraction, and rotation. Fieldings and Hawkins provided a classification system for AAD.[43] Type I AAD is rotatory fixation without anterior displacement of the atlas. Type II AAD is rotatory fixation with less than 5 mm of anterior displacement of the atlas. Type III AAD is rotatory fixation with greater than 5 mm of anterior displacement of the atlas. Type IV AAD is rotatory fixation with posterior displacement of the atlas. All of these injuries can be associated with concurrent fractures, neurologic deficits, or vertebral artery injuries.

The classic "Jefferson fracture" is the result of a compressive force to C1, usually from a blow to the vertex of the head, resulting in fractures at the junctions of the anterior and posterior arches with the lateral masses. Although only one anterior and one posterior arch fracture is necessary to meet diagnostic criteria, any combination of anterior and posterior arch fractures can occur. On radiography, the key view is the open-mouth odontoid view, which may show displacement of the C1 lateral masses. However, CT provides a more comprehensive assessment to define the full extent of the fracture, document other fractures (eg, C2), and to identify bone fragments in the spinal canal (**Fig. 3**).[44] Atypically, fractures limited to the lateral mass of C1 may occur because of a lateral tilt or eccentric axial loading. Isolated fractures of the anterior or posterior arch of C1 should be considered separate from the classic Jefferson fracture because they are stable. Isolated fractures can sometimes be difficult to distinguish from developmental clefts (**Fig. 4**).

Hangman's fracture, or traumatic spondylolisthesis of the axis (C2), gained its name from the pattern of injury that used to occur with judicial hanging.[45] Traumatic hangman's fracture most commonly occurs in instances where there is rapid deceleration of the head such as when the head is forced against the dashboard in a motor vehicle accident. The transmitted force passes through the weakest part of C2, the interarticular segments of the pedicles, resulting in bilateral pars or isthmic fractures. Fortunately, spinal cord damage is uncommon because the spinal canal is wider at

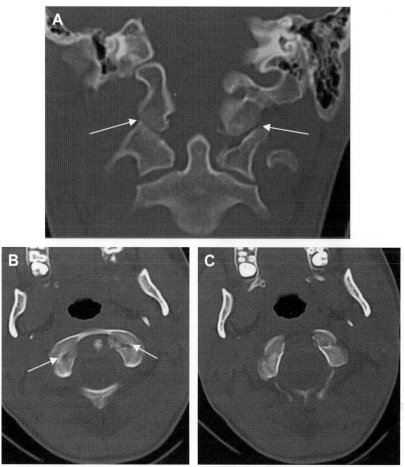

Fig. 1. Type I occipital condyle fracture. (*A*) Coronal reformatted CT demonstrates bilateral fractures through the occipital condyles (*white arrows*). (*B, C*) Axial CT of the same patient shows the fractures extending through both occipital condyles with minimal displacement (*white arrows*).

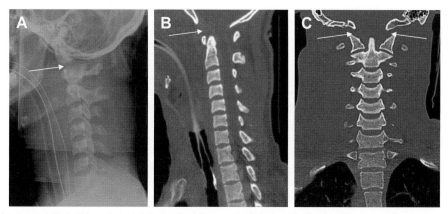

Fig. 2. Atlanto-occipital dislocation. (*A*) Lateral radiograph of the cervical spine demonstrates increased separation of the basion (midpoint of the anterior margin of the foramen magnum on the occipital bone) and the superior tip of the dens in an intubated patient (*white arrow*). (*B, C*) Sagittal and coronal CT reformats again show increased basion to dens distance and superior dislocation of the occipital condyles with respect to the superior surfaces of C1 (*white arrows*).

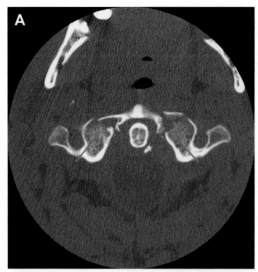

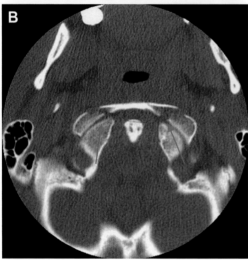

Fig. 3. Jefferson burst fracture. (A, B) Axial CT at the level of the anterior arch demonstrates bilateral fractures through the anterior arch of C1 at the junctions of the anterior arch with the lateral masses (red arrows).

this level and because the injury is decompressive.[46,47] A classification system of the hangman's fracture was devised by Effindi and colleagues and modified by Levins and Edwards.[48] A type I hangman's fracture is an isolated hairline fracture, with less than 3 mm fragment displacement, less than 15° angle at the fracture site, and a normal C2-C3 disc space. There is no disruption of the anterior or posterior longitudinal ligaments or the C2-C3 disc space with this fracture. A type II hangman's fracture is an isolated hairline fracture, with greater than 3 mm fragment displacement, greater than 15° angle at the fracture site, and an abnormal C2-C3 disc space. There is slight

disruption of the anterior longitudinal ligament, and significant disruption of the posterior longitudinal ligament and C2-C3 disc. A type IIA hangman's fracture subtype demonstrates no anterior displacement but severe angulation at the fracture site, resulting in disruption of the C2-C3 disc space. A type III hangman's fracture consists of the type II changes and a C2-C3 articular facet dislocation. Radiography demonstrates anterior displacement of C2 on C3. CT better demonstrates the pattern and extent of injury. MR cervical spine may be necessary if neurologic symptoms develop, and MRA/CTA (MR angiography/CT angiography) of the neck and head may be necessary to look for a vertebral artery dissection if the fracture extends into the foramen transversarium (**Figs. 5** and **6**).

Fractures of the dens or the odontoid process occur through several mechanisms. The classic imaging appearance is of a lucent linear defect, usually through the base of the dens with posterior displacement of the dens arch of C1 relative to the C2 body and arch. The classification system proposed by Anderson and D'Alonso is used to describe dens fractures. A type I fracture is an avulsion of the tip, and needs to be distinguished from an os odontoideum, which is a well-corticated ossification center above a rudimentary dens. Controversy exists as to whether this type is a true consequence of trauma. A type II fracture, the most common, is a transverse fracture through the base of the dens (**Figs. 7** and **8**). This fracture is the most likely to go on to nonhealing, and a primary surgical fusion procedure may be necessary to prevent cervical myelopathy A type III fracture extends into the body of C2 (**Fig. 9**).[49] An isolated C2 lateral body fracture is a rare occurrence but may happen, and is distinguished from dens fractures.

Lower Cervical Spine Injuries

Hyperflexion injuries

The clay shoveler fracture is an oblique avulsive fracture of a lower spinous process, most commonly C6-T1. This fracture gained its name from laborers who sustained this pattern of injury when performing activities involving lifting weights rapidly with the arms extended, for example, shoveling soil, rubble, or snow over the head backward. It is not a common fracture and is more likely to occur in the trauma setting nowadays. The clay shoveler fracture is a stable fracture (**Fig. 10**).[50]

Anterior subluxation occurs in the cervical spine when the posterior ligament complex is disrupted but the anterior longitudinal ligament remains intact. There is no associated bone injury, and

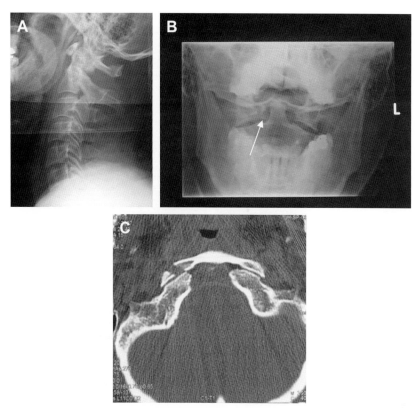

Fig. 4. Atypical Jefferson fracture, isolated fracture through the right anterior arch of C1. (*A*) Lateral cervical spine radiograph demonstrates normal cervical spine alignment and no evidence of fracture. (*B*) Open-mouth view demonstrates asymmetry of the lateral masses with medial displacement on the right side (*white arrow*). (*C*) CT demonstrates a unilateral fracture through the right anterior arch of C1.

the facet joints may be subluxed. For this injury radiological diagnosis can be difficult, but detection is important because of a reported 20% to 50% incidence of failed ligamentous healing leading to instability (**Figs. 11** and **12**).[51]

A simple wedge compression fracture occurs from a flexion injury with loss of height of the anterior vertebral body and buckling of the anterior cortex.

Bilateral interfacetal dislocation (BID) is an extreme form of hyperflexion injury that occurs following a severe flexion force to the head and neck, causing significant anterior displacement of the spine and ligamentous disruption at the level

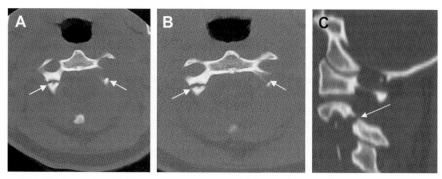

Fig. 5. Hangman's fracture. (*A, B*) Axial CT demonstrates bilateral pars interarticularis fractures of C2 (*white arrows*). (*C*) Sagittal CT reformat shows a minimally displaced fracture through the right pars interarticularis without significant fracture displacement (*white arrow*).

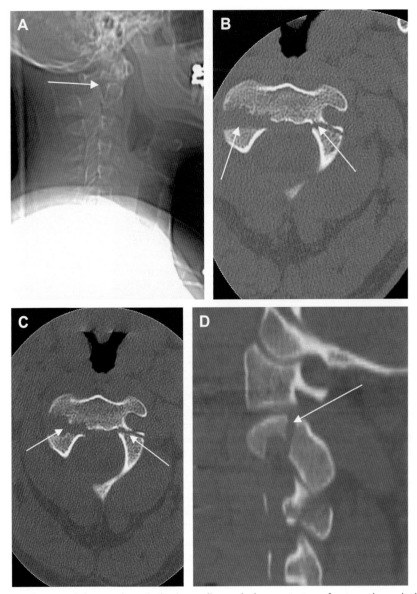

Fig. 6. Hangman's fracture. (*A*) Lateral cervical spine radiograph demonstrates a fracture through the pars inter-articularis of C2 with angulation and displacement at the fracture site (*white arrow*). (*B, C*) Axial CT shows bilateral pars interarticularis fractures with posterior displacement on the right side (*white arrows*). (*D*). Sagittal CT reformat confirms the posterior displacement (*white arrow*).

of the injury. Both inferior articular facets from one vertebral body can dislocate anterior to the superior facets of the subjacent vertebra, implying disruption of the major support ligaments of the anterior, middle, and posterior columns. The facets can be subluxed, perched, or locked. BIDs are often associated with compression fractures of the subjacent vertebra and/or disc herniation at the level of the injury, and these are highly unstable injuries. BIDs are more common in the lower cervical spine (**Figs. 13** and **14**).[52]

The flexion teardrop fracture is the most severe cervical spine injury with a severe flexion force, resulting in a fracture dislocation of the cervical spine, most commonly at C5. This fracture is a devastating injury with complete disruption of all the soft tissues at the level of the injury, including the anterior longitudinal ligament, the intervertebral disc, and the posterior longitudinal ligament. There is a substantial axial force component, which causes the impacted vertebral body to literally "explode." There is typically a large

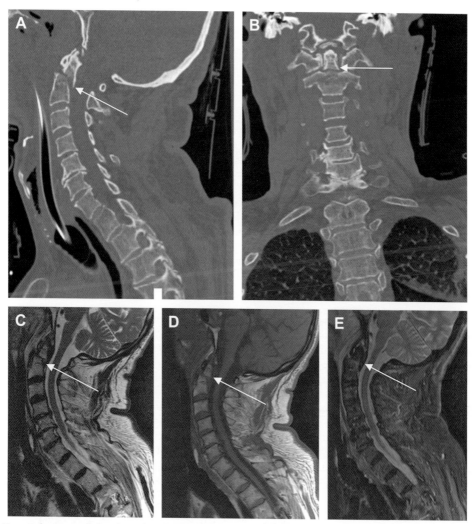

Fig. 7. Type II fracture of the dens. (*A, B*) Sagittal and coronal reformats of the cervical spine in this intubated patient show a mildly displaced type II fracture of the dens (*white arrows*). (*C*) T2, (*D*). T1, and (*E*) short-tau inversion recovery (STIR) sagittal MR sequences show mild bowing but preservation of the posterior longitudinal ligament and no compression of the spinal cord at this level (*white arrows*).

triangular fragment of the anteroinferior margin of the upper cervical vertebra, the teardrop fragment. The retropulsed posterior cortex affects the ventral dura and spinal cord, and patients classically present with the "acute anterior cord syndrome" with quadriplegia and loss of the anterior column senses but preservation of the posterior column senses (**Fig. 15**).[53]

Flexion rotation injuries
A combination of flexion and rotation may result in dislocation of one facet, with the inferior articular process of the dislocated facet displaced in front of the superior articular process of the subjacent vertebra and tearing the posterior ligaments. MR imaging is warranted to assess for cord injury in

patients who manifest neurologic symptoms (**Fig. 16**).[4]

Extension injuries
Hyperextension injuries occur when there is forceful posterior displacement of the head or upper cervical spine, usually from trauma to the face or mandible and/or sudden deceleration, such as when the head is suddenly halted from forward motion by the steering wheel or dashboard in a motor vehicle accident. In general, extension injuries affect the lower cervical spine, although the extension teardrop fracture typically involves the C2 body. Extension mechanism injuries are more common in patients with ankylosing spondylitis, diffuse idiopathic skeletal hyperostosis

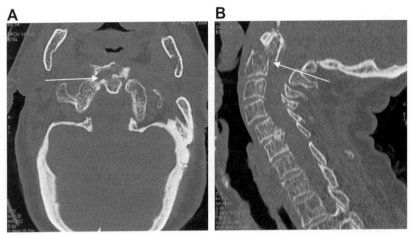

Fig. 8. Type II fracture of the dens. (*A, B*) Axial CT with sagittal reformat shows a type II fracture through the dens (*white arrows*). The bones are osteopenic in this elderly patient. C2 fractures are more common in elderly patients because of osteopenia and degenerative changes.

(DISH), or congenital or acquired spinal stenosis.[54] Hyperextension sprain and hyperextension dislocation are injuries to the soft tissues from a hyperextension injury including the longus colli and capitis muscles, the anterior longitudinal ligament, the intervertebral disc, and the posterior longitudinal ligament. Hyperextension fracture dislocation more commonly occurs in elderly patients with disruption of the articular pillars, the posterior vertebral body, the laminae, the spinous processes, or the pedicles (**Fig. 17**).[55]

Patients with ankylosing spondylitis or DISH are particularly prone to extension type fractures because of the loss of flexibility from ossification of the ligamentous complexes and disc spaces. These patients are therefore prone to fractures of

the pathologic anterior calcification that extend obliquely through the disc into the subjacent vertebral body or posteriorly through the disc space (**Fig. 18**).[54]

The extension teardrop fracture usually occurs when a hyperextension force produces an avulsion fracture of the anteroinferior corner of C2. The characteristic radiographic finding is that the vertical height of the avulsed fragment is greater than the horizontal width. These fractures only involve the anterior column, and therefore are stable in flexion and unstable in extension (**Fig. 19**).[56]

Laminar fractures rarely occur in isolation, but when they do it is usually as a result of a hyperextension injury.[57]

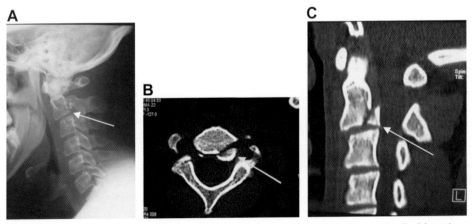

Fig. 9. Type III fracture of the axis. (*A*) Lateral cervical spine radiograph demonstrates minimal subluxation of C2 on C3 but no definite fracture (*white arrow*). (*B, C*) Axial CT and sagittal reformat demonstrate a fracture through the body of C2 with extension into the base of the dens consistent with a type III fracture (*yellow* and *white arrows*).

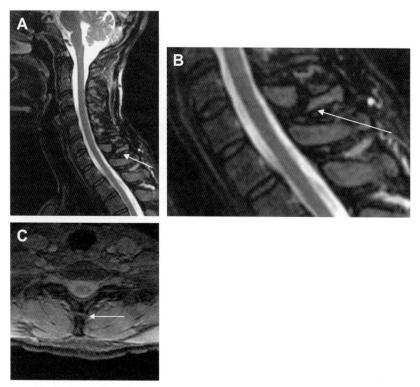

Fig. 10. Clay shoveler fracture. (*A, B*) Sagittal and (*C*) axial MR demonstrate an osseous defect through the spinous process of C7 consistent with a clay shoveler fracture (*white arrows*).

Extension rotation injuries

An articular pillar fracture is a fracture through a lateral mass caused by impaction of the articular mass above during a hyperextension and rotational injury. This fracture usually extends into the transverse process or the lamina and is a stable fracture (**Fig. 20**).[58]

The isolated articular pillar fracture can occur with a simultaneous fracture through the lamina and ipsilateral pedicle.

Burst fractures of the cervical spine

Burst fractures are much more common in the thoracolumbar spine, but can also occur in the

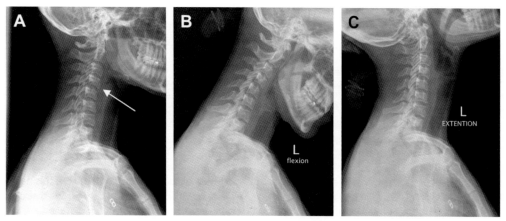

Fig. 11. Anterior subluxation. (*A*) Lateral cervical spine radiograph demonstrates mild anterior subluxation of C4 on C5 (*white arrow*). (*B, C*) Flexion and extension radiographs demonstrate no increased subluxation or kyphosis.

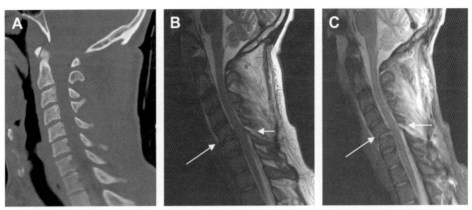

Fig. 12. Anterior subluxation. (*A*) Sagittal reformat CT demonstrates normal cervical alignment with no fracture. (*B, C*) The patient had MR of the cervical spine 40 minutes after the CT scan, which demonstrates mild anterior subluxation of C5 on C6 with subluxation of the facet joints at C5-C6 (*white arrows*).

cervical spine. An axial compression force applied to the cervical intervertebral disc can result in the liquid nucleus pulposus imploding through the vertebral end plate into the center of the vertebral body with retropulsion of bony fragments into the spinal canal, which may cause neurologic compromise (**Fig. 21**). This situation typically results in combined sagittal and coronal splits in the vertebral body from dissipation of axial directed forces.[59]

THORACOLUMBAR SPINE INJURIES

Thoracolumbar spinal fractures are more common than cervical spinal fractures.[2–4] Nearly 90% of all thoracolumbar fractures occur at the thoracolumbar junction, between T11 and L4. This region is vulnerable because of the change in the curvature of the spine from a kyphotic thoracic spinal curvature to a lordotic lumbar spinal curvature.[21,22] The major types of thoracolumbar spine injury are described according to the mechanism of injury: compression or wedge, burst, flexion distraction or chance, and fracture dislocation.

Anterior Wedge Compression Fracture

Anterior wedge compression fractures account for nearly 50% of all thoracolumbar fractures. The classic imaging finding is of a wedge-shaped vertebral body compressing the anterior cortex and sparing the middle and posterior columns. These fractures may occur at multiple vertebral levels. Plain radiographs usually show a focal kyphotic deformity with cortical end plate buckling of the anterosuperior end plate, resulting in a wedge-shaped vertebral body. However, the exact amount of loss of vertebral body height

and the fracture line may be difficult to see on plain film. Radiologic stability is best assessed by CT, which will better delineate the aforementioned features and prove the absence of posterior cortical displacement or middle column involvement. The injury may not be appreciated on axial CT images, as the plane of imaging is parallel to the fracture line, but they are well demonstrated on the sagittal reformatted images. MR imaging will demonstrate marrow edema as a secondary indicator of fracture in addition to any associated soft tissue injuries (**Fig. 22**). The mechanism of injury is an axial loading with or without a flexion component. The 2 population groups in whom this fracture occurs are young patients with a major trauma and osteoporotic patients with an insufficiency fracture. The superior vertebral end plate usually is affected in traumatic and benign insufficiency fractures whereas involvement of the inferior vertebral end plate raises suspicion for a pathologic fracture. Because 20% of vertebral compression fractures are multiple (**Fig. 23**), it is often recommended that the entire spinal axis be screened if a fracture is discovered.[4,60]

Lateral Compression Fracture

A lateral wedge compression fracture is characterized radiologically by a lateral wedge deformity of the vertebral body. This fracture occurs most commonly at the thoracolumbar junction followed by the midthoracic regions at T6-T7. Frontal radiographs may be suitable to establish the diagnosis showing the lateral extension of the fracture. CT confirms the diagnosis by showing an intact posterior vertebral body wall and no fragment retropulsion. The main risk factor is osteoporosis,

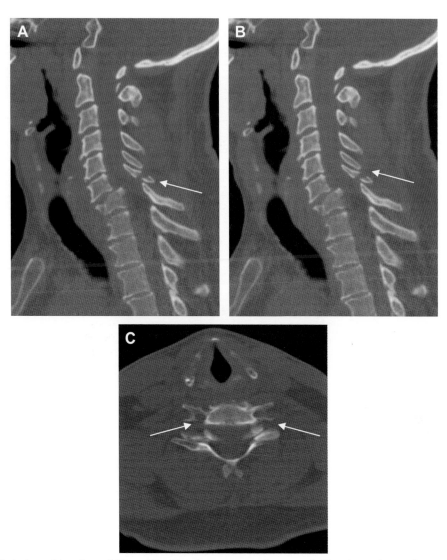

Fig. 13. Anterior subluxation of C6 on C7 with spinous process fracture of C6 and anterior wedge compression fracture of C7. (*A, B*) Sagittal reformatted CT demonstrates approximately 25% anterolisthesis of C6 on C7 with subluxation of the facet joints at C6-C7 (*white arrows*). There is an oblique fracture through the spinous process of C6 and there is loss of stature of the anterior body of C7 secondary to a compression fracture. (*C*) Axial CT confirms the bilateral facet subluxation (*white arrows*).

with many patients complaining of severe and pro-longed pain (**Fig. 24**).[4]

Burst Fracture

A burst fracture is typically produced by pure axial loading mechanism, and is distinguished from an anterior wedge compression fracture by the comminuted fracture of the vertebral body extending through both the superior and inferior vertebral end plates. The mechanism of injury is typically a vertical force such as jumping or falling from a height. Because of the mechanism of injury, burst fractures are often associated with bilateral calcaneal fracture, the so-called lovers' leap fracture. A varying degree of rotation and comminution of the fracture fragments may occur. The requisite imaging feature of the burst injury is retropulsion of the posterior aspect of the vertebral body (ie, the middle column) into the spinal canal or posterior bowing of the posterior vertebral margin. Radiography usually shows a wedge-shaped vertebral body with widened pedicles. CT is superior in evaluating the burst fracture, demonstrating a comminuted vertebral body best seen on axial views. CT shows the degree of posterior retropulsion and

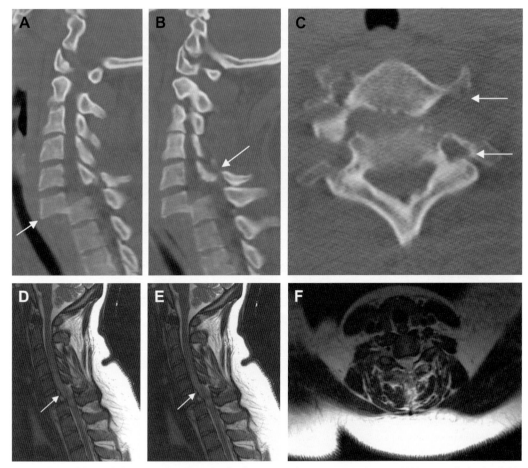

Fig. 14. Bilateral facet dislocation. (*A, B*) Sagittal reformat CT demonstrates almost 100% anterolisthesis of C6 on C7 (*white arrow*) with jumped or locked facet joints (*white arrow*). (*C*) Axial CT at C6-C7 shows bilateral facet dislocation with the "double vertebral body sign" (*white arrows*). (*D–F*) T2 and STIR sagittal and T2 axial MR sequences show abnormal signal consistent with disruption of the anterior longitudinal, the posterior longitudinal, and interspinous ligaments at C6-C7. There is abnormal T2 hyperintense signal throughout the cord from C5 to C7 consistent with spinal cord edema (*white arrows*).

any posterior displacement of bone fragments into the spinal canal. Burst fractures most commonly occur at the thoracolumbar junction, especially T12 and L1. In these regions, retropulsion of bony fragments can cause significant neurologic compromise. In patients with burst fractures with minimal trauma, an underlying cause such as osteoporosis or malignancy should be considered. There is also an increased incidence of sacral and pelvic fractures. Neurologic stability has been defined as spinal canal stenosis of greater than 50%. Surgical versus nonsurgical treatment of burst fractures without neurologic sequelae has been debated recently. There is a body of literature advocating a conservative, nonsurgical approach, with surgical intervention reserved for cases of delayed instability or pain. These options include bed rest or immobilization with or without casting/bracing. There are few good long-term follow up data for simple burst fractures, likely because of the variable management approach. At present, the choice between conservative management and surgery for burst fractures depends on the practice patterns of the surgeon and clinical status of the patient (**Figs. 25–27**).[4,61–64]

Chance Fracture

A Chance fracture involves compression of the anterior column with distraction of the middle and posterior columns. The term "distraction" refers to a complete separation of bone fragments in a craniocaudal direction. The classic Chance or lap-belt injury has decreased in incidence in recent

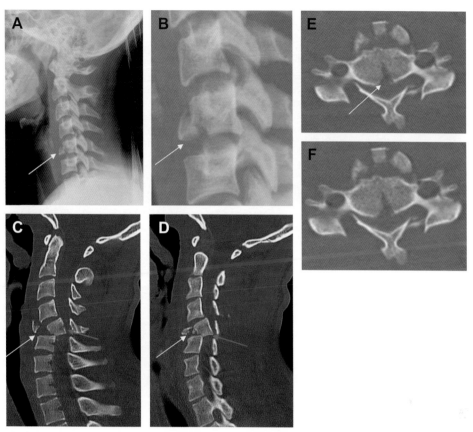

Fig. 15. Flexion teardrop fracture. (*A, B*) Lateral radiographs and (*C, D*) sagittal CT reformats of the cervical spine demonstrate a typical flexion teardrop injury with an anterior triangular fracture fragment (the teardrop) of the anteroinferior aspect of the vertebral body of C5 (*white arrows*) and retropulsion of its posterior vertebral body fragment into the spinal canal with localized kyphotic angulation at C5-C6 (*red arrows*). (*E, F*) Axial CT images demonstrate a sagittal fracture of the vertebral body (*white arrow*).

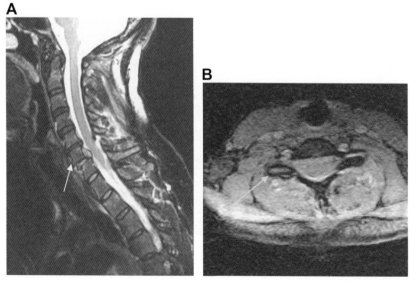

Fig. 16. Unilateral facet dislocation. (*A*) Sagittal T2-weighted MR shows mild anterolisthesis of C6 on C7 (*white arrow*). (*B*) There is unilateral right-sided facet joint dislocation (*yellow arrow*).

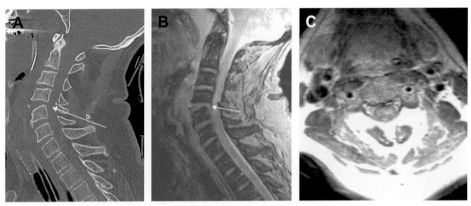

Fig. 17. Hyperextension dislocation. (*A*) Sagittal reformat CT demonstrates mild posterior displacement of C4 on C5 with distraction of the anterior and middle columns (*white arrow*). (*B, C*) T2-weighted sagittal and axial MR confirm these findings and demonstrate widening of the C4-C5 disc space (*white arrow*).

times with the routine use of conventional 3-point restraint.[65] A classic Chance fracture is a horizontal fracture through the spinous process, the lamina, the pedicles, the intervertebral disc space, and the posterior longitudinal, supraspinous, and intraspinous ligaments. The anterior longitudinal ligament is generally intact but may be disrupted in severe injuries. Chance fracture most commonly occurs at L1-L3. It is an acutely unstable injury and is associated with a high rate of abdominal viscera injury.[66] On radiography the findings may be subtle, and include wedging of the anterior vertebral body and increased interspinous distance, that is, posterior element distraction, disc widening, and/or a horizontal fracture through the vertebra. CT is more sensitive, with the sagittal reformatted image showing a horizontally oriented fracture extending across the posterior elements and continuing into the vertebral body with more separation of the fragments posteriorly. The management of these patients depends on the neurologic damage and/or the degree of extraspinal injuries. Due to the extensive degree of soft tissue disruption, the majority of patients do

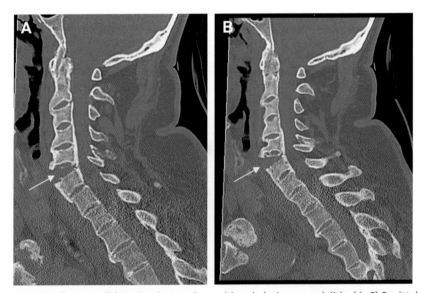

Fig. 18. Hyperextension fracture dislocation in a patient with ankylosing spondylitis. (*A, B*) Sagittal CT reformats demonstrate squaring of the vertebral bodies, syndesmophytes, and calcification of the anterior and posterior longitudinal ligaments, producing a "bamboo spine" appearance. There is a fracture through the calcified anterior longitudinal ligament at C5-C6 extending through and widening the C5-C6 disc space, consistent with a hyperextension fracture dislocation (*white arrows*).

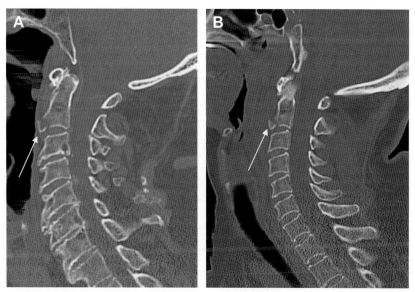

Fig. 19. Hyperextension teardrop fracture. (*A, B*) Sagittal CT reformats demonstrate a fracture through the anteroinferior corner of C2 with the vertical dimension of the fracture greater than the transverse dimension. There is an avulsed triangular fragment of bone from the anterior aspect of C2, a "teardrop segment" (*white arrows*).

require surgery with correction of the deformity (**Figs. 28** and **29**).[67]

Fracture Dislocation

A variety of fracture dislocations of the thoracolumbar spine can occur as a result of combined shearing and flexion forces. With severe hyperflexion injuries, dislocation occurs anteriorly. With flexion rotation injuries, dislocation of the facet joints may occur, with traumatic spondylolisthesis. With severe hyperextension injuries, usually from a blow to the back, there is classically posterior element impaction with fractures of the spinous process, lamina, or facet. Instability results from anterior ligament injuries, with

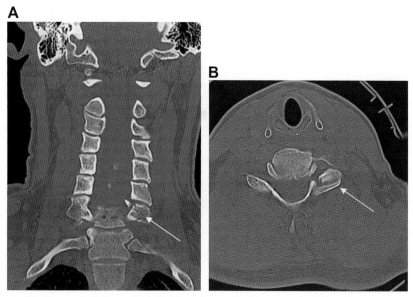

Fig. 20. Isolated pillar fracture of C7 on the left. (*A, B*) Coronal reformat and axial CT demonstrate a comminuted fracture of the lateral articular mass of C7 (*white arrows*).

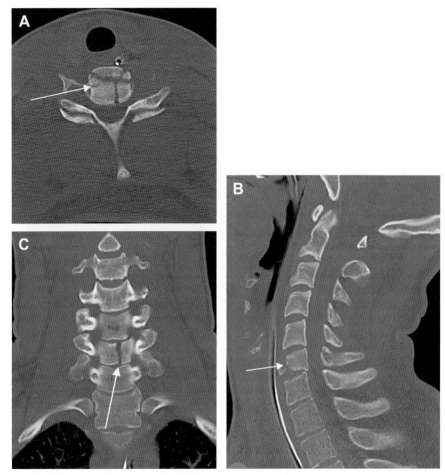

Fig. 21. Cervical burst fracture. (*A*) Axial CT demonstrates a comminuted fracture of a cervical vertebral body with mild retropulsion posteriorly (*white arrow*). (*B*) Sagittal reformat CT demonstrates a burst type fracture of C6 (*white arrow*). (*C*) Coronal reformat CT demonstrates the vertical course of the fracture (*white arrow*).

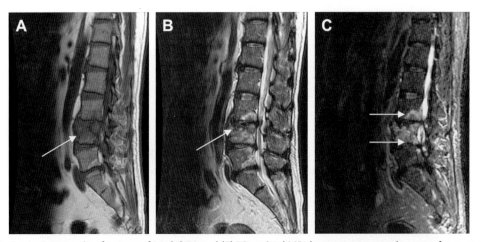

Fig. 22. Acute compression fracture of L4. (*A*) T1 and (*B*) T2 sagittal MR demonstrate a wedge-type fracture deformity of the anterior body of L4 (*white arrows*). (*C*) STIR sagittal MR demonstrates bone marrow edema changes in the inferior vertebral end plate of L3 and throughout the body of L4, indicating that this is an acute fracture (*white arrows*).

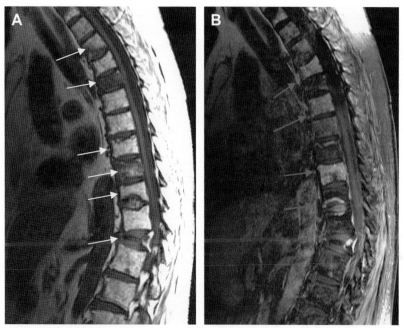

Fig. 23. Multiple thoracolumbar compression fractures. (*A*) T1 and (*B*) STIR sagittal sequences demonstrate multiple insufficiency type vertebral body fractures of varying ages (*white arrows*). There is hyperintense signal within several the vertebral bodies on the STIR sequence, indicating bone marrow edema consistent with more recent or acute fractures (*red arrows*).

widening of the anterior intervertebral disc space and retrolisthesis. There is frequently spinal cord injury (**Fig. 30**).[68]

Other Fractures of the Thoracolumbar Spine

Fractures of the transverse processes of the thoracolumbar spine can and do occur. These fractures can be missed on plain radiography, with CT being more sensitive for detection. The presence of a transverse process fracture increases the likelihood of other injuries including additional transverse process fractures, additional vertebral fractures, and/or abdominal viscera injury (**Fig. 31**).[69] Other fractures that can occur include spinous process fractures or pars interarticularis fractures.

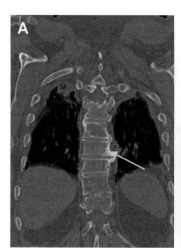
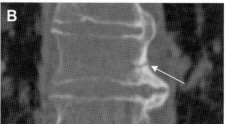

Fig. 24. Lateral T8 cortex fracture. (*A*, *B*) Coronal reformat CT demonstrates a linear nondisplaced fracture through the left lateral cortex of T8 (*yellow* and *white arrows*).

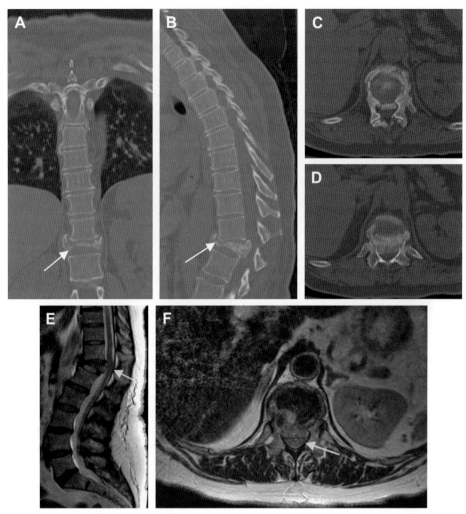

Fig. 25. Burst fracture of T12. (*A, B*) Coronal and sagittal CT reformats of the thoracolumbar spine demonstrate a burst type fracture of T12 with near complete loss of height of the T12 vertebral body, buckling of the posterior cortex of the T12 vertebral body, and posterior bony retropulsion, causing bony canal narrowing (*white arrows*). (*C, D*) Axial CT demonstrates the comminuted nature of the fracture. (*E, F*) Sagittal and axial T2-weighted MR demonstrate the spinal canal narrowing caused by the fracture (*yellow arrows*).

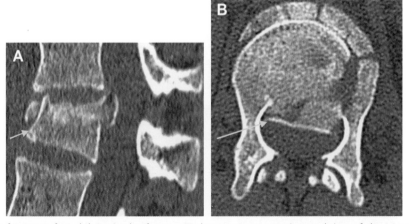

Fig. 26. Burst fracture of L1. (*A*) Sagittal reformat CT demonstrates anterior wedging of the L1 vertebral body with posterior bony retropulsion into the bony canal (*yellow arrow*). (*B*) Axial CT demonstrates the comminuted pattern of the fracture and the degree of retropulsion (*yellow arrow*).

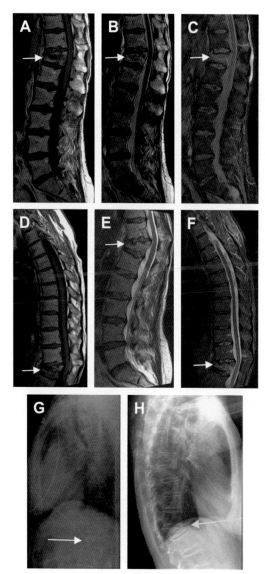

Fig. 27. Failure of conservative management of a T12 burst fracture. (A–C) T1, T2, and STIR sagittal MR demonstrate a burst fracture of T12 with approximately 30% to 40% loss of height anteriorly (*white arrows*). (D–F) T1, T2, and STIR sagittal MR performed 3 months later following conservative treatment with a back brace demonstrate progressive wedging of the T12 vertebral body with approximately 50% loss of height anteriorly (*white arrows*). Plain films at diagnosis (G) and 3 months later (H) demonstrate the interval change (*white and yellow arrows*).

SACRAL FRACTURES

High-velocity injuries of the pelvis can result in traumatic sacral fractures. The best radiographic clue is disruption of the sacral arcuate lines. Approximately 95% of these fractures are vertical

or oblique and 5% are horizontal. Approximately 95% occur in association with other pelvic fractures, and the symptoms can be masked by concurrent injuries at higher levels. There are 3 classic appearances: the first is the "open book," which is a vertically oriented fracture; the second is a "T-bone injury," which is an impacted vertically oriented fracture producing a sclerotic line; and the third is a "vertical shear," which is a vertically oriented fracture with vertical displacement and/ or fractures of the L5 transverse processes. Lumbar spine fractures will be present in up to 30% of patients with sacral fractures. The Denis system is used to classify sacral fractures; zone 1 is lateral to the neural foramina, zone 2 is through the neural foramina, and zone 3 is through the spinal canal. A fracture confined to the sacrum only is considered a stable fracture, but fracture involving the sacrum and another component of the bony pelvis (ie, 2 fractures) is considered an unstable fracture (**Fig. 32**).[4,5,70]

A sacral insufficiency fracture is a stress fracture from normal physiologic force on demineralized bone, most commonly occurring in patients with osteoporosis. This fracture can sometimes be overlooked on an MR image of the lumbar spine. The MR signs are of unilateral or bilateral T1 hypointensity and T2/short-tau inversion recovery hyperintensity in the sacrum. The classic "Honda sign" on bone scan is produced by a characteristic H-shaped pattern of radiotracer uptake in the sacrum (**Fig. 33**).[71]

MR IMAGING OF SPINAL TRAUMA

MR imaging has revolutionized the diagnosis of spinal cord injury and provides the best imaging evaluation of the intervertebral discs, the ligaments, and the spinal cord. Plain radiography and CT are the most appropriate, quickest, and cost-effective methods of assessing for spinal injury, particularly fractures, in the initial acute diagnostic stage. MR imaging, however, has replaced myelography and CT myelography as the primary imaging modality in assessing for epidural hematoma, ligamentous injury, traumatic disc herniation, and spinal cord compression. However, these modalities are reserved only for patients in whom MR imaging is contraindicated.

At a minimum, T1 and T2 sagittal imaging of the spine should be obtained. The T1 sequences provide information on basic anatomy. The T2 sequences are the best for visualizing spinal cord injury, ligamentous edema/disruption, marrow edema, and traumatic disc herniation. A sagittal proton density sequence is useful for confirming ligamentous disruption and/or identifying epidural

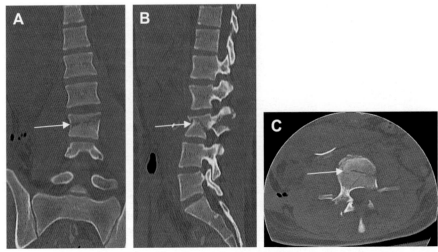

Fig. 28. Chance fracture. (*A*) Coronal, (*B*) sagittal, and (*C*) axial CT images of the thoracolumbar spine demonstrate a comminuted fracture of the posterior vertebral body with a horizontal or split component extending into the pedicles, the bases of the transverse processes, the laminae, and into the spinous process (*white arrows*).

blood/fluid collections. A sagittal gradient echo sequence is useful for detection of spinal cord hemorrhage. Axial T2 sequences are useful to confirm spinal cord signal abnormality identified on the sagittal sequence. An axial T1 with fat saturation is useful to identify vascular dissection. The area of interest, the cervical, thoracic, or lumbar spine, should be imaged first and, depending on the patient's clinical status, the MR findings, and patient cooperation, MR of the additional spinal levels can be obtained. Limited surveys can be obtained if the examination needs to be rapidly terminated.[72]

At present, MR imaging does not offer any advantage over CT in spinal osseous injuries. CT, or at least plain radiography when CT is not available, should first be obtained to assess for osseous fractures. MR imaging is less sensitive than CT in fracture detection but can demonstrate bone marrow edema related to compressive injuries (**Fig. 34**).

MR imaging directly visualizes changes to the anterior longitudinal ligament, the posterior longitudinal ligament, the ligamentum flava, and the interspinous ligaments. Ligamentous rupture is visualized as focal discontinuity with or without associated hematoma. Widening of the facet joints with increased fluid signal can be demonstrated, suggesting a distraction injury (**Fig. 35**).

Posttraumatic disc herniation is more common in the cervical and thoracic regions, unlike degenerative disc herniations. Posttraumatic disc injuries on MR imaging can be classified as either disc injury or disc herniation. Traumatic disc injury manifests as narrowing or widening of the disc

space with T2 hyperintense signal abnormality, usually reflecting tearing of the disc substance. Traumatic disc herniation has a similar MR appearance to nontraumatic disc herniation (**Fig. 36**).

Epidural hematoma is frequently seen in spinal cord injury. Fortunately, it is generally asymptomatic. The imaging characteristics vary with the oxidative state of the hemorrhage and the clot retraction. The incidence of posttraumatic epidural hematoma is greater in patients with ankylosing spondylitis (**Fig. 37**).[73]

Dissection of the vertebral artery is more common than dissection of the carotid artery because the vertebral arteries are fixed in location by the foramina transversaria. Prior data suggest the incidence of vertebral artery dissection in cervical spinal trauma to be as high as 40%, with a large subclinical cohort. Early recognition of this injury is crucial because of its associated morbidity. Neck MRA with 2-dimensional time-of-flight and T1 fat saturation axial sequences are used to screen for this potential complication (**Fig. 38**).

Spinal cord injury without radiographic abnormality (SCIWORA) is defined as spinal cord injury with normal plain radiographs. SCIWORA occurs in children and adults. It usually occurs in the cervical spine following a rear-end motor vehicle accident or direct facial trauma, resulting in a hyperextension sprain or dislocation, sometimes on superimposed cervical spondylosis. Plain radiographs are frequently normal. MR imaging is of particular diagnostic value because it depicts many abnormalities that cannot be seen on plain

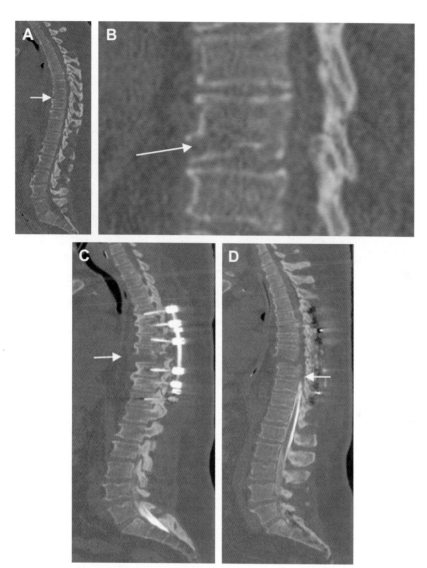

Fig. 29. Chance distraction type fracture. (*A, B*) Sagittal reformat CT demonstrates a horizontal fracture through the inferior vertebral end plate of T8 extending into the posterior elements (*white arrows*). The patient underwent posterior thoracolumbar fusion but his symptoms progressed. (*C*) Sagittal reformat CT myelographic images demonstrate a fracture through the inferior vertebral end plate of T8 with widening of the fracture in the craniocaudal direction (distraction) (*white arrow*). (*D*) Sagittal reformat CT myelographic images demonstrate contrast opacification from the sacrum to T9, where there is a myelographic block (*white arrow*).

radiography, including separation of the intervertebral disc, rupture of the anterior longitudinal ligament, prevertebral hemorrhage, and/or parenchymal spinal cord injury.[74]

MR IMAGING FINDINGS IN SPINAL CORD INJURY

MR imaging is the best imaging modality in evaluation of the spinal cord injury, providing information that helps determine prognosis and potential for patient recovery. MR is the best imaging modality for depicting the internal architecture of the spinal cord. However, it can be difficult to distinguish spinal gray matter from white matter, particularly on the sagittal sequences. The central gray matter is uniformly hyperintense to white matter on all pulse sequences, which is attributed to the higher spin density of gray matter. These image characteristics are usually lost after

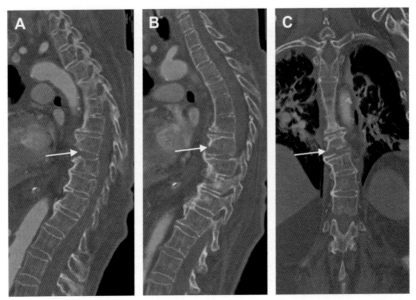

Fig. 30. Fracture distraction. (*A, B*) Sagittal CT reformats and (*C*) coronal CT of the thoracolumbar spine reconstructed from a postcontrast CT of abdomen and pelvis demonstrates a fracture through the anteroinferior body of T7 with distraction (*white arrows*).

spinal cord injury because of accumulation of edema and hemorrhage with swelling of the cord parenchyma.[75]

Spinal cord hemorrhage, as a manifestation of spinal cord injury, usually occurs in the central gray matter of the cord at the point of maximal mechanical impact. Pathologic studies have shown that the underlying lesion is usually hemorrhagic necrosis. In the acute phase following injury the blood products are in the deoxyhemoglobin state, manifesting as hypointensity on T2 and gradient echo images. Deoxyhemoglobin evolves into methemoglobin (animal studies have suggested a time period of up to 8 days), which manifests as hyperintensity on T2 images. Many studies have shown that parenchymal hemorrhage develops rapidly in the cord following trauma. MR imaging can detect the anatomic location and the extent of the hemorrhage. The presence of frank hemorrhage carries a poorer prognosis.[76]

Spinal cord edema, as a manifestation of spinal cord injury, is best demonstrated on T2-weighted sequences as abnormal T2 hyperintense signal within the affected cord segment (**Fig. 39**). Spinal cord edema reflects a focal accumulation of intracellular and interstitial fluid in response to injury, involves a variable length of the cord above and below the level of the injury, and is invariably associated with a degree of swelling. It usually occurs in association with spinal cord hemorrhage, but

not always; spinal cord edema without hemorrhage carries a more favorable prognosis.[77]

Spinal cord swelling, as a manifestation of spinal cord injury, is a focal increase in the caliber of the spinal cord centered at the level of the injury. The cord is normally uniform in caliber with minimal changes at the lower cervical and lower thoracic levels. Abnormal cord swelling is best demonstrated on T1-weighted sequences. The swelling can occur in association with spinal cord hemorrhage and/or edema, and is by itself an indicator of spinal cord injury but not a predictor of the degree of underlying spinal cord dysfunction.[78]

INITIAL ASSESSMENT OF SPINAL CORD TRAUMA

The initial management of a patient with suspected spinal cord injury consists of resuscitating and stabilizing the patient. In the immediate management of any patient with a suspected cervical spine injury, complete cervical spine immobilization is mandatory.[79] Further assessment with a neurologic examination is used to make diagnoses and treatment decisions for the patient. However, it is often difficult to perform an accurate and/or complete neurologic examination of the patient because of a variety of factors including the urgency for medical stabilization, surgical interventions, and factors limiting patient

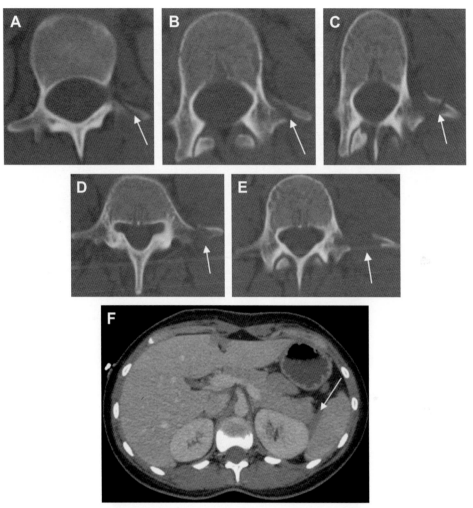

Fig. 31. Transverse process fractures. Axial CT demonstrates acute fractures through the left transverse processes of L1 (*A*), L2 (*B*), L3 (*C*), L4 (*D*), and L5 (*E*) (*white arrows*). Axial postcontrast CT (*F*) demonstrates a small hematoma in the splenic hilum (*white arrow*).

cooperation such as pain, analgesics, alcohol, and drugs. Often, a repeat neurologic examination performed 3 to 7 days after the injury is a better indicator of prognosis than the initial examination.[80,81]

The most frequently used scale to classify spinal cord injury is the American Spinal Injury Association (ASIA) impairment scale (AIS), a 5-point scale from A to E; where AIS A is complete loss of motor and sensory function below the neurologic level including the sacral dermatomes (S4-S5), AIS B is complete loss of motor power with sparing of sensation in the sacral dermatomes (eg, S4-S5), AIS C and AIS D represent motor incomplete injuries differentiated by motor strength, and E is normal.[82,83]

Another clinical parameter that has a significant impact on patient diagnosis, neurologic function, and potential to recover neurologic function is the neurologic level of injury (NLI). The NLI is determined from assessing the motor power and sensory function for myotomes and dermatomes that are innervated by adjacent spinal cord segments. The most caudally intact myotome or dermatome is determined in order to determine the NLI. By inference, the NLI obtained from clinical examination determines the location of the lesion in the spinal cord. Many studies have shown high concurrence rates between the NLI and MR imaging signal changes.[84]

MEDICAL MANAGEMENT OF SPINAL CORD INJURY INCLUDING MEDICAL COMPLICATIONS

Many patients with spinal cord injuries are trauma patients. The initial management of these patients

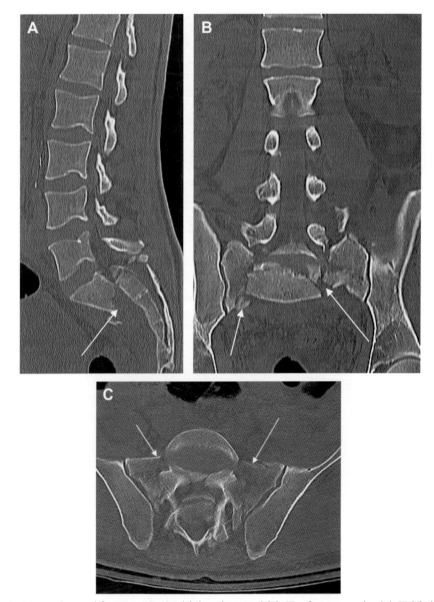

Fig. 32. Acute traumatic sacral fractures. Sagittal (*A*) and coronal (*B*) CT reformats and axial CT (*C*) demonstrate bilateral comminuted fractures of the sacral ala with anterior displacement of the fractured proximal sacral segment (*white arrows*).

consists of basic life support, with full attention to airway management and breathing and circulation parameters. A full primary and secondary survey is necessary, as these patients may have distracting injuries.

Following medical stabilization, determination of approximate level and extent of spinal cord injury, and surgical assessment, pharmacotherapy with methylprednisolone is considered. The use of methylprednisolone in the treatment of acute spinal cord injury is controversial with regard to indication, dosage, and timing. However, most trauma centers will use it at up to 8 hours after injury.[85]

The initial and subsequent medical management of spinal cord injury patients is directed toward prevention of the many medical complications that patients with spinal cord injury are prone

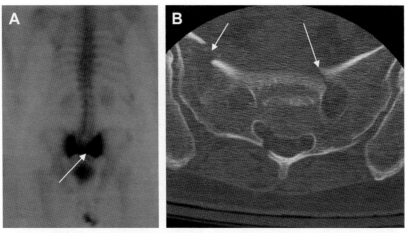

Fig. 33. The Honda sign with a sacral insufficiency fracture. (*A*) A nuclear medicine bone scan demonstrates diffuse uptake of radiotracer throughout the sacrum in an H shape, the Honda sign (*white arrow*). (*B*) Axial CT demonstrates bilateral sacral fractures and osteopenia (*white arrows*).

to develop. These complications include urinary tract infections, pressure ulcers, pain, depression, spasticity, pneumonia, autonomic dysreflexia, deep venous thrombosis with occasional subsequent pulmonary emboli, renal and bladder stones, renal failure, and heterotopic ossification.[1,86] Deep venous thrombosis with or without subsequent pulmonary emboli occur in 47% to 100% of patients with spinal cord injury, and is a life threatening complication.[87] The use of antithrombotic compression stockings is standard.

Several clinical guidelines support the use of low-dose subcutaneous or low molecular weight heparin as prophylaxis.[88] This prophylactic treatment should last for 2 to 3 months. Despite several case series in the literature, at present the literature does not support the use of prophylactic inferior vena cava filters.[89] If contraindications to anticoagulation exist in a patient with a proven deep venous thrombosis or pulmonary embolism, then an inferior vena cava filter is indicated.[90] The aim of management is to prevent recurrent

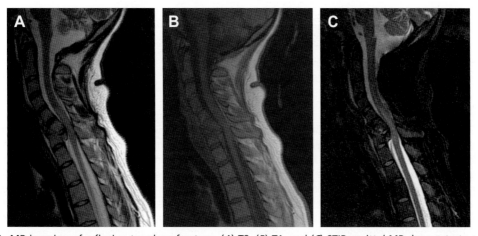

Fig. 34. MR imaging of a flexion teardrop fracture. (*A*) T2, (*B*) T1, and (*C*) STIR sagittal MR demonstrate a hypointense band through the anteroinferior body of C6 with STIR hyperintensity throughout C6 consistent with a fracture. MR is less sensitive than CT in fracture detection but can be diagnosed, as in this case. Additional findings include posterior subluxation of C6 compressing the spinal cord with T2 hyperintense signal from C5 to C7, consistent with spinal cord edema.

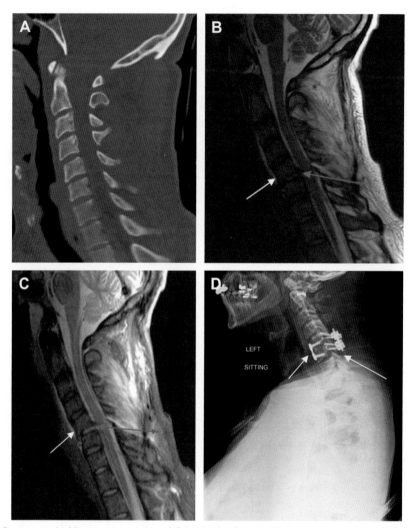

Fig. 35. MR of acute cervical ligamentous injury. (*A*) Sagittal reformat CT demonstrates normal alignment with no fracture. (*B*) T2 and (*C*) STIR sagittal MR demonstrates anterior subluxation of C5 on C6 (*white arrows*) with signal abnormality in the posterior longitudinal ligament and spinous ligaments at C5-C6 (*red arrows*). (*D*) The patient was surgically stabilized with a C5-C6 anterior and posterior fusion (*white arrows*).

pulmonary emboli.[91] Patients with a neurologic level above T6 are at risk for a life-threatening condition called autonomic dysreflexia, in which noxious stimuli can cause malignant hypertension leading to cardiovascular compromise.[92] There are clinical guidelines regarding autonomic dysreflexia, and it is prudent to be aware of this potential complication when managing a patient with a spinal cord injury.[93] Pulmonary complications are the leading cause of mortality in the first year of recovery from a spinal cord injury as well as in long-term survivors.[86] As such, attention must be given to reducing all risk factors for respiratory

complications in patients. Depending on the level of the spinal cord injury, patients may require temporary or permanent ventilator support.[94] Because of immobility and absence of sensation, pressure ulcers or decubiti can form, which can lead to more severe sequelae such as sepsis and osteomyelitis. Prevention of decubiti requires vigilance regarding regular patient turning/repositioning, adequate nutrition, regular assessment of parameters such as albumin, and prompt consultation with a wound care specialist when a pressure ulcer develops.[95] Neurogenic bowel and bladder dysfunction are also common in patients

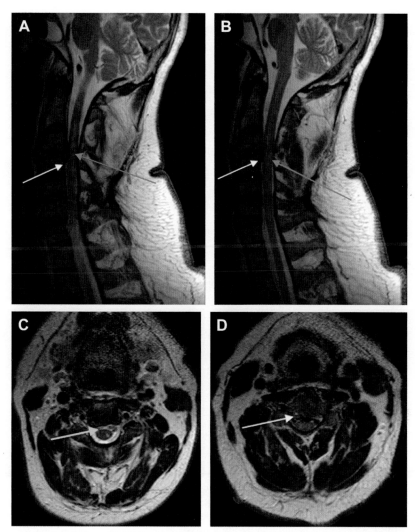

Fig. 36. Traumatic disc herniation. (*A*, *B*) T2 sagittal MR of the cervical spine demonstrates an extrusion type disc herniation at C3-C4 (*white arrows*) displacing the posterior longitudinal ligament and compressing the spinal cord with diffuse T2 hyperintense cord signal from C2 to C5 (*red arrows*). T2 axial MR above the level of the extrusion (*C*) demonstrates normal subarachnoid space anterior to the cord (*yellow arrow*). T2 axial MR at the level of the extrusion (*D*) demonstrates an extruded disc that compresses the cord and causes diffuse T2 hyperintense signal, consistent with cord edema (*white arrow*).

with spinal cord injury. Without proper care, this can lead to recurrent urinary tract infections and sepsis. Close attention needs to be maintained to prevent these complications with regard to diet, stool softeners, and urinary catheterization.[96]

SURGICAL TREATMENT OF SPINAL CORD INJURY

Surgical management of spinal cord injuries can vary from simple external bracing with limitation of activity to complex instrumentation of the spine.

The approach to management can vary from center to center, but the overall aim is to use the least invasive technique to stabilize the injured segment and prevent long-term complications.

Numerous spinal braces are available for the treatment of spinal injuries. The principle of bracing is to reduce motion at the injured spinal area in order to improve the likelihood of healing and reduce the potential for spinal cord injury from an unstable injury. For cervical spine injury, bracing ranges from soft and hard collars (eg, the Miami J collar; Ossur, Foothill Ranch, CA, USA)

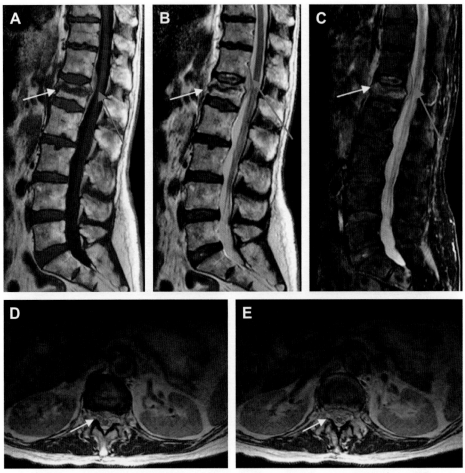

Fig. 37. Epidural hematoma. Sagittal MR of the lumbar spine demonstrates a burst fracture of L1 (*white arrows*) with (*A*) T1 hyperintense, (*B*) T2 isointense, and (*C*) STIR hyperintense, extra-axial material posterior to T12-L2, consistent with blood products (*red arrows*). (*D, E*) T2 axials confirm the epidural location of the blood products, confirming that this is an epidural hematoma (*white arrows*).

to bracing (eg, the Minerva brace) to halo vest immobilization. A simple cervical collar is the least cumbersome but comes at a cost in that it does allow a very limited range of motion. A brace is more cumbersome but allows less movement. Halo vest immobilization provides the most rigid immobilization by fixating a halo ring around the head and securing the halo ring to a thoracic vest with rods.

The upper thoracic spine is a difficult region to immobilize with external orthosis, and requires a long thoracic vest. Spinal fractures from T6-L2 are easier to immobilize with bracing. Casting is another option for lumbar and lumbosacral immobilization.

Surgical intervention in spinal trauma is required to decompress the neural elements in cases of neurologic deficit, to prevent spinal cord injury from potentially unstable injuries, to correct and prevent deformity that could cause long-term adverse neurologic sequelae, and to provide for early mobilization. Anterior, posterior, and combined approaches can be taken operatively. All approaches require a form of spinal instrumentation, defined as a means of straightening and stabilizing the spine using hooks, rods, or wires. An anterior approach is favored when a herniated disc or bone fragment compresses the spinal cord. A posterior approach with instrumentation is favored when deformities are present. A combined anterior and posterior approach is favored for fracture-dislocation injuries when anterior-posterior instrumentation increases the success rate for a surgical stabilization procedure.[4]

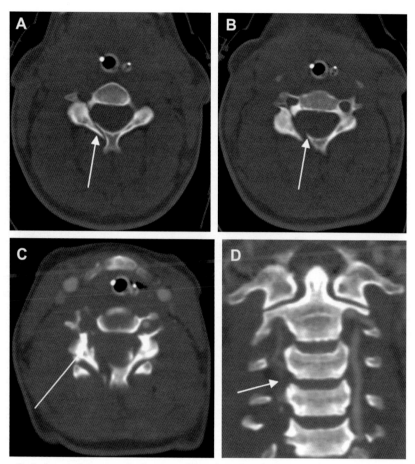

Fig. 38. Traumatic induced right vertebral artery dissection. (*A, B*) Axial CT images in this intubated patient demonstrate a fracture through the right lamina of C4 extending into the right pedicle and through the posterior wall of the right foramen transversarium (*white arrows*). (*C*) CT angiogram through the neck demonstrates no flow in the right vertebral artery at C4 (*white arrow*). (*D*) Coronal CT angiogram reformat through the neck demonstrates no flow in the right vertebral artery at C3-C4 with marked attenuation of the C2-C3 segment of the vessel, reflecting acute dissection (*white arrow*).

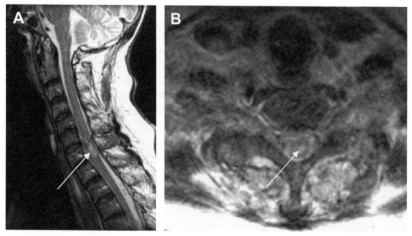

Fig. 39. Spinal cord edema. (*A*) Sagittal and (*B*) axial T2-weighted MR through the cervical cord demonstrate diffuse T2 hyperintense signal at C6, reflecting spinal cord edema (*white arrows*).

SUMMARY

Spine trauma is a complex diagnostic area in which the radiological assessment is crucial. Plain radiography is often used as the initial diagnostic modality. However, stabilization of the acutely injured spine is a primary concern. In this respect, CT is vastly superior to plain film in terms of speed and accuracy. CT requires much less patient mobilization than plain film. In many trauma centers, CT has replaced plain film as the primary modality for evaluation of spinal trauma. MR imaging is not indicated for all cases of spinal trauma but provides detailed information about soft tissue structures including the intervertebral disc, the ligaments, the epidural space, the blood vessels, and the spinal cord. MR imaging provides information on these structures not obtained from other modalities. Patients with spinal cord injury may suffer devastating long-term neurologic deficits, so prompt and efficient spinal imaging guidelines are necessary in all trauma centers. Both the radiologist and the physician need to be aware of the patterns of injury and the implications of these injuries.

REFERENCES

1. National Spinal Cord Injury Statistical Center. Spinal cord injury: facts and figures at a glance. Available at: www.spinalcord.uab.edu. Accessed December 17, 2009.
2. DeVivo MJ. Epidemiology of traumatic spinal cord injury. In: Kirshblum S, Campagnolo DI, DeLisa JA, editors. Spinal cord medicine. Philadelphia: Lippincott, Williams & Wilkins; 2002. p. 69–81.
3. Krause JS, Kewman D, DeVivo MJ, et al. Employment after spinal cord injury: an analysis of cases from the model spinal cord injury systems. Arch Phys Med Rehabil 1999;80:1492–500.
4. Schwartz ED, Flanders AE. Spinal trauma: imaging, diagnosis and management. Lipincott; 2007. p. 23–4.
5. Weissledder R, Wittenberg J, Harisinghani MG. Primer of diagnostic imaging. Mosby; 2002. p. 370-8.
6. Greenspan A. Orthopedic radiology. A practical approach. Philadelphia: Lippincott-Raven; 2000.
7. Sekhon LH, Fehlings MG. Epidemiology, demographics, and pathophysiology of acute spinal cord injury. Spine 2001;26(Suppl 24):S2–12.
8. Heinemann U, Freund M. Diagnostic strategies in spinal trauma. Eur J Radiol 2006;58:76–88.
9. Hu R, Mustard CA, Burns C. Epidemiology of incident spinal fracture in a complete population. Spine (Phila Pa 1976) 1996;21(4):492–9.
10. Cooper C, Atkinson EJ, O'Fallon WM, et al. Incidence of clinically diagnosed vertebral injuries: a population based study in Rochester, Minnesota, 1985-1989. J Bone Miner Res 1992;7:221–7.
11. Foster MR. C1 Fractures. In: JF. Kellam, editor. eMedicine, 19 Dec 2003. Medscape 22 Dec 2008.
12. Boyarsky I, Godorov G. C2 Fractures. In: JF Kellam, et al, editors. eMedicine. 30 Jun 2003. Medscape 11 Oct 2004.
13. Hertner GL, Stewart NJ. Cervical spine acute bony injuries. In: JP Ertl, et al. editors. eMedicine. 9 Jan 2004. Medscape. 11 Oct 2004.
14. Grossman MD, Reilly PM, Gillett D. National survey of the incidence of cervical spine injury and approach to cervical spine clearance in US trauma Centers. J Trauma 1999;47:684–90.
15. Liebermann IH, Webb JK. Cervical spine injuries in the elderly. J Bone Joint Surg Br 1994;76:877–81.
16. Lomoschitz F, Blackmore C, Mirza S, et al. Cervical spine injuries in patients 65 years and older: epidemiological analysis regarding the effects of age and injury mechanism on distribution, type, and stability of injury. AJR Am J Roentgenol 2002;178:573–7.
17. Bub L, Blackmore C, Mann F, et al. Cervical spine fractures in patients 65 years old: a clinical prediction rule for blunt trauma. Radiology 2005;234:143–9.
18. Viccellio P, Simon H, Pressman B, et al. A prospective multicenter study of cervical spine injury in children. Pediatrics 2001;108:e20.
19. Adelgais KM, Grossman DC, Langer SG, et al. Use of helical computed tomography for imaging the pediatric cervical spine. Acad Emerg Med 2004;11:228–36.
20. Kokoska E, Keller M, Rallo M, et al. Characterestics of pediatric cervical spine injuries. J Pediatr Surg 2001;36:100–5.
21. Nadalo LA, Moody JA. Thoracic spine, trauma. In: Bruno MA, et al, editors. eMedicine. 23 March 2009. Medscape. 11 Nov 2008.
22. Lane JM, Johnson CE, Khan SN, et al. Minimally invasive options for the treatment of osteoporotic vertebral compression fractures. Orthop Clin North Am 2002;33(2):431–8.
23. Leahy M, Rahm M. Thoracic spine fractures and dislocations. In: LH Riley, et al. editors. eMedicine. 12 Dec 2007. Medscape 26 Jan 2009.
24. Levi AD, Hurlbert RJ, Anderson P, et al. Neurologic deterioration secondary to unrecognized spinal instability following trauma-a multicenter study. Spine (Phila Pa 1976) 2006;31(4):451–8.
25. Hoffman JR, Mower WR, Wolfson AB, et al. Validity of a set of clinical criteria to rule out injury to the cervical spine in patients with blunt trauma. National emergency x-radiography utilization group. N Engl J Med 2000;343:94–9.
26. Stiell IG, Wells GA, Vandemheen KL, et al. The Canadian C-spine rule for radiography in alert and stable trauma patients. JAMA 2001;286:1841–8.

27. Sliker CW, Mirvis SE, Shanmuganathan K. Assessing cervical spine stability in obtunded blunt trauma patients: review of the medical literature. Radiology 2005;234:733–9.

28. Platzer P, Jaindl M, Thalhammer G, et al. Clearing the cervical spine in critically injured patients: a comprehensive C-spine protocol to avoid unnecessary delays in diagnosis. Eur Spine J 2006;15(12): 1801–10.

29. Woodring JH, Lee C. Limitations of cervical radiography in the evaluation of acute cervical trauma. J Trauma 1993;34:32–9.

30. Nunez DB, Ahmad AA, Coin GC, et al. Clearing the cervical spine in multiple trauma victims: a time effective protocol using helical CT. Emerg Radiol 1994;1:273–8.

31. Blackmore CC, Ramsey SD, Mann FA, et al. Cervical spine screening with CT in trauma patients; a cost effective analysis. Radiology 1999; 212:117–25.

32. Chiu W, Haan J, Cushing B, et al. Ligamentous injuries of the cervical spine in unreliable blunt trauma patients: incidence, evaluation, and outcome. J Trauma 2001;50:457–64.

33. Knopp R, Parker J, Tashjian J, et al. Defining radiographic criteria for flexion extension studies of the cervical spine. Ann Emerg Med 2001;38:31–5.

34. Insko EK, Gracias VH, Gupta R, et al. Utility of flexion and extension radiographs of the cervical spine in the acute evaluation of blunt trauma. J Trauma 2002;53:426–9.

35. Salfuddin A. MRI of acute spinal trauma. Skeletal Radiol 2001;30:237–46.

36. Frankel HL, Rozycki GS, Ochsner GM, et al. Indications for obtaining surveillance thoracic and lumbar spine radiographs. J Trauma 1994;37:673–6.

37. Sheridan P, Peralta R, Rhea J, et al. Reformatted visceral protocol helical computed tomographic scanning allows conventional radiographs of the thoracic and lumbar spine to be eliminated in the evaluation of blunt trauma patients. J Trauma 2003; 55:665–9.

38. Denis F. The three column spine and its significance in the classification of acute thoracolumbar spinal injuries. Neurosurg Clin N Am 1997;8: 499–507.

39. Bohlman HH. Treatment of fractures and dislocations of the thoracic and lumbar spine. J Bone Joint Surg Am 1985;67:165–9.

40. Harris JH Jr. Mechanistic classification of acute cervical spine injuries. In: Harris JH Jr, Mirvis SE, editors. The radiology of acute cervical spine trauma. 3rd edition. Baltimore (MD): Williams and Wilkins; 1996. p. 213–44.

41. Anderson PA, Montesano PX. Morphology and treatment of occipital condyle fractures. Spine (Phila Pa 1976) 1988;13:731–6.

42. Fisher CG, Sun JC, Divorak M. Recognition and management of atlanto-occipital dislocation: improving survival from an often fatal condition. Can J Surg 2001;44:412–20.

43. Fielding JW, Hawkins RJ. Atlantoaxial rotatory fixation. J Bone Joint Surg Am 1977;59:37–44.

44. Harris JH Jr, Mirvis SE. Vertical compression injuries. In: Harris JH Jr, Mirvis SE, editors. The radiology of acute cervical spine trauma. third edition. Baltimore (MD): Williams and Wilkins; 1996. p. 340–65.

45. Lachman E. Anatomy of the judicial hanging. Res Staff Phys 1972;46:54.

46. Elliot JM, Rogers LF, Wissinger JP, et al. The hangmans fracture. Radiology 1972;104:303–7.

47. Li XF, Dai LY, Lu H, et al. A systematic review of the management of hangman's fractures [review]. Eur Spine J 2006;15(3):257–69.

48. Levine AM, Edwards CC. The management of traumatic spondylolisthesis of the axis. J Bone Joint Surg Am 1985;67:217–26.

49. Anderson LD, D'Alonzo RT. Fractures of the odontoid process of the axis. J Bone Joint Surg Am 1974;56:1663–74.

50. Cancelmo JJ Jr. Clay shovellers fracture. A helpful diagnostic sign. Am J Roentgenol Radium Ther Nucl Med 1972;115(3):540–3.

51. Bohlman HH. Acute fractures and dislocations of the cervical spine-an analysis of 300 hospitalized patients and a review of the literature. J Bone Joint Surg Am 1979;61:1119–42.

52. Doran SE, Papadopoulos SM, Ducker TB, et al. Magnetic resonant imaging documentation of co-existent traumatic locked facets of the cervical spine. J Neurosurg 1993;79(3):341–5.

53. Torg JS, Pavlov H, O'Neill MJ, et al. The axial load teardrop fracture. A biomechanical, clinical and roentgenographic analysis. Am J Sports Med 1991;19(4):355–64.

54. Murray GC, Persellin RH. Cervical fracture complicating ankylosing spondylitis: a report of eight cases and a review of the literature. Am J Med 1981;70(5): 1033–41.

55. Scher AT. Hyperextension trauma in the elderly: an easily overlooked spinal injury. J Trauma 1983;23(12):1066–8.

56. Korres DS, Zoubos AB, Kavadias K, et al. The "tear drop" or avulsed fracture of the anterior inferior angle of the axis. Eur Spine J 1994;3(3):151–4.

57. Cimmino CV, Scott DW. Laminar avulsion in a cervical vertebra. AJR Am J Roentgenol 1977;129(1):57–60.

58. Shanmuganathan K, Mirvis SE, Dowe M, et al. Traumatic isolation of the cervical articular pillar: imaging observations in 21 patients. AJR Am J Roentgenol 1996;166(4):897–902.

59. Bensch FV, Koivikko MP, Kiuru MJ, et al. The incidence and distribution of burst fractures. Emerg Radiol 2006;12(3):124–9.

60. Campbell SE, Phillips CD, Dubrovsky E, et al. The value of CT in determining potential instability of simple wedge compression fractures of the lumbar spine. AJNR Am J Neuroradiol 1995;16: 1385–92.

61. Angtuaco EJ, Binet EF. Radiology of thoracic and lumbar fractures. Clin Orthop Relat Res 1984;189: 43–57.

62. Petersilge CA, Emery SE. Thoracolumbar burst fracture: evaluating stability. Semin Ultrasound CT MR 1996;17:105–13.

63. Petersilge CA, Pathria MN, Emery SE, et al. Thoracolumbar burst fractures: evaluation with MR imaging. Radiology 1995;194:49–54.

64. Wilcox RK, Boerger TO, Allen DJ, et al. A dynamic study of thoracolumbar burst fractures. J Bone Joint Surg Am 2003;85(11):2184–9.

65. Liu YJ, Chang MC, Wang ST, et al. Flexion distraction injury of the thoracolumbar spine. Injury 2003; 34:920–3.

66. Tyroch AH, McGuire EL, McLean SF, et al. The association between chance fractures and intraabdominal injuries revisited: a multicenter review. Am Surg 2005;71(5):434–8.

67. Ball ST, Vaccaro AR, Albert TJ, et al. Injuries of the thoracolumbar spine associated with restraint use in head on motor vehicle accidents. J Spinal Cord Med 2004;27:269–72.

68. Denis F, Burkus JK. Shear fracture dislocations of the thoracic and lumbar spine associated with forceful hyperextension (lumberjack paraplegia). Spine (Phila Pa 1976) 1992;17(2):156–61.

69. Miller CD, Blyth P, Civil ID. Lumbar transverse process fractures—a sentinel marker of abdominal organ injuries. Injury 2000;31:773–6.

70. Montana MA, Richardson ML, Kilcoyne RF, et al. CT of sacral injury. Radiology 1986;161(2):499–503.

71. Hunter JC, Brandser EA, Tran KA. Pelvic and acetabular trauma. Radiol Clin North Am 1997;35(3): 559–90.

72. Provenzale J. MR imaging of spinal trauma. Emerg Radiol 2007;13:289–97.

73. Gonzalez-Beicos A, Nunez D, Fung A, et al. Trauma to the ankylotic spine: imaging spectrum of vertebral and soft tissue injuries. Emerg Radiol 2007;14: 371–8.

74. Yucesoy K, Yuksel KZ. SCIWORA in MRI era. Clin Neurol Neurosurg 2008;110(5):429–33.

75. Croul SE, Flanders A. Neuropathology of spinal cord injury. Adv Neurol 1997;72:317–23.

76. Ramon S, Dominguez R, Ramirez L, et al. Clinical and magnetic resonance imaging correlation in acute spinal cord injury. Spinal Cord 1997;35(10): 664–73.

77. Marciello M, Flanders A, Herbison GJ, et al. Magnetic resonance imaging related to neurologic outcome in cervical spinal cord injury. Arch Phys Med Rehabil 1993;74:940–6.

78. Flanders A, Schaefer DM, Doan HT, et al. Acute cervical spine trauma: correlation of MRI imaging findings with degree of neurologic deficit. Radiology 1990;177(1):25–33.

79. Radiographic assessment of the cervical spine in symptomatic trauma patients. Neurosurgery 2002; 50(Suppl 3):S36–43.

80. Maynard FM, Reynolds GG, Fountain S, et al. Neurological prognosis after traumatic quadriplegia. Three year experience of California regional spinal cord injury care system. J Neurosurg 1979; 50(5):611–6.

81. Burns AS, Lee BS, Ditunno JF Jr, et al. Patient selection for clinical trials: the reliability of the early spinal cord injury examination. J Neurotrauma 2003;20(5): 477–82.

82. American Spinal Injury Association. International standards for the neurological classification of spinal cord injury. Chicago: American Spinal Injury Association; 2002.

83. American Spinal Injury Association. Reference manual for the international standards for neurological classification of spinal cord injury. Chicago: American Spinal Injury Association; 2003.

84. Kingwell SP, Curt A, Dvorak MF. Factors affecting neurological outcome in traumatic conus medullaris and cauda equina injuries [review]. Neurosurg Focus 2008;25(5):e7.

85. Short DJ, El Masry WS, Jones PW. High dose methylprednisolone in the management of acute spinal cord injury—a systematic review from a clinical perspective. Spinal Cord 2000;38(5): 273–86.

86. DeVivo MJ, Krause JS, Lammertse DP. Recent trends in mortality and causes of death among persons with spinal cord injury. Arch Phys Med Rehabil 1999;80(11):1411–9.

87. Geerts WH, Pineo GF, Heit JM, et al. Prevention of venous thromboembolism: the seventh ACCP conference on antithrombotic and thrombolytic therapy. Chest 2004;126(Suppl 3):338S–40S.

88. Hebbeler SL, Marciniak CM, Crandall S, et al. Daily vs twice daily enoxaparin in the prevention of venous thromboembolic disorders during rehabilitation following acute spinal cord injury. J Spinal Cord Med 2004;27(3):236–40.

89. Consortium for Spinal Cord Medicine Clinical Practice Guidelines. Prevention of thromboembolism in spinal cord injury. J Spinal Cord Med 1997;20(3): 259–83.

90. Looby S, Given MF, Geoghegan T, et al. Gunther tulip retrievable inferior vena caval filters: indications, efficacy, retrieval, and complications. Cardiovasc Intervent Radiol 2007;30(1):59–65.

91. Scarvelis D, Anderson J, Davis L, et al. Hospital mortality due to pulmonary embolism and an evaluation of the usefulness of preventative interventions. Thromb Res 2009;125(2):166–70.

92. Kuric J, Hixon AK. Clinical practice guidelines: autonomic dysreflexia. Jackson Heights (NY): Eastern Paralyzed Veterans Association; 1996.

93. Consortium for Spinal Cord Medicine. Acute management of autonomic dysreflexia: individuals with spinal cord injury presenting to health care facilities. J Spinal Cord Med 2002;25(Suppl 1):S67–88.

94. Wicks AB, Mentor RR. Longterm outlook in quadriplegic patients with initial ventilator dependency. Chest 1986;90(3):406–10.

95. Consortium for Spinal Cord Medicine Clinical Practice Guidelines. Pressure ulcer prevention and treatment following spinal cord injury: a clinical practice for healthcare professionals. J Spinal Cord Med 2001;24(Suppl 1):S40–101.

96. Consortium for Spinal Cord Medicine. Neurogenic bowel management in adults with spinal cord injury: clinical practice guidelines. Washington, DC: Paralyzed Veterans of America; 1998.

Head and Neck Infection and Inflammation

Rich S. Rana, MD[a], Gul Moonis, MD[b,c],*

KEYWORDS

• Head and neck • Inflammation • Infection • Abscess

This article discusses the imaging manifestations of infectious and inflammatory conditions of the head and neck. Special attention is paid to the sites, routes of spread, and complications of neck infections. Because the clinical signs and symptoms and the complications of these conditions are often determined by the precise anatomic site involved, anatomic considerations are stressed. Familiarity with the fascial layers and spaces of the neck and the contents of each space is helpful for this discussion.[1] The fascial layers of the neck are important barriers to infection, and once infection is established, the fascial layers play a part in directing its spread.

SUPERFICIAL NECK INFECTIONS

The superficial cervical fascia underlies the skin and is composed of the adipose tissue, superficial neurovascular structures, lymphatics, and platysma muscle (**Fig. 1**). Infection in the superficial space usually manifests as cellulitis, lymphadenitis, or abscess.

As opposed to cervical lymphadenopathy, which simply refers to the enlargement of the lymph nodes in the neck, cervical lymphadenitis is defined as the enlarged, inflamed, and tender lymph nodes of the neck. Cervical lymphadenitis is common in children, and the most common cause is an upper respiratory illness. Because cervical lymphadenitis is typically self-limited, the exact incidence is difficult to ascertain and imaging is usually not performed. Common sites of cervical lymphadenitis are the submandibular and deep cervical nodes because these nodes filter much of the lymphatic fluid from the head and neck. Acute bilateral cervical lymphadenitis is the most common form and is usually caused by a viral upper respiratory tract infection.[2] Acute unilateral cervical lymphadenitis is the next most common form and is usually caused by bacterial infection, with the most common causative organisms being *Staphylococcus aureus* and *Streptococcus pyogenes*.[3] The incidence of methicillin-resistant *S aureus* has increased in the recent years.[4] Acute unilateral cervical lymphadenitis in older children or adults with a history of periodontal disease is usually caused by an infection with anaerobic bacteria. Superficial neck abscesses usually begin as lymphadenitis, which then progresses from phlegmon to abscess (**Fig. 2**).

DEEP NECK INFECTIONS

The deep cervical fascia is divided into 3 layers (superficial, middle, and deep) that enclose the contents of the head and neck and give rise to the deep spaces of the neck (see **Fig. 1**).

Intrinsic or deep neck space infections (DNSIs) usually represent the overgrowth of the normal flora of the contiguous mucosal surfaces from

a Department of Radiology, Beth Israel Deaconess Medical Center, Harvard Medical School, 330 Brookline Avenue, E/CC-455, Boston, MA 02215, USA
b Department of Radiology, Massachusetts Eye and Ear Infirmary, 243 Charles Street, Boston, MA 02114, USA
c Department of Radiology, Beth Israel Deaconess Medical Center, Harvard Medical School, 330 Brookline Avenue, WCCB-90, Boston, MA 02215, USA
* Corresponding author. Department of Radiology, Beth Israel Deaconess Medical Center, Harvard Medical School, 330 Brookline Avenue, WCCB-90, Boston, MA 02215.
E-mail address: gmoonis@bidmc.harvard.edu

Radiol Clin N Am 49 (2011) 165–182
doi:10.1016/j.rcl.2010.07.013

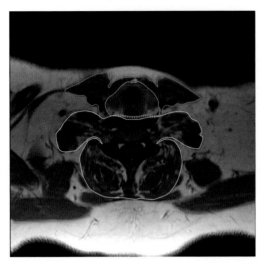

Fig. 1. Layers of deep cervical fascia. The strap muscles and sternocleidomastoid muscle are enclosed by the superficial layer of deep cervical fascia *(pink)*. The visceral space is enveloped by the middle, or visceral, layer of deep cervical fascia *(blue)*. The deep layer of deep cervical fascia *(yellow)* surrounds the paraspinal and prevertebral components of the perivertebral space. From anterior to posterior, the retropharyngeal and danger spaces are separated by the alar fascia *(yellow dashed line)*, which is part of the deep cervical fascia.

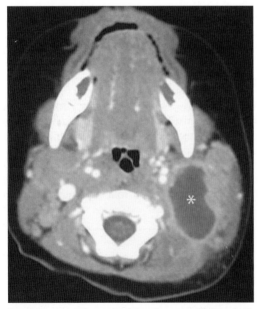

Fig. 2. Suppurative adenitis of a superficial node. Axial contrast-enhanced computed tomography demonstrates an abscess in the left superficial neck resulting from suppurative adenitis *(asterisk)*.

which the infection originated. Most infections are polymicrobial with not only predominantly anaerobic but also facultative oral bacteria.[5] Even in the antibiotic era, life-threatening complications of DNSIs may occur, including airway compromise, venous thrombosis, and mediastinal extension. Diagnosis of the complications of deep space infections may be delayed because many patients with this condition are started on oral antibiotics as outpatients, which may mask local signs such as edema, fluctuation, and pointing of abscess. The most common clinical signs and symptoms are fever, pain, and swelling, which may be present for a variable period, ranging from 1 day to several weeks. Additional symptoms include odynophagia, dysphagia, and trismus. *Streptococcus viridans*, *Klebsiella pneumoniae*, and *Peptostreptococcus* are the most common pathogens that cause neck infections.[6] The most common odontogenic organisms are *S viridans*, *Prevotella*, *Staphylococci*, and *Peptostreptococcus*.[7]

SOURCE AND SITE OF INFECTIONS

Odontogenic infections are the most common source of infections in the head and neck among adults.[8] Other sources include sialadenitis, trauma, intravenous (IV) drug use, and sinusitis. In a large percentage of cases, no source is found.[9,10] In children, the most common source of infection is the tonsils.[3] Comorbidities frequently found in patients with DNSI are diabetes mellitus, old age, alcohol abuse, systemic disease, and immunosuppressed states, such as in patients with AIDS or in those undergoing chemotherapy. Primary head and neck cancer may occasionally present as a DNSI.[11] Recurrent neck infections can also be seen in the setting of developmental lesions such as thyroglossal duct cysts and branchial cleft cysts **(Fig. 3)**.[12]

Odontogenic Spread of Infection

Inflammatory disease of the teeth can be divided into periodontal or endodontal infection.[13] Endodontal infection occurs at the root apex of the tooth. Typically, the infection originates as dental caries, which destroys enamel and dentine, permitting bacteria to enter the pulp chamber containing the neurovascular bundle. The infection then travels down the root canal and out to the apical foramen, with resultant bone resorption. At this point, an acute abscess or a chronic granuloma may form involving the apex of the tooth **(Fig. 4)**.

Periodontal infection originates as gingivitis and travels along the side of the tooth along the

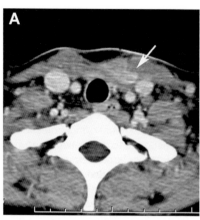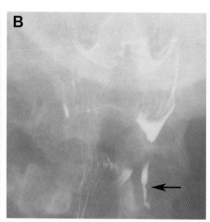

Fig. 3. Fourth branchial cleft cyst causing recurrent perithyroidal inflammation. (*A*) Axial contrast-enhanced computed tomography demonstrates phlegmonous changes anterior to and inseparable from the left lobe of the thyroid gland (*arrow*). (*B*) Barium esophagram demonstrates opacification of a fistulous tract (*arrow*) from the apex of the left pyriform sinus extending into the thyroid bed.

periodontal ligament, causing bone resorption and formation of a periodontal pocket in which infection propagates, which results in a radiolucency along the side of the tooth (see **Fig. 4**).

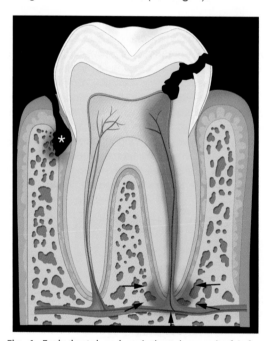

Fig. 4. Endodontal and periodontal spread of infection. On the right side of the image, dental caries allow bacteria to enter the pulp chamber and travel down the root canal to the apical foramen where a periapical lucency corresponds to bone loss (*arrows*). Pressure from the pulpitis compromises the blood supply to the tooth rendering it nonvital. On the left side of the image, gingivitis alongside of tooth (*asterisk*) travels along the periodontal ligament to cause bone resorption and formation of a periodontal pocket in which infection propagates.

The most common paths of spread of maxillary odontogenic infection are to the buccal, masticator, and parapharyngeal spaces.[7] Specifically, infection originating in the maxillary incisors, canines, premolars, and first molars tends to spread to the buccal space, whereas infection originating in the second maxillary molar tends to spread to the masticator space (**Fig. 5**). Infection of the third maxillary molar tends to spread to the parapharyngeal space.[14]

In the mandibular teeth, odontogenic infection originating in the incisors, canines, or first premolars is most likely to spread into the sublingual space. Because the second and third mandibular molar tooth roots extend below the mylohyoid muscle insertion, odontogenic infection originating from these teeth is most likely to spread into the submandibular space (**Fig. 6**).[15] Oroantral fistula can occur as a complication of dental infection with resorption of the tooth root. Because the sinus floor is oriented parallel to the transverse plane, it can be difficult to appreciate this complication on axial imaging; thus coronal or panoramic reformations are key in demonstrating the communication.[16]

Odontogenic sinusitis refers to the secondary infection of the paranasal sinuses originating from dental infection. Although most paranasal sinus infections result from an upper respiratory tract infection, direct spread of the infection from the teeth and associated oral tissues can result in secondary sinusitis, sometimes with a discrete perforation in the wall of the sinus.[15] The maxillary sinus is the main sinus involved because of the proximity of the posterior maxillary teeth. Infection may originate from a periapical abscess or retained tooth fragment after extraction. Symptoms

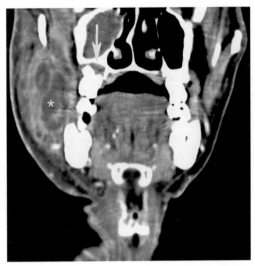

Fig. 5. Masticator space infection. Coronal contrast-enhanced computed tomography demonstrates right masticator space abscess (*asterisk*) originating from an odontogenic infection of the maxillary molar (*arrow*).

include headache, foul discharge, fever, weakness, and drainage. Findings on computed tomography (CT) include thickening of sinus walls, sclerosis, and perforation. Surgery to increase the size of the ostia in the lateral walls of the nasal cavity may help to improve drainage.

Osteomyelitis may complicate odontogenic infection and can demonstrate 4 radiographic patterns[17]: lytic, sclerotic, and mixed forms and a bony sequestrum.

Rarely, odontogenic infections may spread to the orbit and are often clinically unsuspected

(**Fig. 7**). The route of spread may involve the premolar soft tissues, maxillary sinuses, or infratemporal fossa.[18] These cases require dental surgery for the resolution of infection.

Invasive Fungal Sinusitis

Sinusitis may be suspected to be of fungal origin based on atypical clinical presentations, including nonresponse to antibiotics, or on imaging features. Fungal sinonasal disease is typically divided into 4 broad classes based on pathophysiology: acute invasive (fulminant) sinusitis, chronic invasive sinusitis, noninvasive fungal colonization (or mycetoma), and allergic mycotic sinusitis. Fungal hyphal forms are the most common causes of acute invasive sinusitis, with the most frequent being that of *Aspergillus* species. Mucormycosis is the next most common, with especially high prevalence in persons with diabetes, and is caused by the genus *Mucor*, belonging to the class of Zygomycetes. Members of this class thrive in high-sugar environments and are thus also found in decaying fruit. Although less common than hyphal forms, yeast forms occur in immunocompromised hosts and include *Candida*, *Histoplasmosa*, *Cryptococcus*, and *Coccidioides*.

Common CT features of invasive fungal sinusitis include soft tissue changes in the sinus with high-density opacification. In chronic infection, there is often thickened reactive bone, whereas acute invasive sinusitis often demonstrates focal bony erosion.[19] Mycetoma has a characteristic hypointensity on T2-weighted magnetic resonance (MR) images. Mucormycosis has a predisposition for the orbits, cavernous sinuses, and skull base (**Figs. 8** and **9**) and also perineural invasion.

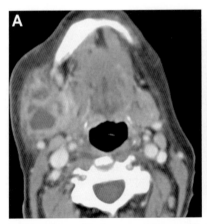
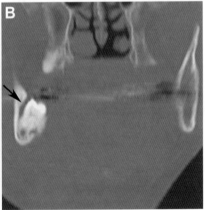

Fig. 6. Odontogenic submandibular space abscess. (*A*) Axial contrast-enhanced computed tomography demonstrates multiple low-density collections in the right submandibular space with circumferential rim enhancement as well as enlargement of the submandibular gland. (*B*) Coronal reformation with the bone window demonstrates the underlying periodontal disease (*arrow*).

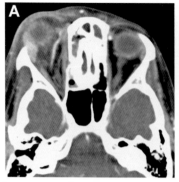
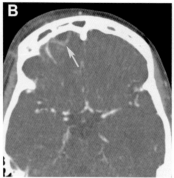
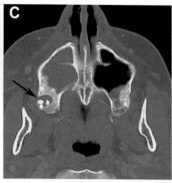

Fig. 7. Odontogenic orbital infection and epidural abscess. (*A*) Axial contrast-enhanced CT (CECT) through the right orbit demonstrates orbital cellulitis and phlegmon. (*B*) Axial CECT demonstrates an epidural abscess of the right frontal lobe (*arrow*). (*C*) Axial CECT demonstrates periapical lucency in a right maxillary molar, which was the source of infection in this patient (*arrow*). This patient also had odontogenic sinusitis of the maxillary sinus.

Sialolithiasis/Sialadenitis

Sialolithiasis refers to salivary gland stones or calculi and is the most common benign condition affecting the salivary glands. The submandibular gland is by far most commonly affected because its secretions are more mucous, alkaline, and viscous than that of the other glands.[20] Most stones are radiopaque, but CT is more sensitive than radiography to demonstrate sialothiasis and its complications, including sialadenitis and abscesses.

Sialadenitis, or glandular inflammation of the salivary glands, is most commonly caused by sialolithiasis. Other inflammatory conditions that cause sialadenitis include mumps, AIDS, influenza, and infection with Coxsackie viruses. Bacterial infections, granulomatous disease, and idiopathic parotitis are less common. On CT, the gland demonstrates enlargement, hypodensity

on precontrast scan, and avid postcontrast enhancement, with adjacent inflammatory stranding and fascial thickening. The salivary duct may be dilated and thick-walled, and an obstructing sialolith is usually seen (**Fig. 10**). On MR imaging, gland enlargement and hyperintensity on T2-weighted images are because of inflammation and edema. Although the sialolith is not as well appreciated, its presence may be inferred if a punctate signal void is seen on all sequences.

Orbital Infection

Orbital subperiosteal abscess is a form of postseptal orbital cellulitis in which there is inflammatory tissue and edema formation beneath the orbital periosteum. This form of orbital cellulitis should be suspected in patients presenting to the emergency department with rhinosinusitis and ocular symptoms. Sinusitis of the ethmoid

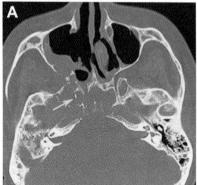
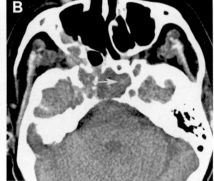

Fig. 8. Fungal sinusitis. (*A*) Axial contrast-enhanced CT in the bone window demonstrates soft tissue opacification of the right maxillary and sphenoid sinus with extensive osseous destruction of the central skull base (*arrow*). There is erosion of the posterior wall of the right maxillary sinus, the pterygopalatine fossa (*asterisk*), the sphenoid bone, the sella, and the right carotid canal. (*B*) Soft tissue window demonstrates hyperdense contents of the sphenoid sinus (*arrow*).

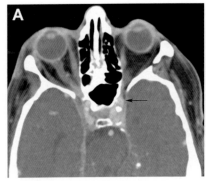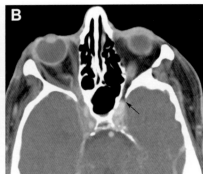

Fig. 9. Fungal sinusitis. (*A*) Axial contrast-enhanced CT (CECT) demonstrates enlargement and enhancement of the left cavernous sinus (*arrow*). (*B*) Axial CECT also demonstrates involvement of the left orbital apex (*arrow*).

sinus is a common predisposing condition, with the lateral aspect of the ethmoid sinus being a commonly involved site.[21] An odontogenic source of infection is a less common cause.[22] CT findings include a soft tissue mass extending from the bony wall of the orbit causing the displacement of the extraocular muscles. There may be a thin strip of preserved extraconal fat separating the abscess from the medial rectus muscle (**Fig. 11**). Clinically, there may be orbital swelling, chemosis, proptosis, and progressive impairment of extraocular motility. If these conditions are allowed to progress, ophthalmic vein thrombosis and cavernous sinus thrombosis are associated complications.

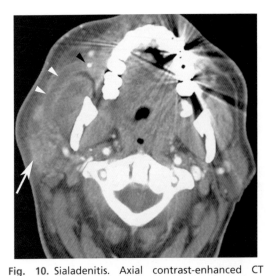

Fig. 10. Sialadenitis. Axial contrast-enhanced CT demonstrates enlargement and hyperenhancement of the right parotid gland (*arrow*), dilation of Wharton duct with ductal wall thickening (*white arrowheads*), and an obstructing sialolith (*black arrowhead*). Also note the adjacent soft tissue inflammatory change and fascial thickening.

Coalescent Mastoiditis

Mastoiditis most commonly occurs as a result of infection of the middle ear, with the route of spread involving the aditus ad antrum, the mastoid antrum, and eventually the mastoid air cells. Mastoiditis can less frequently be the result of the complication of a cholesteatoma. Destruction of the septa of the mastoid air cells signals the transformation of the incipient mastoiditis to the coalescent form, which portends a worse prognosis. In addition, coalescent mastoiditis has several associated complications, including epidural abscess, sigmoid sinus thrombosis, petrous apicitis, subdural empyema, carotid artery spasm or arteritis, and Bezold abscess.[23] On CT, coalescent mastoiditis demonstrates destruction of the mastoid air cell septa. If the mastoid tip suffers osteolysis, phlegmon and eventually abscess may organize with extent into the cervical soft tissues inferiorly; the resultant abscess is termed Bezold abscess (**Fig. 12**).

Malignant Otitis Externa

Necrotizing, or malignant, otitis externa is an entity distinct from the other forms of ear infection. This form affects the external auditory canal (EAC), begins at the cartilaginous/bony junction, and results in purulent drainage. Most cases occur in elderly persons with diabetes, and the causative agent is *Pseudomonas* species. HIV-positive patients are also at an increased risk. It is important to recognize and treat the infection early because it can spread to the nasopharynx, infratemporal fossa, parapharyngeal space, temporomandibular joint, middle and inner ears, and skull base, manifesting as skull base osteomyelitis.

CT is the imaging modality typically performed first for diagnosis.[24] On CT, malignant otitis externa manifests as soft tissue in the EAC, middle ear cavity, and mastoids. There is bony erosion of the

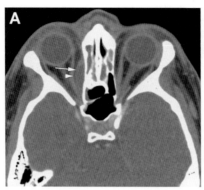
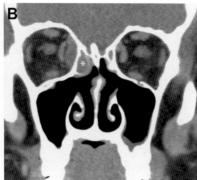

Fig. 11. Orbital subperiosteal abscess. (A) Axial contrast-enhanced CT demonstrates opacification of the ethmoid sinuses and a low-density collection along the medial aspect of the right orbit with a thin peripheral enhancement (*arrow*). Note the sparing of a thin stripe of extraconal fat (*arrowhead*) and lateral deviation of the right medial rectus muscle. (B) Coronal reformation demonstrates the extent of subperiosteal abscess and also a mucocele of the right ethmoid sinus (*asterisk*).

EAC, which, when extensive, may extend to the skull base (**Fig. 13**). On MR imaging, there is extensive edema and fluid in the EAC, middle ear, and mastoid air cells; soft tissue infiltration of the skull base and jugular foramen; and, occasionally, formation of an epidural or prevertebral abscess.

Ludwig Angina

Ludwig angina is a submandibular space infection originally described by von Ludwig[25] in 1836 as a "…gangrenous induration of the connective tissues of the neck which advances to involve the tissues that cover the small muscles between the larynx and the floor of the mouth."

The clinical presentations are usually cellulitis, sublingual/submandibular space fasciitis, and involvement of muscle and connective tissue, but without actual submandibular sialadenitis. There is a tender, firm anterior neck edema without fluctuance. Other signs and symptoms include drooling, tachypnea, dyspnea, and stridor. The cause is odontogenic in 80% to 90% of patients.[26] Although Ludwig angina is a cellulitis with diffuse infiltration, subsequent abscess formation is not uncommon. The mode of spread is typically direct, rather than lymphatic.

Ludwig angina may result in a life-threatening airway compromise. In a review of 210 patients with deep neck abscess, overall 20% of patients required tracheostomy as compared with 75% of patients with Ludwig angina.[27] CT may demonstrate either a diffusely infiltrative process or a more discrete low-attenuation area, reflecting abscess (**Fig. 14**).[28]

Peritonsillar Abscess

Peritonsillar abscess, sometimes referred to colloquially as "quinsy," is the most common deep

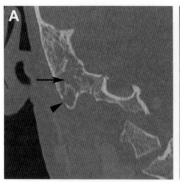
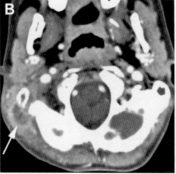
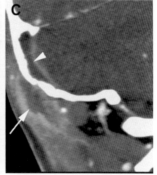

Fig. 12. Coalescent mastoiditis. (A) Coronal bone reformation CT image demonstrates extensive opacification and coalescence of septa within the right mastoid air cells (*arrow*). Note the cortical disruption of the mastoid tip inferiorly (*arrowhead*). (B, C) Axial and coronal contrast-enhanced CT with soft tissue windows demonstrate a low-density fluid collection inferior to the mastoid tip with a rim of enhancement indicating Bezold abscess (*arrows*). Also note right sigmoid sinus thrombosis as a complication of mastoiditis (*arrowhead*).

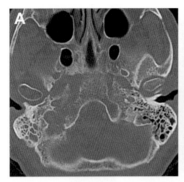
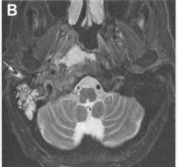
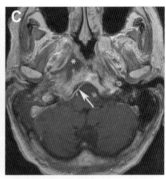

Fig. 13. Malignant otitis externa. (*A*) Axial contrast-enhanced CT with bone windows demonstrates osteomyelitis involving the right skull base. The clivus, right petrous apex, and jugular foramen demonstrate lytic change. (*B*) Axial T2-weighted MR image demonstrates edema involving the right temporal bone, including the EAC (*arrow*), skull base, jugular foramen, and prevertebral space. (*C*) Axial T1 postcontrast MR image demonstrates enhancement of the same regions. There is an abscess in the prevertebral space (*asterisk*). Also note an epidural abscess along the clivus (*arrow*). Inflammatory changes surround the internal carotid artery on the right.

neck infection.[2] Peritonsillar abscess is often polymicrobial. The most common aerobic bacteria are group A *Streptococcus*, *S aureus*, and *Haemophilus influenzae*, whereas the most common anaerobic bacteria are *Fusobacterium*, *Peptostreptococcus*, and pigmented *Prevotella*.[29] The presentation often includes fever, malaise, dysphagia, odynophagia, trismus, and "hot-potato" voice. On physical examination, bulging of the superior tonsillar pole and soft palate and deviation of the uvula are often seen. Inflammation of the tonsils is referred to as tonsillitis, which causes a typically striated appearance with the enhancement of the mucosa and submucosal edema (**Fig. 15**). Anatomically, peritonsillar abscess represents an infection between the tonsillar capsule and superior constrictor muscle (**Fig. 16**) and is usually a complication of

acute tonsillitis. Recently, inflammation of the Weber glands,[29] which are approximately 2 dozen mucous salivary glands in the soft palate just superior to the tonsil, has also been implicated in the pathogenesis of peritonsillar abscess. Thus, peritonsillar abscess is also possible in patients who have had tonsillectomy. If infection spreads outside the constrictor ring, it represents a parapharyngeal abscess (**Fig. 17**).

Retropharyngeal and Danger Space Abscess

The retropharyngeal space extends from the skull base to approximately T3-T4 and is bounded anteriorly by the slip of the middle layer of the deep cervical fascia known as the visceral layer. Posteriorly, the retropharyngeal space is bound by a slip of the deep layer of the deep cervical fascia known

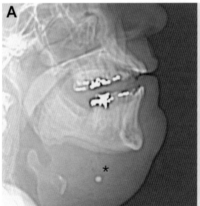
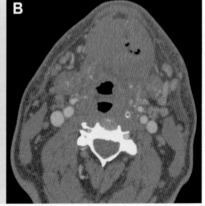

Fig. 14. Ludwig angina. (*A*) Scout CT view demonstrates submandibular space soft tissue swelling and small locules of gas (*asterisk*). (*B*) Axial contrast-enhanced CT demonstrates diffuse infiltration of the sublingual and submandibular spaces, small locules of gas, and thickening of platysma and fascial planes. The airway is mildly effaced. No discrete abscess is seen.

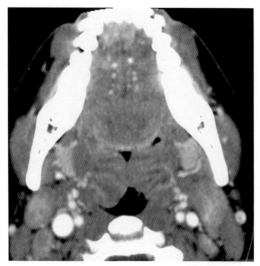

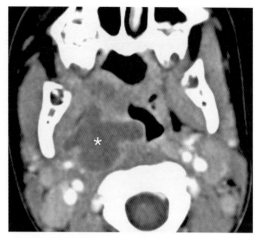

Fig. 15. Tonsillitis. Axial contrast-enhanced CT demonstrates enlargement of the palatine tonsils, with a striated appearance representing mucosal enhancement. Low-density areas between the striations represent parenchymal edema.

Fig. 17. Parapharyngeal abscess. Axial contrast-enhanced CT demonstrates a low-density collection of the right parapharyngeal space (*asterisk*) caused by peritonsillar abscess, which has extended beyond the constrictor ring.

as the alar fascia. Immediately posterior to the alar fascia is the danger space (see **Fig. 1**), which extends inferiorly into the posterior mediastinum. An infectious process in these compartments can be seen in a spectrum ranging from phlegmon to suppurative adenitis/frank abscess (**Fig. 18**). It is not possible to differentiate the retropharyngeal space from the danger space on imaging (**Fig. 19**), and danger space infection can be inferred only if

the infection spreads below the T4 level. Retropharyngeal abscess may extend posteriorly to involve the danger and prevertebral spaces as well as cause osteomyelitis of the spine.

Unlike peritonsillar abscess, which is medial to the constrictor ring, parapharyngeal and retropharyngeal abscesses are lateral. The most common sources for retropharyngeal abscess in children is suppurative adenitis.[30] Cervical spine surgery is another potential cause of infection of

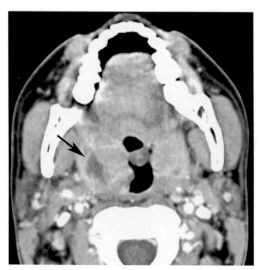

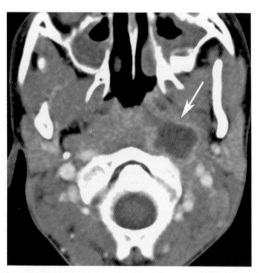

Fig. 16. Peritonsillar abscess. Axial contrast-enhanced CT demonstrates a low-density fluid collection with rim enhancement along the lateral tonsillar wall on the right (*arrow*).

Fig. 18. Suppurative adenitis of a retropharyngeal node. Axial contrast-enhanced CT demonstrates a low-density lymph node (*arrow*) in the left retropharyngeal space indicating suppurative adenitis causing abscess.

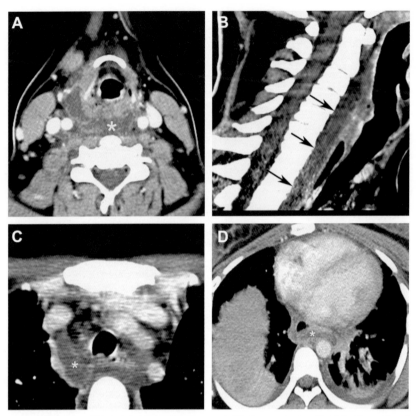

Fig. 19. Danger space abscess. (*A*) Axial contrast-enhanced CT demonstrates fluid in the retropharyngeal and danger spaces at the level of the hyoid bone (*asterisk*). (*B*) Sagittal reformation through the midline subglottic neck demonstrates the cervical danger space abscess (*arrows*). (*C, D*) Axial CT images at the level of the aortic arch and diaphragm demonstrate the most inferior extent of the abscess, with both right paratracheal and posterior mediastinal components (*asterisks*).

the prevertebral/retropharyngeal spaces. It is difficult to differentiate suppurative adenitis of the retropharyngeal nodes from frank abscess (see the section Abscess vs Phlegmon).

Calcific tendonitis affecting the longus coli muscle was first described by Hartley[31] in 1964. The clinical presentation for this condition is varied, but there is generally no history of head/neck infection and no cervical lymphadenopathy. There may be a mild leukocytosis and/or an elevated erythrocyte sedimentation rate.[32] The classic radiographic description is an amorphous calcification anterior to the C1-C4 vertebral bodies with prevertebral soft tissue swelling. However, radiography is unreliable for the diagnosis, and CT has long been considered the preferred modality.[33] On CT, an amorphous calcification is seen moreclearly, is localized to the prevertebral space, and is reliably differentiated from an avulsed fracture (**Fig. 20**). A diffuse edema or discrete effusion can be differentiated with MR imaging,[34] although this distinction is usually not necessary. However, differentiating this entity

from a retropharyngeal abscess is necessary to avoid drainage or surgery. After treatment with nonsteroidal antiinflammatory drugs, this condition is self-limited in about 1 to 2 weeks.[35]

Necrotizing Fasciitis

Necrotizing fasciitis is an aggressive infection of both the superficial and deep soft tissues of the neck. Both aerobic and anaerobic bacteria can act as so-called flesh-eating bacteria. Skin, mucosal, dental, or tonsillar sites of origin may be identified, and overall necrotizing fasciitis occurs more frequently in immunocompromised patients. Complications include sepsis, making prompt surgical exploration necessary. At times, it may be difficult to differentiate necrotizing fasciitis from a less-aggressive infection, but the presence of gas-forming organisms is a clue.

Diffuse thickening of the cutis and subcutis and reticulation of fat indicate cellulitis. Enlargement, thickening, and enhancement of fasciae indicate fasciitis. Enlarged edematous muscle indicates

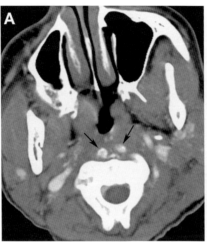
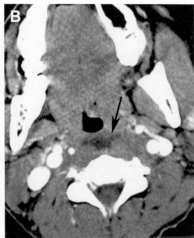

Fig. 20. Calcific tendonitis of the longus colli tendon. (*A*) Axial contrast-enhanced CT image demonstrates amorphous calcification of the longus colli tendon (*arrows*). (*B*) There is an associated effusion in the retropharyngeal space, without enhancement (*arrow*).

myositis. Fluid collections in multiple spaces indicate soft tissue necrosis (**Fig. 21**).[36] Airway compromise can occur with severe infection.

The visceral layer of the deep cervical fascia surrounds the thyroid, trachea, anterior wall of the esophagus, and thyroid cartilage to the superior mediastinum, defining the anterior visceral space. Most infections involving this space result from the perforation of the esophagus, with risk factors being instrumentation, foreign body, or trauma. Infection of the visceral space portends an increased risk of mediastinitis and airway compromise.

Although the most common cause of acute mediastinitis is esophageal rupture, descending necrotizing fasciitis from DNSI traveling along the retropharyngeal space, danger space, carotid space, prevertebral space, or anterior visceral space can also spread into the mediastinum (see **Fig. 19**B). The most common source of descending cervical mediastinitis is odontogenic infection.[37] Comorbid conditions such as diabetes may make certain patients highly susceptible to spreading cellulitis. Mediastinitis may also result from direct extension from an adjacent source of infection, including osteomyelitis of the sternoclavicular joint, pulmonary infections, and spread of granulomatous disease from mediastinal lymph nodes. The treatment is IV antibiotics, and because mediastinitis is a surgical emergency, surgical debridement, drainage, and airway management are typically necessary.[37]

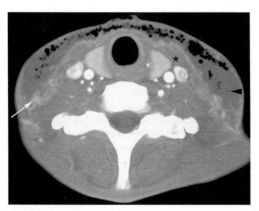

Fig. 21. Necrotizing fasciitis. Axial contrast-enhanced CT at the level of the thyroid gland demonstrates subcutaneous gas in the anterior neck with low-density appearance of the sternocleidomastoid muscle indicating myositis (*asterisk*) as well as enhancement of the fascia (*arrow*) and fluid collections (*arrowhead*).

Epiglottitis

Acute epiglottitis in adults is a cellulitis of the epiglottis, aryepiglottic folds, and adjacent tissues (**Fig. 22**). If not treated promptly, this condition can progress to a life-threatening airway obstruction. Epiglottitis results from bacteremia or direct invasion of the epithelial layer by the pathogenic organism, which typically travels from the posterior nasopharynx. Although the incidence of epiglottitis in children has decreased because of the *H influenzae* type b (Hib) vaccination, this bacterium is still the most common causative organism.[38] The incidence of epiglottitis in adults appears to be increasing.[39,40] Adult epiglottitis may represent a distinct form of epiglottitis because the supraglottic tissues are involved in most cases, and culture yields are uniformly lower

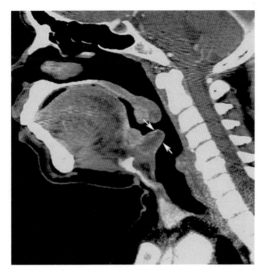

Fig. 22. Epiglottitis. Sagittal contrast-enhanced CT demonstrates edema and swelling of the epiglottis compatible with epiglottitis (*arrows*). (*Courtesy of Dr Robert Morales University of Maryland Medical Center, Baltimore, MD.*)

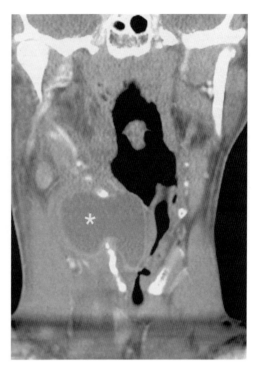

Fig. 23. Laryngopyocele. Coronal contrast-enhanced CT demonstrates a mixed internal and external laryng-opyocele (*asterisk*) with rim enhancement and edema of the glottis and supraglottis.

in cases of this condition than in traditional pediatric cases of acute epiglottitis. Other causative organisms are *Streptococcus* and *Staphylococcus* in immunocompetent hosts and *Pseudomonas* and *Candida* in immunocompromised hosts.

Laryngopyocele

Laryngopyocele represents infection of a dilated laryngeal ventricle. This entity is thought to arise in a preexisting laryngocele with stasis, resulting in secondary infection. The incidence is low and has been reported as 1 in 2.5 million in the United Kingdom.[41] Although a rare diagnosis, laryngopyocele can present as an acute airway emergency,[42] and thus it is important to recognize this condition early. Clinical presentation may include odynophagia, aspiration, and respiratory compromise. Intubation or tracheostomy, use of broad-spectrum antibiotics, and needle or surgical decompression are considered necessary in the treatment of laryngopyocele. CT demonstrates a fluid or missed fluid-air density collection emanating from the laryngeal ventricle, with extension superolaterally into the paraglottic fat. Thick rim enhancement of the walls indicates inflammation (**Fig. 23**).

VASCULAR COMPLICATIONS OF HEAD AND NECK INFECTIONS

Head and neck infections can also result in numerous vascular complications, especially when the infection involves the parapharyngeal space. Major vascular complications include Lemierre syndrome, cavernous sinus thrombosis, and arterial complications, such as vasospasm, arteritis, pseudoaneurysm, and carotid blowout.

Lemierre Syndrome

In 1936, Andre Lemierre reported a syndrome of anaerobic septicemia that resulted from infection in 1 of 6 possible sites and caused septic thrombophlebitis and metastatic abscesses. The first of these sites was the "...nasopharynx, particularly tonsillar and peritonsillar abscesses."[43] Although other sites were as remote as the endometrium in postpartum women, the term Lemierre syndrome has since been used to describe a narrower clinical syndrome resulting from head and neck infections in which venous thrombophlebitis and septicemia occur with or without metastatic abscesses. Most cases that Lemierre described in Paris in the 1930s were caused by *Bacillus funduliformis* (now *Fusobacterium necrophorum*), but he also described "...several species of anaerobic organisms which are specifically distinct from one another." Lemierre's original description of the progression of infection was "...thrombophlebitis of the tonsillar and peritonsillar veins which can spread to the internal jugular vein or even to the facial vein."

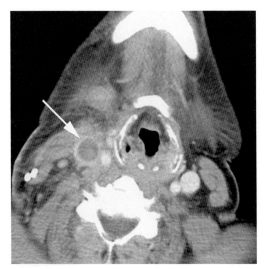

Fig. 24. Lemierre syndrome. Axial contrast-enhanced CT demonstrates septic thrombophlebitis of the right internal jugular vein with thickening and enhancement of the walls of the thrombosed vein and surrounding tissues (*arrow*).

Because Lemierre syndrome was thought to be uncommon in the postantibiotic era, it was termed in 1984 as the "forgotten disease".[44] However, recent reviews of the literature suggest an increasing incidence.[45,46]

Often, those affected are previously healthy immunocompetent adolescents and young adults, with a male predominance. The offending organism is most commonly *Fusobacterium* anaerobic gram-negative bacilli, which are part of the normal flora of the mouth. Predisposing factors include trauma, edema, anoxia, or tissue

destruction after dental disease. A typical lag time is 4 to 8 days between the primary event and septicemia.[43] Imaging demonstrates enlargement and thrombosis of the internal jugular vein, with enhancement of the walls of the vein and perivenular soft tissues (**Fig. 24**). Metastatic abscesses may also occur with superficial thrombophlebitis without frank internal jugular vein thrombophlebitis (**Fig. 25**).

Cavernous Sinus Thrombosis

The cavernous sinus is a venous space, which is part of the anteroinferior group of dural venous sinuses. The cavernous sinus drains the insular cortex and parenchyma around the sylvian fissure via the sphenoparietal sinus. Each cavernous sinus communicates with the contralateral side and the pterygoid plexus as well as the superior ophthalmic vein. Because these sinuses anastomose with the facial veins, which are valveless, paranasal sinal, odontogenic, and facial infections (eg, a furuncle that was manipulated) can spread into the cavernous sinus (**Fig. 26**). Patients with cavernous venous sinus thrombosis often have a history of midface infection for 5 to 10 days. Presenting signs and symptoms include headache, fevers, and cranial nerve signs. The patient may have orbital pain, visual disturbances, and fullness with periorbital edema or discrete abscess. Other symptoms include confusion, drowsiness, and coma as a result of central nervous system involvement and/or sepsis. Although there are only small series that compare CT with MR imaging for diagnosing cavernous sinus thrombosis,[47] CT venography seems to be superior to

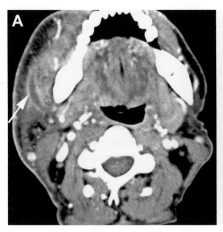
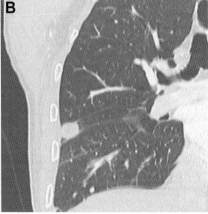

Fig. 25. Odontogenic septic thrombophlebitis without internal jugular vein (IJV) thrombosis. (*A*) Axial contrast-enhanced CT demonstrates odontogenic masticator and parotid space infection with septic thrombophlebitis of the retromandibular vein (*arrow*). (*B*) Coronal reformation with lung windows demonstrates resulting septic pulmonary embolus. Note that these complications may occur without demonstrated IJV thrombosis as in this case.

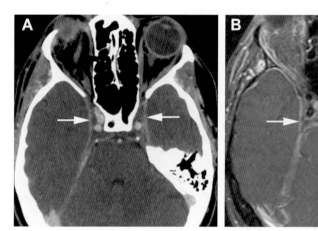

Fig. 26. Cavernous sinus thrombosis. (*A, B*) Axial postcontrast CT and T1-weighted MR images demonstrate enlargement and filling defects (*arrows*) in the cavernous sinuses bilaterally, indicating cavernous sinus thrombosis. There is enlargement of the right superior ophthalmic vein, indicating ophthalmic vein thrombosis with edema and proptosis of the right orbit.

MR venography in the identification of the cerebral venous sinuses and at least equivalent in the diagnosis of cerebral venous sinus thrombosis.[48] Matched mask bone elimination may help further automate CT venography and improve cavernous sinus evaluation.[49] In the authors' experience, CT venography or routine CT of the skull base with a contrast is a reliable tool for the evaluation of cavernous venous sinus thrombosis. Findings include the enlargement of the cavernous sinus and presence of filling defects representing thrombosis (see **Fig. 26**). The superior ophthalmic vein may also be enlarged and thrombosed.

Arterial Complications

Vasospasm is a common finding in which there is narrowing of the ipsilateral internal carotid artery related to the retropharyngeal lymphadenitis and abscess (**Fig. 27**). However, this condition has not been associated with neurologic deficits and is generally regarded as benign.[50]

True arterial complications of head and neck infection were reported more frequently before the 1930s, with a dramatic decrease of these complications in the more recent literature.[51] Arteritis represents an inflammation of the internal carotid artery but is not associated with narrowing. The only histologically reported confirmation of arteritis due to deep neck infection does not include a description of the layers involved.[52]

If pseudoaneurysm complicates arteritis, the patient may develop a pulsatile mass, pain, and cranial neuropathies. *Salmonella* and *Klebsiella* produce elastase and may facilitate the formation of pseudoaneurysms (**Fig. 28**).[53]

Carotid blowout represents a life-threatening hemorrhage of the internal carotid artery as a complication of deep neck infection.[54] The traditional therapies are carotid ligation or balloon occlusion. More recently, stent-graft therapy has been attempted and may be a temporizing measure, but the long-term safety and patency of this therapy are not established. Also, many of the published data are in patients with a history of head and neck cancer who have undergone radiation therapy.[55]

ABSCESS VERSUS PHLEGMON

One limitation of CT examination is in distinguishing phlegmon versus abscess. An abscess is defined as a drainable cavity of infected debris,

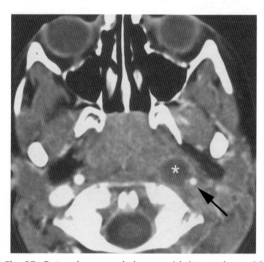

Fig. 27. Retropharyngeal abscess with internal carotid artery (ICA) spasm. Axial contrast-enhanced CT demonstrates retropharyngeal abscess (*asterisk*) on the left with associated narrowing of the left ICA (*arrow*).

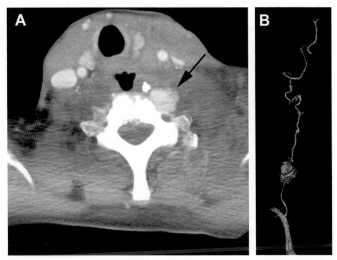

Fig. 28. Vertebral artery pseudoaneurysm. (*A*) Axial CT angiography source image demonstrates a left vertebral artery pseudoaneurysm (*arrow*) resulting from a neck abscess in a patient with perforated Zenker diverticulum. CT performed 1 week prior had shown a normal-caliber vertebral artery. (*B*) Volume-rendered image helps delineate the extent of pseudoaneurysm.

whereas a phlegmon is an infected tissue without necrosis and therefore without a drainable fluid collection. A fluid-attenuation collection with peripheral rim enhancement has been considered as the classic imaging finding for abscess on CT examination, whereas phlegmon has been described as a low-density edematous tissue without discrete peripheral enhancement. However, the use of these criteria is expected to

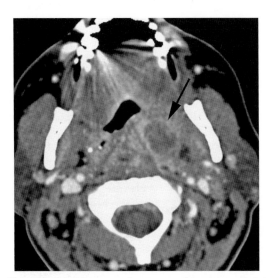

Fig. 29. Parapharyngeal space phlegmon. Axial contrast-enhanced CT demonstrates a low-density fluid collection with partial rim enhancement in the left parapharyngeal space (*arrow*) with a mass effect on the airway. Although the appearance suggested abscess, no pus was aspirated.

result in significant false-positive results (**Fig. 29**). The positive predictive value of these features has been reported as 71% to 83%.[3,56,57] Therefore, CT offers the most value when used to exclude abscess because negative predictive values are uniformly high if those in whom no pus was obtained or who recovered without surgical management are considered not to have had clinically relevant abscess. Thus, the decision for drainage should be made clinically. However, information useful in guiding drainage procedures can be obtained, and the presence of complications can be assessed by CT. Indications for drainage include continued fevers, lack of improvement or worsening clinically, and continued leukocytosis despite antibiotics. One study analyzed the false-positive results of CT by size and found that they all occurred in collections less than 3.5 cm.[58] Therefore, a low-density collection of more than 3.5 cm with rim enhancement should confidently suggest the presence of drainable pus at surgery.

SUMMARY

The signs, symptoms, and complications of the infectious and inflammatory disorders of the head and neck are determined largely by the anatomic compartment of origin. The fascial layers serve as important barriers to infection and often determine the path of the spread of infection. Cervical lymphadenitis is common in children and is the usual origin of superficial neck abscesses. Adults are more likely than children to have a DNSI, with odontogenic infection being the most common source. There are specific risk factors that can raise the suspicion for DNSI. Multiple routes of spread are possible from odontogenic infection, which can commonly result in the involvement of the buccal, masticator, parapharyngeal, submandibular, and sublingual spaces. Odontogenic sinusitis, osteomyelitis, and orbital infections are additional potential complications of odontogenic infection.

Invasive fungal sinusitis may be suspected clinically or based on imaging features. Mucormycosis has a special predisposition for orbital, cavernous sinus, skull base, and perineural involvement. Sialolithiasis is the most common cause of sialadenitis, which by far most commonly involves the submandibular gland, with diagnostic imaging findings. Orbital subperiosteal abscess should be suspected when rhinosinusitis occurs with ocular symptoms, with the medial orbit being a commonly affected site. The coalescent form of mastoiditis must be recognized, which has specific associated complications with characteristic imaging features. Malignant otitis externa is distinct from other forms of ear infection and has specific patterns of spread and several known complications, which can be evaluated on CT or MR imaging.

Ludwig angina is a submandibular/sublingual space infection, which is also usually odontogenic. Peritonsillar abscess is the most common DNSI and can also result in parapharyngeal abscess. Retropharyngeal and danger space infections have similar imaging findings, but danger space infection can be inferred when there is spread of infection below T4. Longus colli calcific tendonitis can mimic retropharyngeal abscess but has specific imaging findings that should allow its differentiation. Necrotizing fasciitis is a serious infection often signaled by the presence of gas-forming organisms and requires early recognition and treatment. Mediastinitis usually results from esophageal rupture but can also be a complication of DNSI and in either case can result in a life-threatening airway compromise. Epiglottitis is a cellulitis of the epiglottis and aryepiglottic folds, which can lead to a life-threatening airway obstruction. Epiglottitis in adults may be a distinct form, and its incidence appears to be increasing despite the decreased pediatric incidence as a result of the Hib vaccination. Laryngopyocele is a rare but serious infection in a preexisting laryngocele and is differentiated by clinical data and an enhancing rim with inflammatory change.

Lemierre syndrome has a range of presentations and imaging findings, and despite once being referred to as the forgotten disease, the incidence of this condition is increasing. Cavernous sinus thrombosis is a serious complication of DNSI, for which CT venography or routine CT of the skull base with contrast is appropriate for evaluation. Although less common than in the preantibiotic era, arterial manifestations of DNSI include vasospasm, arteritis, pseudoaneurysm, and carotid blowout. With the exception of vasospasm, these manifestations are potentially serious complications that require early recognition.

Although a useful tool in the evaluation of DNSI, contrast-enhanced CT is expected to yield up to a 25% false-positive rate for the diagnosis of abscess. This rate is lower when larger fluid collections are considered, and essentially all abscesses greater than 3.5 cm can be reliably differentiated from phlegmon.

REFERENCES

1. Craven J. Anatomy of the naso- and oropharynx. Anaesth Intensive Care Med 2005;6:217–52.
2. Healy C, Baker CJ. Cervical lymphadenitis. In: Feigin R, Cherry JD, Demmler-Harrison GJ, et al, editors. Textbook of pediatric infectious diseases. Philadelphia: Saunders; 2009. p. 185.
3. Ungkanont K, Yellon RF, Weissman JL, et al. Head and neck space infections in infants and children. Otolaryngol Head Neck Surg 1995;112:375–82.
4. Guss J, Kazahaya K. Antibiotic-resistant *Staphylococcus aureus* in community-acquired pediatric neck abscesses. Int J Pediatr Otorhinolaryngol 2007;71:943–8.
5. Roscoe DL, Hoang L. Microbiologic investigations for head and neck infections. Infect Dis Clin North Am 2007;21:283–304, v.
6. Huang TT, Liu TC, Chen PR, et al. Deep neck infection: analysis of 185 cases. Head Neck 2004;26:854–60.
7. Rega AJ, Aziz SR, Ziccardi VB. Microbiology and antibiotic sensitivities of head and neck space infections of odontogenic origin. J Oral Maxillofac Surg 2006;64:1377–80.
8. Larawin V, Naipao J, Dubey SP. Head and neck space infections. Otolaryngol Head Neck Surg 2006;135:889–93.
9. Lee JK, Kim HD, Lim SC. Predisposing factors of complicated deep neck infection: an analysis of 158 cases. Yonsei Med J 2007;48:55–62.
10. Wang LF, Kuo WR, Tsai SM, et al. Characterizations of life-threatening deep cervical space infections: a review of one hundred ninety-six cases. Am J Otolaryngol 2003;24:111–7.
11. Wang CP, Ko JY, Lou PJ. Deep neck infection as the main initial presentation of primary head and neck cancer. J Laryngol Otol 2006;120:305–9.

12. Nusbaum AO, Som PM, Rothschild MA, et al. Recurrence of a deep neck infection: a clinical indication of an underlying congenital lesion. Arch Otolaryngol Head Neck Surg 1999;125:1379–82.

13. Abrahams JJ. Dental CT imaging: a look at the jaw. Radiology 2001;219:334–45.

14. Obayashi N, Ariji Y, Goto M, et al. Spread of odontogenic infection originating in the maxillary teeth: computerized tomographic assessment. Oral Surg Oral Med Oral Pathol Oral Radiol Endod 2004;98:223–31.

15. Fehrenbach MJ. Spread of dental infection. Practical Hygiene 1997;6:13–9. Available at: http://www.mmcpub.com/pdf/1997jph/199705jph_pdf/97jphv6n5p13.pdf. Accessed July 22, 2010.

16. Abrahams JJ, Berger SB. Oral-maxillary sinus fistula (oroantral fistula): clinical features and findings on multiplanar CT. AJR Am J Roentgenol 1995;165:1273–6.

17. Yoshiura K, Hijiya T, Ariji E, et al. Radiographic patterns of osteomyelitis in the mandible. Plain film/CT correlation. Oral Surg Oral Med Oral Pathol 1994;78:116–24.

18. Kaban LB, McGill T. Orbital cellulitis of dental origin: differential diagnosis and the use of computed tomography as a diagnostic aid. J Oral Surg 1980;38:682–5.

19. Moonis G. Imaging of sinonasal anatomy and inflammatory disorders. Crit Rev Comput Tomogr 2003;44:187–228.

20. Yousem DM, Kraut MA, Chalian AA. Major salivary gland imaging. Radiology 2000;216:19–29.

21. Handler LC, Davey IC, Hill JC, et al. The acute orbit: differentiation of orbital cellulitis from subperiosteal abscess by computerized tomography. Neuroradiology 1991;33:15–8.

22. Caruso PA, Watkins LM, Suwansaard P, et al. Odontogenic orbital inflammation: clinical and CT findings—initial observations. Radiology 2006;239:187–94.

23. Vazquez E, Castellote A, Piqueras J, et al. Imaging of complications of acute mastoiditis in children. Radiographics 2003;23:359–72.

24. Grandis JR, Curtin HD, Yu VL. Necrotizing (malignant) external otitis: prospective comparison of CT and MR imaging in diagnosis and follow-up. Radiology 1995;196:499–504.

25. von Ludwig F. Medrcmischescorrespondenz. Blatt des Wurttembergrschen Arztlrchen Vereins 1836;6:21–5 [in German].

26. Srirompotong S, Art-Smart T. Ludwig's angina: a clinical review. Eur Arch Otorhinolaryngol 2003;260:401–3.

27. Parhiscar A, Har-El G. Deep neck abscess: a retrospective review of 210 cases. Ann Otol Rhinol Laryngol 2001;110:1051–4.

28. Weber AL, Siciliano A. CT and MR imaging evaluation of neck infections with clinical correlations. Radiol Clin North Am 2000;38:941–68, ix.

29. Galioto NJ. Peritonsillar abscess. Am Fam Physician 2008;77:199–202.

30. Shefelbine SE, Mancuso AA, Gajewski BJ, et al. Pediatric retropharyngeal lymphadenitis: differentiation from retropharyngeal abscess and treatment implications. Otolaryngol Head Neck Surg 2007;136:182–8.

31. Hartley J. Acute cervical pain associated with retropharyngeal calcium deposit. A case report. J Bone Joint Surg Am 1964;46:1753–4.

32. Offiah CE, Hall E. Acute calcific tendinitis of the longus colli muscle: spectrum of CT appearances and anatomical correlation. Br J Radiol 2009;82:e117–21.

33. Hall FM, Docken WP, Curtis HW. Calcific tendinitis of the longus coli: diagnosis by CT. AJR Am J Roentgenol 1986;147:742–3.

34. Eastwood JD, Hudgins PA, Malone D. Retropharyngeal effusion in acute calcific prevertebral tendinitis: diagnosis with CT and MR imaging. AJNR Am J Neuroradiol 1998;19:1789–92.

35. Chung T, Rebello R, Gooden EA. Retropharyngeal calcific tendinitis: case report and review of literature. Emerg Radiol 2005;11:375–80.

36. Becker M, Zbaren P, Hermans R, et al. Necrotizing fasciitis of the head and neck: role of CT in diagnosis and management. Radiology 1997;202:471–6.

37. Kiernan PD, Hernandez A, Byrne WD, et al. Descending cervical mediastinitis. Ann Thorac Surg 1998;65:1483–8.

38. Hafidh MA, Sheahan P, Keogh I, et al. Acute epiglottitis in adults: a recent experience with 10 cases. J Laryngol Otol 2006;120:310–3.

39. Cheung CS, Man SY, Graham CA, et al. Adult epiglottitis: 6 years experience in a university teaching hospital in Hong Kong. Eur J Emerg Med 2009;16:221–6.

40. Ng HL, Sin LM, Li MF, et al. Acute epiglottitis in adults: a retrospective review of 106 patients in Hong Kong. Emerg Med J 2008;25:253–5.

41. Khan NW, Watson G, Willat D. Pyolaryngocoele: management of an unusual cause of odynophagia and neck swelling. Clinical Medicine Insights: Ear, Nose and Throat 2008;1:1–4. Available at: http://www.la-press.com/pyolaryngocoele-management-of-an-unusual-cause-of-odynophagia-and-neck-article-a857. Accessed July 22, 2010.

42. Mace AT, Ravichandran S, Dewar G, et al. Laryngopyocoele: simple management of an acute airway crisis. J Laryngol Otol 2009;123:248–9.

43. Lemierre A. On certain septicaemias due to anaerobic organisms. Lancet 1936;227:701–3.

44. Moore-Gillon J, Lee TH, Eykyn SJ, et al. Necrobacillosis: a forgotten disease. Br Med J (Clin Res Ed) 1984;288:1526–7.

45. Karkos PD, Asrani S, Karkos CD, et al. Lemierre's syndrome: a systematic review. Laryngoscope 2009;119:1552–9.

46. Jones C, Siva TM, Seymour FK, et al. Lemierre's syndrome presenting with peritonsillar abscess

and VIth cranial nerve palsy. J Laryngol Otol 2006; 120:502—4.

47. Ozsvath RR, Casey SO, Lustrin ES, et al. Cerebral venography: comparison of CT and MR projection venography. AJR Am J Roentgenol 1997;169:1699—707.

48. Linn J, Ertl-Wagner B, Seelos KC, et al. Diagnostic value of multidetector-row CT angiography in the evaluation of thrombosis of the cerebral venous sinuses. AJNR Am J Neuroradiol 2007;28:946—52.

49. Majoie CB, van Straten M, Venema HW, et al. Multisection CT venography of the dural sinuses and cerebral veins by using matched mask bone elimination. AJNR Am J Neuroradiol 2004;25:787—91.

50. Hudgins PA, Dorey JH, Jacobs IN. Internal carotid artery narrowing in children with retropharyngeal lymphadenitis and abscess. AJNR Am J Neuroradiol 1998;19:1841—3.

51. Reisner A, Marshall GS, Bryant K, et al. Endovascular occlusion of a carotid pseudoaneurysm complicating deep neck space infection in a child. Case report. J Neurosurg 1999;91:510—4.

52. Hogarth TB. Intra-pharyngeal haemorrhage from the internal carotid artery. Report of a case and arteriographic findings. J Laryngol Otol 1959;73:764—7.

53. Constantinides H, Passant C, Waddell AN. Mycotic pseudoaneurysm of common carotid artery mimicking parapharyngeal abscess. J Laryngol Otol 2000;114: 796—7.

54. Waggie Z, Hatherill M, Millar A, et al. Retropharyngeal abscess complicated by carotid artery rupture. Pediatr Crit Care Med 2002;3:303—4.

55. Chang FC, Lirng JF, Luo CB, et al. Carotid blowout syndrome in patients with head-and-neck cancers: reconstructive management by self-expandable stent-grafts. AJNR Am J Neuroradiol 2007;28: 181—8.

56. Smith JL 2nd, Hsu JM, Chang J. Predicting deep neck space abscess using computed tomography. Am J Otolaryngol 2006;27:244—7.

57. Vural C, Gungor A, Comerci S. Accuracy of computerized tomography in deep neck infections in the pediatric population. Am J Otolaryngol 2003;24: 143—8.

58. Freling N, Roele E, Schaefer-Prokop C, et al. Prediction of deep neck abscesses by contrast-enhanced computerized tomography in 76 clinically suspect consecutive patients. Laryngoscope 2009;119: 1745—52.

Multidetector and Three-Dimensional CT Evaluation of the Patient With Maxillofacial Injury

Laura L. Avery, MD[a],*, Srinivas M. Susarla, MD, DMD, MPH[b], Robert A. Novelline, MD[a]

KEYWORDS

- Maxillofacial injury • Facial fractures • Multidetector CT
- Facial trauma

Interpretation of images associated with the traumatically injured face is challenging. The complexity of facial anatomy, coupled with the superimposition of numerous bony structures on plain radiographs, poses specific obstacles to accurate interpretation of facial injury. Although plain radiographs can be helpful in cases of isolated injuries, CT is the most useful modality for evaluating facial injury. When compared with radiographs, CT can be acquired faster (6 seconds) with easy patient positioning and minimal dependence on patient cooperation. Interpretation is simplified by the use of multidetector CT with two- and three-dimensional reformations, which allows for accurate and efficient diagnosis of the hard and soft tissues of the maxillofacial region.[1-9] In addition, surgical planning is facilitated by the use of CT, which allows for an accurate assessment of skeletal stability, rotation, and displacement of bony fragments. Multidetector CT also has the notable advantage of rapid image acquisition, with less motion-artifact, and two-dimensional reformations in multiple planes (axial, coronal, and sagittal).[10] The creation of three-dimensional images is relatively straightforward from multidetector CT source images and has been shown to aid in the diagnosis and management of complex, multiplanar facial injuries.[11-15] Although isolated mandibular fractures have often been accurately diagnosed using plain film techniques, notable limitations include sagittal fractures of the mandibular condyle and anterior displacement of the condyle (often seen with subcondylar fractures), both of which are more easily visualized on CT.[16,17] Finally, in the intubated trauma patient with suspected facial injuries, direct examination is often limited and over 50% of the facial fractures may not be apparent from clinical evaluation alone.[18]

This article reviews facial anatomy as it pertains to traumatic injury, emphasizes the clinical findings associated with various types of facial injury, and simplifies the diagnosis of facial injury on CT.

TECHNIQUE

Acquisition of high-resolution images is imperative for proper diagnosis of fractures on facial CT. Slice thickness should be narrow (eg, 0.625 mm on a 64 slice scanner). The field of view should extend

[a] Department of Radiology, Division of Emergency Radiology, Massachusetts General Hospital, 55 Fruit Street, FND210A, Boston, MA 02114, USA
[b] Department of Oral and Maxillofacial Surgery, Massachusetts General Hospital, Harvard Medical School, WACC230, Boston, MA 02114, USA
* Corresponding author.
E-mail address: lavery@partners.org

Radiol Clin N Am 49 (2011) 183–203
doi:10.1016/j.rcl.2010.07.014

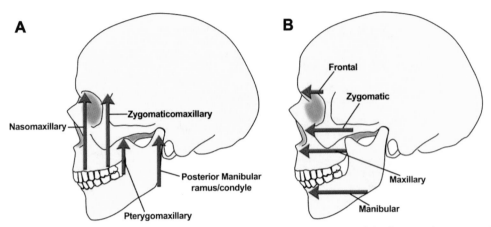

Fig. 1. Vertical and horizontal buttresses of the face. (*A*) The vertical buttresses of the face are the nasomaxillary, zygomaticomaxillary, pterygomaxillary, and ramus/condyle of the mandible. (*B*) The horizontal buttresses of the face include the frontal, zygomatic, maxillary, and mandibular.

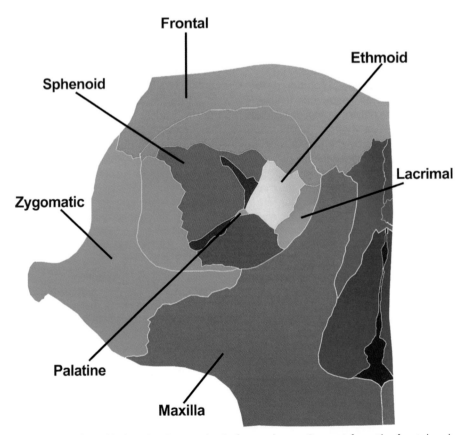

Fig. 2. Orbital region. The orbital region is comprised of seven bones. Support from the frontal and zygomatic buttresses gives the orbital rims increased strength. The thinner bones of the internal orbit are subject to fracture and are commonly involved in fractures that propagate through the orbital floor (eg, isolated orbital floor blowout fractures, Lefort II and Lefort III fractures).

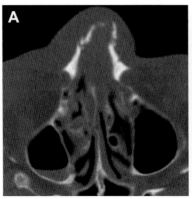
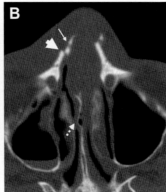

Fig. 3. Nasal fractures. (A) Axial image of the nasal region demonstrates comminuted, laterally displaced fractures of the paired nasal bones. (B) A more inferior axial image demonstrates a fracture through the right frontal process of the maxilla (*arrowhead*), posterior to the nasomaxillary suture (*small arrow*). A fracture of the nasal septum/vomer is visualized more posteriorly (*dotted arrow*).

from the frontal sinuses through the mandible. Axial images should be reconstructed in both bone and soft tissue algorithms at a 1.25-mm slice thickness for standard viewing. Coronal and sagittal reformats should be performed on all cases. A 0.625-mm source image should be used to produce three-dimensional images in all cases of fracture.

RELEVANT ANATOMIC CONCEPTS

Although the finer anatomy of the face is complex and often overwhelming, there are organizational principles for facial anatomy that can help guide the radiologist evaluating facial injury. The face can be organized into five distinct anatomic regions: (1) nasal, (2) orbital, (3) zygomatic, (4) maxillary, and (5) mandibular. Injuries to the face can be classified as those related to a single region; disparate regions; or multiple contiguous regions (eg, midface smash or panfacial fractures).

A second concept that is helpful in evaluating imaging associated with facial trauma is the buttress concept. The face is composed of the five previously mentioned regions, which in turn are supported by horizontal and vertical buttresses (**Fig. 1**). Forces directed toward the face are distributed along these buttresses, giving rise to characteristic fracture patterns. The vertical buttresses of the face include the connections between the maxilla and nasal bones (nasomaxillary), zygoma (zygomaticomaxillary), and pterygoid plates (pterygomaxillary), as well as the ramus/condyle unit of the mandible. The horizontal buttresses of the face, also known as the "anterior-posterior buttresses", include the frontal, zygomatic, maxillary, and mandibular buttresses.

The nasal region, which is comprised of the paired nasal bones, lacrimal bones, frontal processes of the maxillae, the nasal septae (cartilaginous and bony), and the ethmoid sinuses, is supported vertically by the nasomaxillary buttress and medial orbital wall and horizontally by the zygomatic buttress and infraorbital rim.

The orbital region, defined as the conically shaped bony structure that holds the globe, is composed of seven bones (**Fig. 2**). The maxillary, zygomatic and frontal bones comprise the bulk of the external orbital skeleton. The internal orbit, in particular the orbital walls, is supported by the lacrimal, palatine, ethmoid, and sphenoid bones. The orbit is supported horizontally by the frontal and zygomatic buttresses, as well as the supra- and infra-orbital rims and zygomatic body. Because of the bulky skeletal support of the orbit

Table 1 Classification of nasal fractures		
Type		**Characteristics**
I	Simple	Unilateral
II		Bilateral
III	Comminuted	Unilateral
		Bilateral
		Including frontal process of maxilla
IV	Complex	Associated with septal hematoma
		Associated with open nasal laceration
V		Associated with NOE fracture/midface fracture

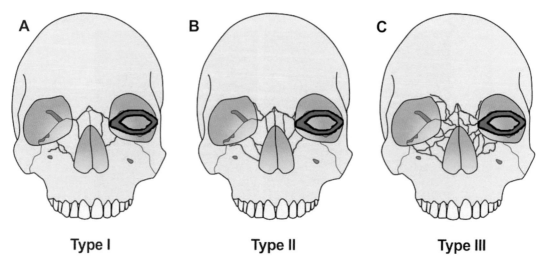

Fig. 4. NOE fracture classification system. NOE fractures are classified by the degree of comminution of the central fragment of the lower two thirds of the medial orbital rim and the involvement of the medial canthal tendon (MCT) insertion. (*A*) Type I fractures: there is a single large central fragment that bears the MCT. (*B*) Type II fractures: there is comminution of the central fragment, but the MCT is attached to a fragment large enough to be stabilized. (*C*) Type III fractures: comminution extends beneath the insertion of the canthal ligament, and reconstruction of the canthal insertion point is necessary.

by these buttresses, it does not easily separate from the surrounding skeletal structures in the absence of high-energy injury. The internal orbital skeleton, however, which is primarily responsible for determining orbital volume, is composed of smaller and thinner bones that are more likely to fracture.

The zygomatic region is supported vertically by the zygomatic process of the frontal bone, lateral orbital rim, lateral zygomatic body and the zygomaticomaxillary buttress (zygomatic process of the maxilla). It is supported horizontally by the zygomatic arch, infraorbital rim, and the zygomatic body (zygomatic buttress). This region serves as a conduit connecting the temporal, maxillary, sphenoid, and frontal bones. Fractures of the zygoma complex disrupt these connections.

The maxillary region of the face includes the dentate region of the maxilla (the alveolar process) and the bony components of the hard palate: the palatine process of the maxilla and the palatine bones. This region is supported vertically by the nasomaxillary, zygomaticomaxillary and pterygomaxillary buttresses and horizontally by the maxillary buttress.

The final region of the face, the mandibular region, is comprised of the mandible and the temporomandibular joint. The mandible has both a vertical buttress (by the posterior mandibular ramus/condyle unit) and a horizontal buttress. It is notable for being the only portion of the facial skeleton (viscerocranium) that is mobile. As such, it shares no direct connection to other bones of the face and remains a self-contained unit, supported by the associated buttresses, masticatory muscles, and temporomandibular joint apparatus.

TYPES OF FACIAL FRACTURES

Facial fractures can involve one or more regions and one or many facial bones. As such, it is often difficult to classify facial fractures simply on the basis of the bones involved. Instead, the radiologist should be familiar with the classical patterns of facial fractures, the bones they involve, and the regions included in a given fracture pattern.

Nasal Fractures and Naso-orbito-ethmoid Fractures

Fractures of the nasal region generally involve the nasal bones in isolation or the naso-orbit-ethmoid (NOE) complex, which includes the bones of the medial orbit and the medial canthal tendon. Because of the prominence of the nasal dorsum and its relatively weak bony support, relatively little

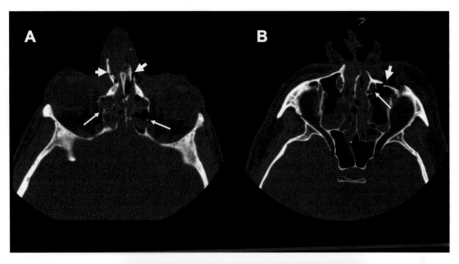

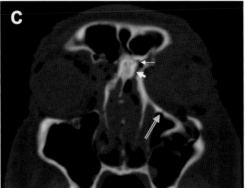

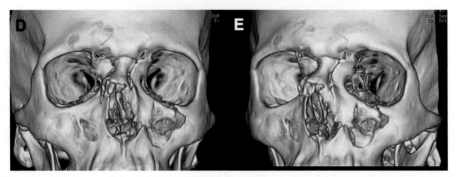

Fig. 5. Bilateral NOE fractures. (*A*) Axial images demonstrate bilateral nasal fractures (*arrowheads*) and impacted fractures of the ethmoid sinuses with disruption of both orbital laminae (laminae papyracea) (*arrows*). (*B*) On the left side, the nasolacrimal (*large arrow*) duct appears posteriorly displaced relative to the right. There is a fracture of the anterior wall of the maxillary sinus (*arrowhead*). (*C*) Coronal image demonstrates fracture through the nasofrontal suture (*small arrow*) and nasomaxillary suture (*arrowhead*). A fracture through the inferior orbital rim is seen (*yellow arrow*). (*D, E*) Three-dimensional reformations give a summary representation of nasal displacement and fracture of the orbital rim. Note the well-demonstrated medial orbital fractures on the oblique image (*E*).

Table 2
Classification of NOE fractures

Type	Characteristics
I	Single fracture of the central fragment, no medial canthal tendon involvement
II	Comminuted central fragment, no medial canthal tendon involvement
III	Comminuted central fragment with medial canthal tendon involvement

energy is required to fracture the nasal bones. As such nasal bone fractures are among the most common facial fractures.[19–21] The clinical history often includes nasal deformity, tenderness over the nasal dorsum, nasal or medial orbital edema, epistaxis, nasal instability, or crepitus. It should be noted, however, that these features are often transient and their absence does not exclude nasal injury in the appropriate context (ie, there is a low negative predictive value).[22] Relevant information useful for diagnosis includes the

mechanism of injury and the force and direction of the blow. Lateral forces account for most nasal fractures, with displacement occurring inferiorly or laterally. Concomitant displacement of the nasal septum and frontal processes of the maxillae may also occur (**Fig. 3**).[23] Occasionally, the anterior maxillary spine, located at the base of the nose, may be fractured and when avulsed is often associated with disruption of the cartilaginous septum. Rohrich and Adams[20] have devised a simple classification scheme to aid the treating clinician (**Table 1**).

More complex fractures involving the nasal region include NOE fractures (**Fig. 4**). The NOE complex includes skeletal structures that are shared by both the nasal and orbital regions. Specifically, the nasal bones, ethmoid bones, and inferior orbital rims are involved. Fractures commonly involve posterior displacement of the anterior nasal structures into the medial orbital rim and ethmoid sinuses (telescoping) (**Fig. 5**). Clinical findings generally are consistent with those of neighboring facial fractures, although there are some findings unique to NOE fractures. Increased intercanthal and interpupillary distance (telecanthus), flattening of the nasal dorsum, or disruption in the medial canthal tendon insertion (positive "traction test" or "bowstring sign") should

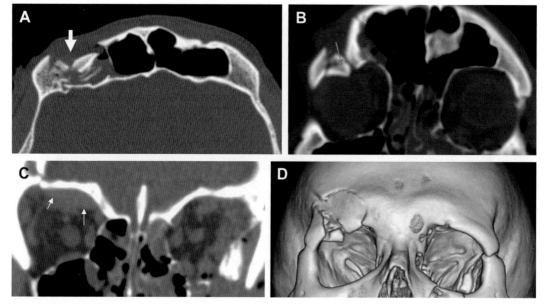

Fig. 6. Superior orbital rim fracture with extension to the orbital roof and frontal sinus. (*A*) Axial image demonstrates impacted superior orbital rim resulting from a direct narrow impact (*arrow*). (*B*) Coronal images demonstrate bony fragments of the orbital rim, which impresses on the globe when compared with the contralateral side (*green arrow*). (*C*) Coronal image in soft tissue demonstrates an extraconal hematoma associated with the fracture (*arrows*). Rapid expansion of the hematoma can lead to compartment syndrome. (*D*) Three-dimensional images nicely demonstrate depressed fracture fragments extending into the orbit.

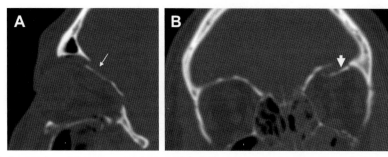

Fig. 7. Left-sided orbital roof fracture with intact orbital rim. (*A*) Sagittal image through the orbit demonstrates mild inferior displacement of an orbital roof fracture fragment (*arrow*). (*B*) Coronal image demonstrates orbital roof fracture with mild mass effect on the adjacent extraocular muscles (*arrowhead*).

raise suspicion for a NOE fracture. Because of the abundance of vital soft tissue structures in this region, such symptoms as epiphora (excessive tearing), bilateral periorbital ecchymoses ("raccoon eyes"), or cerebrospinal fluid rhinorrhea should alert the radiologist to search for additional injuries to the nasolacrimal apparatus, anterior cranial fossa, or nasofrontal duct, respectively.[4,24,25] NOE fractures are clinically classified according to the integrity of the central bone fragment or lower two thirds of the medial orbital rim, the most superior aspect of which is the medial canthal tendon attachment (**Table 2**).[26]

Orbital Fractures

The orbit is composed of numerous bones of varying shapes and sizes and is rigidly attached to the frontal bone, cranial base, and midfacial skeleton. As such, injuries to the forehead, zygoma, maxilla, or nasal region can potentially (and often do) involve the internal or external orbit. For example, it has been estimated that most orbital roof fractures involving the globe (blow-in fractures) are associated with frontal sinus or skull base fractures.[27] Fractures of the orbit do occur in isolation, however, particularly with direct blows to the supraorbital or infraorbital rims (**Fig. 6**). Blow-in fractures are those involving the orbital roof with inferior displacement of the frontal bone into the intraorbital soft tissues thereby decreasing orbital volume (**Fig. 7**). Blow-in fractures usually result from direct impact to the supraorbital rim, in which case the rim is disrupted. Alternatively, forces on the frontal bone may be transmitted to the thinner orbital roof, with collapse of buckling of the roof into the orbit. In these cases, the supraorbital rim is often intact.[27] These orbital roof fractures may extend posteriorly to the orbital apex and compromise the neurologic structures entering the orbit in

this region (CN II, III, IV, V1, and VI), leading to visual acuity changes and ophthalmoplegia (**Fig. 8**).[28] In addition, accumulation of blood and edema within the orbit may result in increased intraorbital pressure and resultant compromise to intraorbital neurovascular structures (orbital compartment syndrome). Orbital roof fractures with concomitant fractures of the anterior cranial fossa or posterior table of the frontal sinus can be associated with pneumocephalus.[29] Ocular injuries are also commonly seen in patients with orbital blow-in fractures.[30]

In contrast, orbital blow-out fractures are those that involve the medial or inferior walls of the orbit and demonstrate displacement of the fractured segment into the ethmoid sinus/nasal cavity or maxillary sinus, respectively (**Fig. 9**). In this regard, CT imaging in both the axial and coronal planes is essential for accurate diagnosis and as an aid to

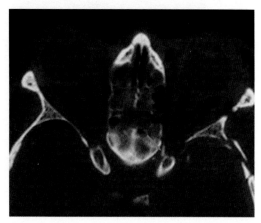

Fig. 8. Complex orbital roof and sphenoid bone fractures with extension to the orbital apex. Axial image through the level of the optic canal demonstrates a fracture fragment (*green arrow*) extending into the canal with resultant nerve injury.

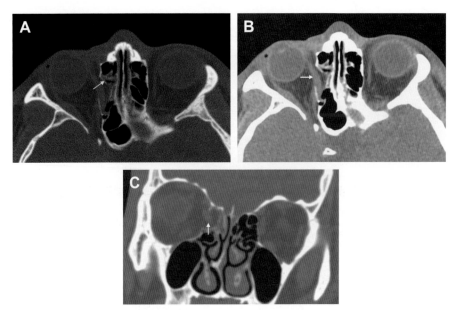

Fig. 9. Blow-out fracture of medial orbital wall. (*A*) Axial image in bone windows demonstrates a fracture of the medial orbital wall through the orbital plate of ethmoid (*yellow arrow*). (*B*) Axial image in soft tissue windows demonstrates herniation of the medial rectus muscle into the fracture defect (*arrow*). (*C*) Coronal image demonstrates blow-out of medial orbital wall with herniation of the medial rectus (*arrow*). Note the honeycomb structure of the numerous bony septa of the contralateral ethmoid sinus, which support the orbital plate of ethmoid, allowing it to withstand the sudden rise in intraorbital hydraulic pressure better than the orbital floor. This is given as a reason for the higher frequency of orbital floor fractures relative to medial orbital fractures.

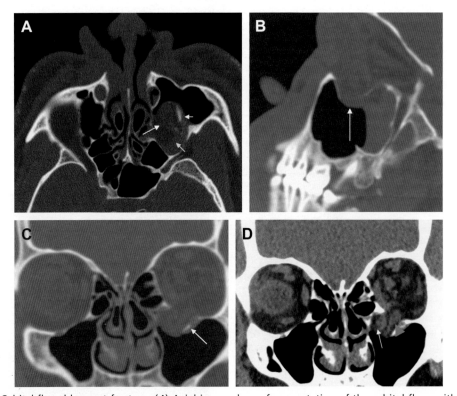

Fig. 10. Orbital floor blow-out fracture. (*A*) Axial image shows fragmentation of the orbital floor with a fallen fragment (*small white arrowhead*), herniated intraorbital fat (*white arrow*), and layering blood (*yellow arrow*). (*B*) Sagittal image demonstrates the large depressed orbital floor fracture with herniation of orbital contents (*arrow*). (*C*) Coronal image in bone windows demonstrates orbital floor fracture with "trapdoor" fragment (*arrow*). (*D*) Coronal image in soft tissue window demonstrates partial herniation of the inferior rectus muscle (*green arrowhead*) along with intraorbital fat and hemorrhage (*white arrow*).

surgical planning.[6,23] A key diagnostic distinction with regard to blow-out fractures is the integrity of the infraorbital rim. By definition, the orbital rim is intact with blow-out fractures. Orbital blow-out fractures result from broad based blows to the orbit that increases intraorbital pressure to the extent that the weakest wall of the orbit (ie, the floor or medial wall, both of which are

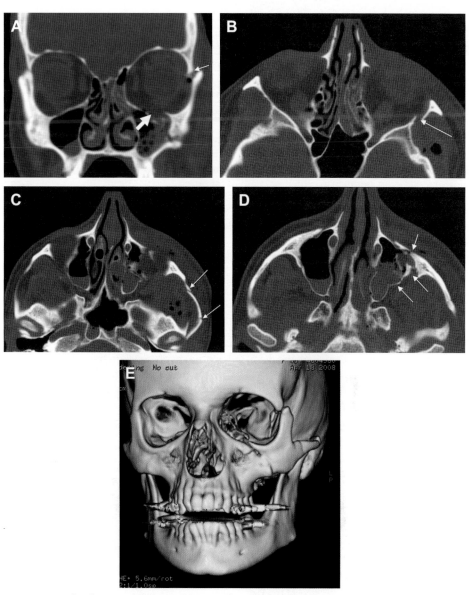

Fig. 11. Zygoma complex fracture. (*A*) Coronal image of a zygoma complex fracture demonstrates diastasis of the zygomaticofrontal suture (*small arrow*). This zygomatic attachment is best seen on coronal reformations. The inferior portion of the fracture is seen propagating from the anterior wall of the maxillary sinus to the orbital floor (*large arrow*). (*B*) A superior axial image through the level of the orbit demonstrates a fracture of the lateral orbital wall at the level of the zygomaticosphenoid suture (*arrow*). (*C*) An inferior axial image demonstrates a comminuted fracture of the zygomatic arch with fracture of the zygomaticotemporal suture (*arrows*). (*D*) An even more inferior axial image demonstrates fracture of the anterior and posterior/lateral walls of the maxillary sinus at the zygomaticomaxillary sutures (*arrows*). (*E*) Slightly oblique three-dimensional image shows depressed zygomatic arch, with lateral displacement of the zygoma (Knight and North Type B).

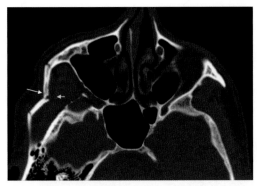

Fig. 12. Isolated zygomatic arch fracture. Axial image demonstrates a typical depressed three part V-shaped fracture of the zygomatic arch (*white arrow*). Compression of the temporalis tendon is seen (*yellow arrow*).

Table 3 Classification of zygoma complex fractures	
Type	**Characteristics**
A	Fracture of only one zygomatic pillar: zygomatic arch, lateral orbital rim, or infraorbital rim
B	Fracture involving all four zygomatic articulations with displacement
C	Multifragment fractures including comminution of the zygoma body

bounded by air filled spaces) collapse outward (**Fig. 10**). The result is an increase in orbital volume and a potential for orbital soft tissue contents to herniate into the adjacent space. When the medial or inferior rectus muscles are involved, by herniation into the ethmoid or maxillary sinuses, respectively, the clinical consequence is globe entrapment. Entrapment is seen with small, narrow fractures, where the muscle can be immobilized in the fracture and is seen on CT scan as an abrupt kink in the muscle.[23] Sagittal reformations are useful for evaluation of inferior rectus position relative to the fractured orbital floor. In contrast, wider fractures of the orbital floor, where the diameter of the fracture allows for partial displacement of the globe, result in enophthalmos.[30] Clinically significant indications for repair include entrapment and enophthalmos. It is important to note whether an orbital floor fracture extends to include the posterior wall of the maxillary sinus, because involvement to this extent increases the difficulty of repair.

Fractures that include the orbital floor and the orbital rim are classified separately. Damage to the orbital rim typically results from a narrowly applied force with a direct blow to the rim or a high-energy blow that results in an orbital floor fracture with an orbital rim component. It is important to distinguish between this type of injury and a blow-out fracture, which spares the orbital rim. The involvement of the infraorbital rim in this context has implications for surgical repair and must be noted. Finally, given the relatively rigid structure of the external orbital ring (composed of the maxilla, zygoma, and frontal bone), a seemingly isolated fracture of the orbital rim must be evaluated carefully for concomitant fracture to other segments of the orbit.

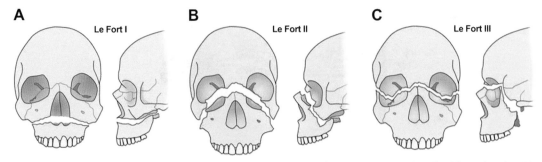

Fig. 13. Lefort fractures, levels I–III. This figure depicts the classic fracture patterns described by Lefort in 1901. (*A*) Lefort I level fracture: the horizontal plane of the fracture extends between the pterygoid plates of the sphenoid bone to the piriform aperture and lateral nasal wall. The Lefort I fracture involves the maxilla, including the maxillary sinus. (*B*) Lefort II fracture: the fracture propagates from the pterygoid plates posteriorly, through the orbital floor, to the nasofrontal suture. In bilateral cases, this gives rise to the classic "pyramidal" pattern. (*C*) Craniofacial disjunction, or the Lefort III fracture: involves total separation of the midfacial structures from the cranial base. This level of fracture propagates from the pterygoid plates, through the lateral orbital wall (frontozygomatic suture), by the orbital floor, to the nasofrontal suture.

Zygomatic Fractures

A direct blow to the lateral midface (the zygomatic region) can result in disruption of the zygoma from its anatomic connections to the temporal, sphenoid, frontal, and maxillary bones. This type of fracture is known as a "zygoma" or "zygomatic complex" fracture (**Fig. 11**). Three large connections that are disrupted are the zygomaticofrontal (either by the zygomaticofrontal suture or the frontal process of the zygoma); zygomaticomaxillary (propagating through the infraorbital rim and orbital floor); and zygomaticotemporal (often seen as a zygomatic arch fracture). The zygomaticosphenoid attachment

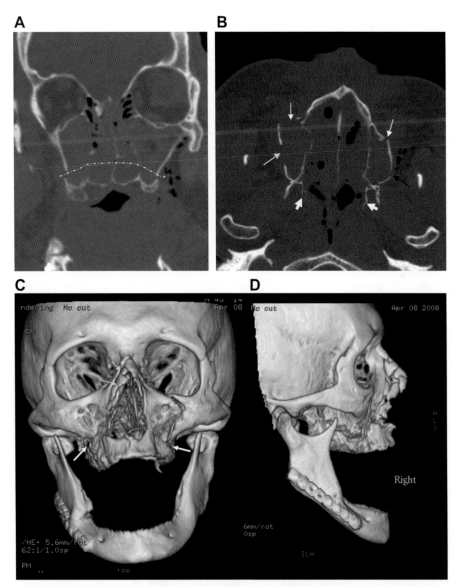

Fig. 14. Lefort I fracture with comminuted nasal and frontal process of maxilla fractures. (*A*) Coronal image through the mid maxillary sinus demonstrates a horizontally oriented fracture propagating just above the alveolar process of the maxilla through the bases of the sinuses (*dotted line*). Note fracture through the nasal septum. (*B*) Axial image through the level of the inferior maxillary sinuses and pterygoid plates. Note fracture through the anterior (*white arrows*) and posterolateral (*yellow arrows*) walls of the maxillary sinuses. Fractured pterygoid plates are also present (*arrowheads*). (*C*) Three-dimensional image beautifully demonstrates the fracture through the maxilla just superior to the alveolar process (*white arrows*). It is easy to imagine the "free floating" nature of the hard palate with this fracture pattern. Note is made of comminuted nasal fractures (*yellow arrows*). (*D*) Three-dimensional lateral image demonstrates propagation of the fracture through the base of the pterygoid pates posteriorly (*yellow arrows*).

located along the lateral orbital wall may rarely propagate to involve the orbital apex.[23] Clinical signs and symptoms include cheek depression; infraorbital nerve paresthesia; or globe entrapment (with significant orbital floor involvement) or visual acuity changes and ophthalmoplegia (with orbital apex involvement). With involvement of the zygomatic arch, depression of the arch and compression of the temporalis tendon at its insertion point on the coronoid process of the mandible manifests clinically as trismus (limited mouth opening) (**Fig. 12**).[23,31] The presence of significant displacement, trismus, entrapment, orbital apex involvement, or CNV2 paresthesia are indications for operative intervention.[32] Zygoma complex fractures are classified according to the direction and magnitude of displacement, and bony integrity of the zygoma, as originally described by Knight and North using plain films.[33] This classification scheme organized fractures into six groups: Group I (non-displaced fractures), Group II (isolated zygomatic arch injury), Group III (depressed, non-rotated body fractures), Group IV (medially rotated body fractures), Group V (laterally rotated fractures), and Group VI (complex, comminuted fractures with additional fracture lines across the main fragment). Though system was originally based on fracture stability after reduction, with groups II and V fractures

generally stable following reduction without fixation and groups III, IV and VI requiring some form of fixation for stability, it is now generally accepted that all displaced fractures require open reduction and fixation.[24,25,31,33] A more recent classification system, based on CT imaging, is helpful for establishing the necessity for surgical treatment (**Table 3**).[24]

Maxillary Fractures

Among the most well-described facial fractures are those involving the maxilla at the Lefort I, II, and III levels (**Fig. 13**).[34] In addition, fractures involving the nasal, orbital, and zygomatic regions often involve the maxilla. The clinical examination for fractures involving the dentate regions of the face (maxilla and mandible) often is significant for dental malocclusion. Given the proprioceptive sensitivity of the masticatory system, even nondisplaced fractures may present clinically with a complaint of malocclusion.[24,35] In the context of this clinical history, careful exploration for maxillary fractures is necessary.

The common feature of Lefort maxillary fractures is the involvement of the pterygoid plates. The classification of Lefort I, II, and III can be easily determined based on the propagation of the

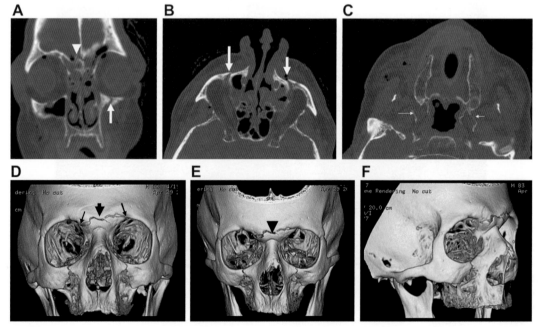

Fig. 15. Lefort II fracture. (*A, B*) Coronal and axial images of this classic Lefort II fracture demonstrates inferior orbital rim fractures (*arrows*) and a horizontal fracture just superior to the nasal-frontal suture (*arrowhead*). (*C*) An inferior axial image at the level of the palate demonstrates comminuted pterygoid plate fractures (*arrows*). (*D, E*) Three-dimensional images demonstrate fracture through the inferior orbital (*green arrows*) and medial orbital rims (*black arrows*). Horizontal fracture just superior to the nasofrontal suture (*arrowheads*). (*F*) Note the propagation of the fracture through the posterior maxilla (*arrows*). The zygomatic arch is intact.

fracture from the level of the posterior maxilla, and on the clinical signs and symptoms.

The Lefort I level fracture involves the segments attaching the alveolar process of the maxilla to the remainder of the face superiorly (**Fig. 14**). In particular, the fracture propagates from the lateral aspect of the piriform rims to the pterygoid plates, also fracturing the anterior wall of the maxillary sinus. Often the nasal septum is fractured. This level of fracture is manifest clinically as a maxilla and hard palate that is distinctly mobile relative to the remainder of the midface.

In a Lefort II level fracture (or pyramidal fracture), the fracture extends from the pterygoid plates to involve the inferior and medial orbital rims, terminating in a fracture of the nasal bones or a diathesis at the nasofrontal suture (**Fig. 15**). The line of fracture includes the lateral and anterior walls of the maxillary sinus, the orbital floor, and the medial orbital wall. This results in a triangular-, or pyramidal-, shaped fracture involving the maxillary, orbital, and nasal regions. Clinically, the maxillary and nasal regions are distinctly separate from the remainder of the face and are mobile. The

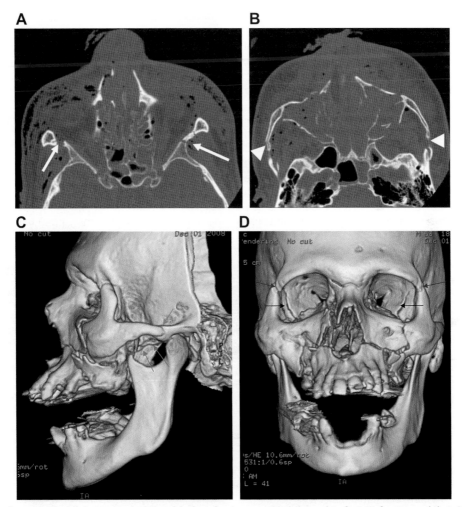

Fig. 16. Complex facial fractures multilevel Lefort fractures, with bilateral Lefort III fractures. (A) Axial image through the level of the orbit demonstrates fractures of the lateral orbital walls at the level of the zygomaticosphenoid sutures (*arrows*). Complex fractures of the ethmoid sinuses and frontal process of maxilla are also identified. (B) Axial image at the level of the frontal sinuses demonstrates comminuted fractures of the zygomatic arches bilaterally (*arrowheads*). Displaced fractures of the anterior and posterior/lateral walls of the maxillary sinuses are identified consistent with Lefort II component. (C) Three-dimensional image in a lateral projection demonstrates the involvement of the pterygoid plates (*red arrows*). A fracture through the zygomatic arch is also identified (*green arrow*). (D) Three-dimensional image shows fracture extending superiorly and laterally to involve the orbital floor (*black arrows*) and the frontozygomatic suture (*blue arrows*). When this pattern occurs bilaterally, the facial skeleton is effectively separated from the cranial base. As such, bilateral Lefort III level fractures are often termed "craniofacial disjunction."

zygomatic bones remain attached to the remainder of the skeleton by their connections to the frontal, temporal, and sphenoid bones.

The highest level Lefort fracture, Lefort III, is often termed "craniofacial disjunction." The fracture line propagates from the pterygoid plates to involve the connection between the upper face and the skull base. Specifically, the fracture involves the pterygoid plates, zygomatic arches, lateral and medial orbital rims, and nasal bones or nasofrontal suture (**Fig. 16**). Disconnections at these areas result in a midfacial and inferior orbital complex that is distinctly mobile relative to the remainder of the superior orbit and upper face.

Although classically described as having bilateral involvement, Lefort fractures may be unilateral or bilateral paired fractures of different levels (eg, left-sided Lefort I with right-sided Lefort II).[36] Surgical approaches are often dependent on the classification of fracture, because fixation is dependent on the presence of a stable, nonfractured skeletal region. In this context, it is vital that midfacial injuries be classified appropriately. For example, a bilateral Lefort II fracture with a right-sided zygoma complex fracture is not the same as a right-sided Lefort III and left-sided Lefort II. In the former case, the orbital rims are involved bilaterally and the orbital floor on the right has a more complex fracture pattern that may need to be rigidly fixed to appropriately restore orbital volume.

The most complex fracture involving the maxillary region is the midfacial smash or crush injury (**Fig. 17**). This type of injury results in severe comminution of the anterior midface, with involvement of multiple facial regions and destabilization of numerous facial buttresses.[23,29] Adequate repair of such injuries requires complete visualization of the fractured segments, only possible with three-dimensional reformatted images. The degree of loss of vertical midfacial height, comminution, and bony discontinuity, most accurately captured in three-dimensional imaging, determines the necessity for autogenous bone grafting to allow for rigid fixation.[13,37]

Another, less common, fracture of the maxilla is the palatal fracture, or sagittal maxillary fracture.[38] This is conceptually similar to a unilateral Lefort I fracture in the sagittal plane, separating the maxilla into right and left symmetric segments or greater and lesser asymmetric segments. If the fracture propagates anteriorly to include the alveolar process, clinical examination reveals a significantly mobile alveolar segment. Additional isolated fractures of the alveolar ridge of the maxillae are common (**Fig. 18**). These fractures usually occur in the context of trauma to the teeth. Teeth may

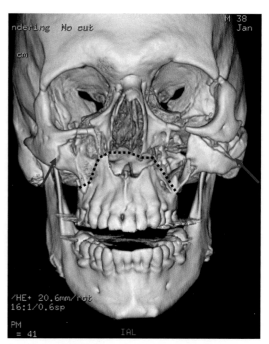

Fig. 17. Smashed face. The three-dimensional image demonstrates a complex injury of the midface that does not conform to a single fracture pattern. Such complex injuries, or "midface smash" injuries, typically are the result of high-energy trauma and may involve multiple soft tissue structures. In this patient, the orbital floors are fractured bilaterally (*red arrows*) and there is bilateral involvement of the zygomaticomaxillary complexes (*blue arrows*). The left zygoma is comminuted and there is a bilateral Lefort I level fracture of the maxilla (*dashed line*). Surgical repair of these injuries is complicated and the radiologist should be aware of potential injuries to surrounding soft tissue structures, including large soft tissue lacerations and injuries to the facial nerve, parotid duct, and lacrimal apparatus.

be missing or be mobile on physical examination. If missing teeth are not accounted for, a chest radiograph may be warranted to excluded tooth aspiration.

Mandibular Fractures

The mandible is the only mobile bone in the face and is a continuous structure connecting the two temporomandibular joints. As such, mandibular fractures can be among the most complicated type of facial fractures to treat. There are numerous causes of mandibular fractures, the most common being automobile accidents, assaults, and falls.[39] Fractures of the mandible can be classified according to location, pattern, and displacement based on biomechanical factors.

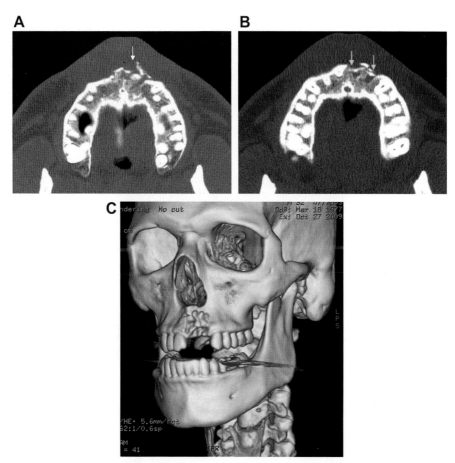

Fig. 18. Isolated fracture of the alveolar ridge. (*A*) Axial image of the alveolar portion of the maxilla demonstrates a comminuted fracture (*white arrow*). (*B*) The fracture extends to the roots of the left central and lateral incisor (*yellow arrows*). (*C*) Three-dimensional reformation demonstrates the isolated alveolar ridge associated with trauma to the teeth with resultant tooth loss.

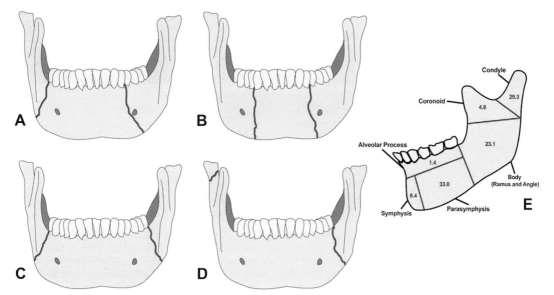

Fig. 19. Illustration of mandibular fracture patterns and prevalence. (*A*) Angle and opposite body. (*B*) Bilateral body. (*C*) Bilateral angle. (*D*) Condyle and opposite angle. (*E*) Percent mandibular fractures by location.

There are six distinct regions of the mandible that are commonly fractured (**Fig. 19**).[1,39] The most common location for mandibular fracture is the mandibular body, which is defined as the region of the mandible between the posterior aspect of the mandibular canine and the posterior aspect of the second molar. Next is the condylar region, followed by the mandibular angle and mandibular symphysis (**Fig. 20**). Isolated coronoid process fractures and isolated alveolar process fractures are rare. Of note, condylar fractures are the most commonly undiagnosed (**Figs. 21** and **22**).[40] This has important implications for treatment, because intracapsular fractures of the mandibular condyle that remain untreated can result in temporomandibular joint ankylosis, requiring future surgical intervention for correction.

Patterns of mandibular fracture of clinical significance are coup-countercoup injuries and fractures resulting in "flail" segments. Common coup-countercoup injuries include angle and contralateral body, bilateral angle, and angle and contralateral condyle. Bilateral symphysis fractures in which the genioglossus muscle attachment is with the fractured segment, destabilize the tongue, resulting in a propensity for airway compromise caused by a "flail segment" (**Fig. 23**).

With regard to biomechanical stresses, mandibular fractures are classified as favorable if the vector forces of the masticatory muscles act to reduce the fracture and unfavorable if such forces displace the fracture. Horizontally favorable fractures include those of the mandibular angle where the fracture is perpendicular to the orientation of the masseteric and medial pterygoid fibers. Likewise, a horizontally unfavorable fracture of the mandibular angle is one in which the fracture line is parallel to the muscle fiber orientation. Vertically favorable fractures are those in which the fracture line, as viewed in the axial plane, is parallel to the orientation of the medial pterygoid fibers (or perpendicular to the orientation of the lateral pterygoid fibers), with unfavorable fractures being perpendicular to the medial pterygoid fibers (or parallel to the lateral pterygoid fibers) in the same plane.

The clinical history consistent with mandibular injury includes dental malocclusion, dental trauma, sublingual hematoma, intraoral hemorrhage, or

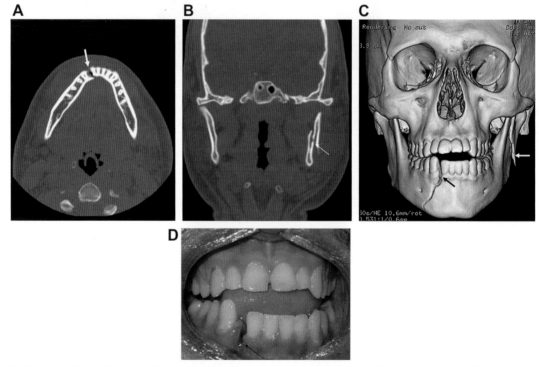

Fig. 20. Mandibular fractures. (*A*) Axial images through the level of the mandible demonstrate a right parasymphyseal fracture (*arrow*). (*B*) Coronal image demonstrates fracture of the left mandibular ramus (*arrow*). (*C*) Three-dimensional image shows a parasymphyseal fracture extending to the alveolar portion of the mandible (*black arrow*). Fracture of the left ramus is also identified (*white arrow*). Three-dimensional imaging is best suited to demonstrate the degree of displacement and rotation of fracture fragments. (*D*) Clinical image of the patient's mouth demonstrates the alveolar portion of the fracture with extension through the gingiva making this an "open" fracture (*arrow*).

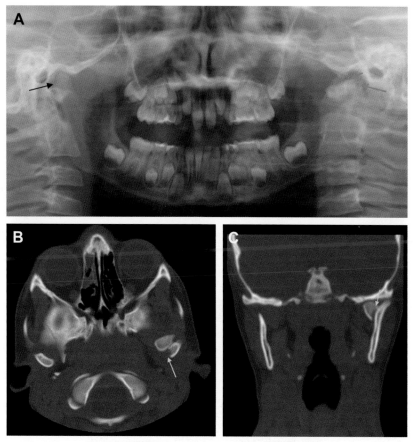

Fig. 21. Left Intracapsular mandibular condyle in an 8 year old who fell on his chin while skateboarding. (*A*) Panorex image in this young patient demonstrates significant motion artifact especially on the left. Normal right mandibular condyle is noted (*black arrow*). Irregularity of the left mandibular condyle is noted with a duplicated appearance (*green arrows*). (*B*) Axial image through the mandibular condyles demonstrates a sagittally oriented left condyle fracture (*yellow arrow*). (*C*) Coronal image demonstrates the isolated intracapsular condyle fracture (*yellow arrow*).

lower lip or chin paresthesia (CNV3 travels within the mandible en route to supply the skin of the lower lip and chin). Fractures involving the temporomandibular joint, best seen with coronal reformations, may also present with injury to the external auditory canal, including otorrhea or otorrhagia.[41]

Although plain film techniques can successfully demonstrate mandibular fractures, it is important to obtain CT imaging, in both the axial and coronal planes, for evaluation of the patient with mandibular trauma. Plain film techniques, such as the panoramic radiograph, may be adequate for evaluation of some types of mandibular fractures, but have limited use for diagnosing midface injury. Given that many patients presenting with mandibular fractures may also have midfacial injury, CT is the ideal modality to completely evaluate the facial skeleton. Clinicians treating mandibular fractures

often monitor treatment progress with plain film imaging, however, and the radiologist should be familiar with such methods.

Frontal Sinus Fractures

Although not technically part of the facial skeleton, the frontal bone is particularly prominent and often injured in the patient with facial trauma and often managed by the facial surgeon (**Fig. 24**). The frontal sinus is bounded anteriorly and posteriorly by bony walls, commonly referred to as the "anterior and posterior tables." The anterior table is adjacent to the soft tissue of the forehead and the posterior table separates the sinus from the anterior cranial fossa. Isolated fractures of the anterior table are the least serious injury and often do not require repair. Fractures involving the

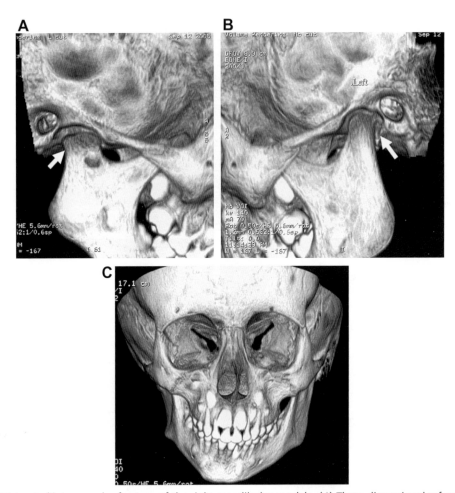

Fig. 22. Untreated intracapsular fracture of the right mandibular condyle. (*A*) Three-dimensional reformation in a patient who suffered an undiagnosed right intracapsular fracture that caused irregularity and foreshortening of the mandibular condyle (*arrow*). (*B*) Three-dimensional image demonstrates the normal appearance of the

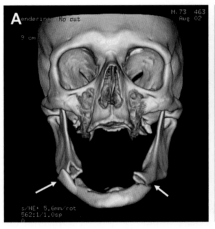

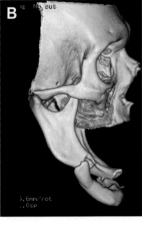

Fig. 23. Flail mandible. (*A*) Three-dimensional image demonstrates bilateral significantly displaced anterior mandible fractures resulting in a "flail segment." The fractures are located at the parasymphyseal-body junction bilaterally (*arrows*). (*B*) Three-dimensional lateral projection demonstrates the significant posterior displacement of the anterior mandibular arch. It is easy to imagine that this degree of displacement would destabilize the anterior supporting structures of the tongue and lead to possible airway compromise.

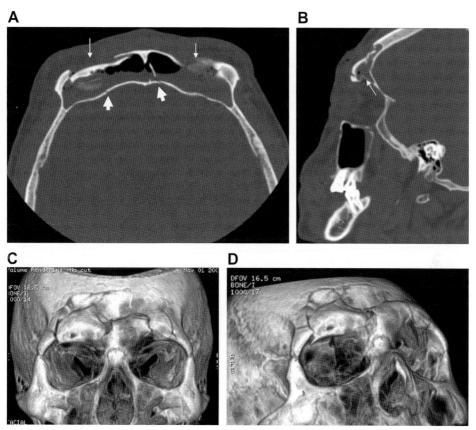

Fig. 24. Frontal sinus fracture. (*A*) Axial image shows comminuted fractures of the anterior wall of the frontal sinus (*arrows*). Nondisplaced posterior wall fractures are also seen (*arrowheads*). (*B*) Sagittal image demonstrates the fracture extending to the orbital roof (*arrow*). (*C, D*) Three-dimensional image beautifully demonstrate the degree of comminution and displacement of the frontal sinus fracture.

anterior and posterior tables are more serious, because there is central nervous system involvement and there are compound skull fractures, requiring, at a minimum, antibiotic treatment. Pneumocephalus is often a key finding suggestive of posterior table fractures. Propagation of the frontal sinus fracture into the anterior cranial fossa, along the cribiform plate, may present clinically as cerebrospinal fluid rhinorrhea. The simplest classification scheme for frontal sinus fractures requires a description of the anterior table, posterior table, and patency of the nasofrontal duct (**Table 4**).[42–44]

MAXILLOFACIAL FRACTURES IN THE PEDIATRIC POPULATION

Because of the timing of craniofacial growth and development of the occlusion, the patterns of facial fractures in children are distinctly different than adults. Although nasal fractures are the most common type of pediatric facial fracture, mandibular fractures remain the most frequent cause of hospitalization and almost always require

treatment.[4,45,46] In addition, the distribution of bony mass in the pediatric facial skeleton results in a higher frequency of condylar fractures in children than adults and a lower frequency of

Table 4 Clinical significance of structural involvement in frontal sinus fractures	
Type	**Significance**
Isolated anterior table	If displacement is greater than width of anterior table, requires open reduction
Posterior table involvement	By definition, compound skull fracture, requires antibiotic treatment at a minimum Consider possible cerebrospinal fluid leak
Nasofrontal duct involvement	If involved, requires operative intervention to obliterate sinus

midfacial fractures in children, because the sinuses are not completely pneumatized.[47,48] When midfacial injuries are detected in children, the fracture patterns do not follow the typical Lefort scheme, but are more obliquely oriented across the injured parts of the face.[49] The relative prominence of the cranium in children results in a greater frequency of frontal bone and orbital roof fractures.[49] Incomplete ossification of the facial bones often results in greenstick or incomplete fractures.[47] Treatment in children is usually performed without delay and accurate diagnosis is paramount.[46] Three-dimensional reconstructions are important in this population, because bony discontinuities have important implications for craniofacial growth and often require primary bone grafting, which is preferable to secondary or alloplastic reconstruction.[46] Finally, children presenting with facial injuries should always be evaluated clinically for distant skeletal and soft tissue injuries consistent with abuse.[50]

MAXILLOFACIAL FRACTURES ASSOCIATED WITH CERVICAL SPINE OR INTRACRANIAL INJURY

It has been well established that patients who present with maxillofacial trauma often have concomitant injuries to the cervical spine and skull base.[51–53] Injuries to these structures are themselves associated with intracranial hemorrhage.[54] Results from large case series suggest that, among patients initially evaluated for facial injury, between 4% and 10% have simultaneous cervical spine injury and almost 50% have concurrent intracranial injury.[51,52] Fractures of the upper facial skeleton (the forehead and superior orbit) are associated with an increased likelihood of lower cervical spine fractures and intracranial injury. Unilateral fractures of the midfacial skeleton (the nasal, orbital, zygomatic, and maxillary regions) are associated with basilar skull fractures and multiple intracranial injuries. Unilateral fractures of the mandible are associated with upper cervical spine injury. Most importantly, severe bilateral midfacial injury is associated with severe skull base fractures and death. These predictable patterns of associated cervical spine and intracranial injury should prompt the radiologist to recommend additional imaging studies in patients who present with facial trauma and undergo maxillofacial CT.

REFERENCES

1. Rhea JT, Rao PM, Novelline RA. Helical CT and three-dimensional CT of facial and orbital injury. Radiol Clin North Am 1999;37(3):489–513.

2. Iinume T, Hirota Y, Ishio K. Orbital wall fractures: conventional views and CT. Rhinology 1994;32:81.

3. Johnson DH Jr, Colman M, Larsson S, et al. Computed tomography in medial maxilla-orbital fractures. J Comput Assist Tomogr 1984;8:416.

4. Laine FJ, Conway WF, Laskin DM. Radiology of maxillofacial trauma. Curr Probl Diagn Radiol 1993; 22:145.

5. Lambert DM, Mirvis SE, Shanmuganathan K, et al. Computed tomography exclusion of osseous paranasal sinus injury in blunt trauma patients: the "clear sinus" sign. J Oral Maxillofac Surg 1997;55:1207.

6. Nolasco FP, Mathog RH. Medial orbital wall fractures: classification and clinical profile. Otolaryngol Head Neck Surg 1995;112:549.

7. Novelline RA. Three-dimensional CT of facial trauma. In: Thrall JH, editor. Current practice of radiology. St. Louis (MO): Mosby-Year Book; 1993. p. 323–35.

8. Novelline RA, Liebig T, Jordan J, et al. Computed tomography of orbital and occular injuries. Emerg Radiol 1994;1:56.

9. Russell JL, Davidson MJ, Daly BD, et al. Computed tomography in the diagnosis of maxillofacial trauma. Br J Oral Maxillofac Surg 1990;28:287.

10. Tello R, Suojanen J, Costello P, et al. Comparison of spiral CT and conventional CT in 3D visualization of facial trauma: work in progress. Comput Med Imaging Graph 1994;18:423.

11. Levy RA, Edwards WT, Meyer JR, et al. Facial trauma and 3D reconstructive imaging: insufficiencies and correctives. AJNR Am J Neuroradiol 1992;13:885.

12. Fox LA, Vannier MW, West OC, et al. Diagnostic performance of CT, MPR and 3DCT imaging in maxillofacial trauma. Comput Med Imaging Graph 1995;19:385.

13. Mayer JS, Wainwright DJ, Yeakley JW, et al. The role of three-dimensional computed tomography in the management of maxillofacial trauma. J Trauma 1988;28:1043.

14. Gillespie JE, Isherwood I, Barker GR, et al. Three-dimensional reformation of computed tomography in the assessment of facial trauma. Clin Radiol 1987;38:523.

15. Rose EH, Norris MS, Rosen JM. Application of high-tech three-dimensional imaging and computer-generated models in complex facial reconstructions with vascularized bone grafts. Plast Reconstr Surg 1993;91:252.

16. Yamaoka M, Furusawa K, Iguchi K. The assessment of fracture of the mandibular condyle by use of computerized tomography: incidence of sagittal split fracture. Br J Oral Maxillofac Surg 1994;32:77.

17. Raustia AM, Pyhtinen J, Oikarinen KS, et al. Conventional radiographic and computed tomographic findings in cases of fracture of the mandibular condylar process. J Oral Maxillofac Surg 1990;48:1258.

18. Rehm CG, Ross SE. Diagnosis of unsuspected facial fractures on routine head computerized tomographic scans in the unconscious multiply injured patient. J Oral Maxillofac Surg 1995;53:522.

19. Reddy LV, Elhadi HM. Nasal fractures. In: Fonseca, Marciani, Turvey, et al, editors. In: Oral and maxillofacial surgery, vol. 2. St. Louis (MO): Saunders; 2009. p. 270–82.

20. Rohrich RJ, Adams WP Jr. Nasal fracture management: minimizing secondary nasal deformities. Plast Reconstr Surg 2000;106(2):266–73.

21. Supriya M, Clement WA, Ahsan F. Satisfaction with cosmesis following nasal manipulation: do previous fractures matter? J Laryngol Otol 2006;120:749–52.

22. Tremolet de Villers Y, Schultz RC. Nasal fractures. J Trauma 1975;15(4):319–27.

23. Pathria MN, Blaser SI. Diagnostic imaging of craniofacial fractures. Radiol Clin North Am 1989;27:839.

24. Manson PN, Markowitz B, Mirvis S, et al. Toward CT-based facial fracture treatment. Plast Reconstr Surg 1990;85:202.

25. Reddy LV, Pagnotto M. Midface fractures. In: Fonseca, Marciani, Turvey, et al, editors. In: Oral and maxillofacial surgery, vol. 2. St. Louis (MO): Saunders; 2009. p. 233–56.

26. Markowitz BL, Manson PN, Sargent L, et al. Management of the medial canthal tendon in nasoethmoid orbital fractures: the importance of the central fragment in classification and treatment. Plast Reconstr Surg 1991;87(5):843–53.

27. Martello JY, Vasconez HC. Supraorbital roof fractures: a formidable entity with which to contend. Ann Plast Surg 1997;38:223.

28. Chirico PA, Mirvis SE, Kelman SE, et al. Orbital "blow in" fractures: clinical and CT fractures. J Comput Assist Tomogr 1989;13:1017.

29. Lawrason JN, Novelline RA. Diagnostic imaging of facial trauma. In: Mirvis SE, Young JWR, editors. Diagnostic imaging in trauma and critical care. Baltimore (MD): Williams & Wilkins; 1992. p. 243.

30. Leone CR Jr. Periorbital trauma. Int Ophthalmol Clin 1995;35:1.

31. Rohrich RJ, Hollier LH, Watumuli D. Optimizing the management of orbitozygomatic fractures. Clin Plast Surg 1992;19:149.

32. Freeman LN, Selff SR, Aguilar GL, et al. Self-compression plates for orbital rim fractures. Ophthal Plast Reconstr Surg 1991;7:198.

33. Knight JS, North JF. The classification of malar fractures: an analysis of displacement as a guide to treatment. Br J Plast Surg 1961;13:325.

34. LeFort R. E'tude experimentale sur les fractures de la machoire superieure. Rev Chir 1901;23:208 [in French].

35. Romano JJ, Manson PN, Mirvis SE, et al. Le Fort fractures without mobility. Plast Reconstr Surg 1990;85:355.

36. Levine RS, Grossman RI. Head and facial trauma. Emerg Med Clin North Am 1985;3:447.

37. Szachowicz EH. Facial bone wound healing. Otolaryngol Clin North Am 1995;28:865.

38. Thompson R, Myer CM III. Sagittal palate fracture. Ann Otol Rhinol Laryngol 1988;97(4 pt 1):432.

39. Coletti DP, Caccamese JF Jr. Diagnosis and management of mandible fractures. In: Fonseca, Marciani, Turvey, et al, editors. In: Oral and maxillofacial surgery, vol. 2. St. Louis (MO): Saunders; 2009. p. 139–61.

40. Assael LA. Clinical aspects of imaging in maxillofacial trauma. Radiol Clin North Am 1993;31:209.

41. Avrahami E, Frishman E, Katz R. CT evaluation of otorrhagia associated with condylar fractures. Clin Radiol 1994;49:877.

42. Strong EB, Pahlavan N, Saito D. Frontal sinus fractures: a 28-year retrospective review. Otolaryngol Head Neck Surg 2006;135:774.

43. Tiwari P, Higuera S, Thornton J, et al. The management of frontal sinus fractures. J Oral Maxillofac Surg 2005;63:1354.

44. Fattahi T. Management of frontal sinus fractures. In: Fonseca, Marciani, Turvey, et al, editors. In: Oral and maxillofacial surgery, vol. 2. St. Louis (MO): Saunders; 2009. p. 256–69.

45. McGrath CJ, Egbert MA, Tong DC, et al. Unusual presentations of injuries associated with the mandibular condyle in children. Br J Oral Maxillofac Surg 1996;34:311.

46. Zimmermann CE, Troulis MJ, Kaban LB. Pediatric facial fractures: recent advances in prevention, diagnosis and management. Int J Oral Maxillofac Surg 2006;35(1):2–13.

47. Koltal PJ, Rabkin D. Management of facial trauma in children. Pediatr Clin North Am 1996;43:1253.

48. Moore MH, David DJ, Cooter RD. Oblique craniofacial fractures in children. J Craniofac Surg 1990;1:4.

49. Karesh JW, Kelman SE, Chirico PA, et al. Orbital roof "blow-in" fractures. Ophthal Plast Reconstr Surg 1991;7:77.

50. Haug RH, Foss J. Maxillofacial injuries in the pediatric patient. Oral Surg Oral Med Oral Pathol Oral Radiol Endod 2000;90(2):126–34.

51. Mithani SK, St-Hilaire H, Brooke BS, et al. Predictable patterns of intracranial and cervical spine injury in craniomaxillofacial trauma: analysis of 4786 patients. Plast Reconstr Surg 2009;123(4):1293–301.

52. Elahi MM, Brar MS, Ahmed N, et al. Cervical spine injury in association with craniomaxillofacial fractures. Plast Reconstr Surg 2008;121(1):201–8.

53. Hills MW, Deane SA. Head injury and facial injury: is there an increased risk of cervical spine injury? J Trauma 1993;34(4):549–53.

54. Kloss F, Laimer K, Hohlrieder M, et al. Traumatic intracranial haemorrhage in conscious patients with facial fractures—a review of 1959 cases. J Craniomaxillofac Surg 2008;36(7):372–7.

Imaging of Nonaccidental Injury and the Mimics: Issues and Controversies in the Era of Evidence-Based Medicine

Patrick D. Barnes, MD

KEYWORDS

- Evidence-based medicine • Nonaccidental injury
- Nonaccidental trauma • Nonaccidental head injury
- Child abuse

Nonaccidental injury (NAI) is reportedly the most frequent cause of traumatic injury in infants (peak incidence age 6 months; 80% of traumatic brain injury deaths under the age of 2 years).[1–4] NAI, nonaccidental trauma (NAT), and nonaccidental head injury are more recently used terms instead of the traditional labels, child abuse, battered child syndrome, and shaken baby syndrome (SBS). The traditional definition of NAI/SBS is intentional or inflicted physical injury to infants characterized by the triad of (1) subdural hemorrhage (SDH), (2) retinal hemorrhage (RH), and (3) encephalopathy (ie, diffuse axonal injury [DAI]) occurring in the context of inappropriate or inconsistent history (particularly when unwitnessed) and commonly accompanied by other apparently inflicted injuries (eg, skeletal).[1–4] This empirical formula is under challenge by evidence-based medical and legal principals.[4–14]

TRAUMATIC BRAIN INJURY

Traumatic brain injury has been categorized in several ways.[1,4] Primary injury directly results from the initial traumatic force and is immediate and irreversible (eg, contusion or shear injury). Secondary injury arises from or is associated with the primary injury and is potentially reversible (eg, swelling, hypoxia-ischemia, seizures, or herniation). Traditional biomechanics describes impact loading as linear forces that produce localized cranial deformation and focal injury (eg, fracture, contusion, or epidural hematoma). Accidental injury (AI) is considered typically associated with impact and, with the exception of epidural hematoma, is usually not life threatening. Impulsive loading refers to angular acceleration/deceleration forces resulting from sudden nonimpact motion of the head on the neck (ie, whiplash) and produces diffuse injury with tissue disruption (eg, bridging vein rupture with SDH and white matter shear with DAI). Young infants are thought particularly vulnerable to the latter mechanism (ie, SBS) because of weak neck muscles, a relatively large head, and an immature brain. SBS is traditionally postulated to result in the triad of primary traumatic injury (ie, SDH, RH, and DAI), which has been reportedly associated with the most severe and fatal CNS injuries. Stated assault mechanisms

Disclosure: Dr Barnes provides expert consultation and testimony in child abuse cases, occasionally with compensation, and including on behalf of the defense.
Department of Radiology, Lucile Packard Children's Hospital, Stanford University Medical Center, 725 Welch Road, Palo Alto, CA 94304, USA
E-mail address: pbarnes@stanford.edu

Radiol Clin N Am 49 (2011) 205–229
doi:10.1016/j.rcl.2010.08.001

in NAI include battering, shaking, impact, shaking-impact, strangulation, suffocation, and combined assaults (shake-bang-choke).[1–4] Although the spectrum of injury in NAI overlaps that of AI, certain patterns have been previously reported as characteristic of or highly suspicious for NAI.[1–4] These include multiple or complex cranial fractures (**Fig. 1**), acute interhemispheric SDH (**Fig. 2**), acute-hyperacute SDH (**Fig. 3**), DAI, chronic SDH, and the combination of chronic and acute SDH (**Fig. 4**). The latter combination is thought indicative of more than one abusive event. Imaging evidence of brain injury may occur with or without other clinical findings of trauma (eg, bruising) or other traditionally higher-specificity imaging findings of abuse (eg, classic metaphyseal lesions or rib fractures) (**Fig. 5**).[1–4] Therefore, clinical and imaging findings of injury out of proportion to the history of trauma and injuries of different ages have been the basis of making a medical diagnosis and offer expert testimony that such "forensic" findings are "proof" of NAI/SBS, particularly when encountered in premobile, young infants.

EVIDENCE-BASED MEDICINE

Evidence-based medicine (EBM) is now the guiding principle as medicine moves from an authoritarian to an authoritative era to overcome bias and ideology.[4,15–20] EBM quality-of-evidence ratings of the literature (eg, classes I–IV) are based on levels of accepted scientific methodology and biostatistical significance (eg, P values) and apply to the formulation of standards and guidelines for every aspect of medicine, including diagnostics, therapeutics, and forensics. EBM analysis reveals that few published reports in the traditional NAI/SBS literature merit a quality-of-evidence rating above class IV (eg, expert opinion alone).[5] Such low ratings do not meet EBM recommendations for standards (eg, level A) or for guidelines (eg, level B). Difficulties exist in the rational formulation of a medical diagnosis or forensic determination of NAI/SBS based on an alleged event (eg, shaking) that is inferred from clinical, imaging, or pathology findings in the subjective context of (1) an unwitnessed event, (2) a noncredible history, or (3) an admission or confession under dubious circumstances.[6] This problem is further confounded by the lack of consistent and reliable criteria for the diagnosis of NAI/SBS and because much of the traditional literature on child abuse consists of anecdotal case series, case reports, reviews, opinions, and position papers.[5,6,10,11,21,22] Many reports include cases having impact injury, which

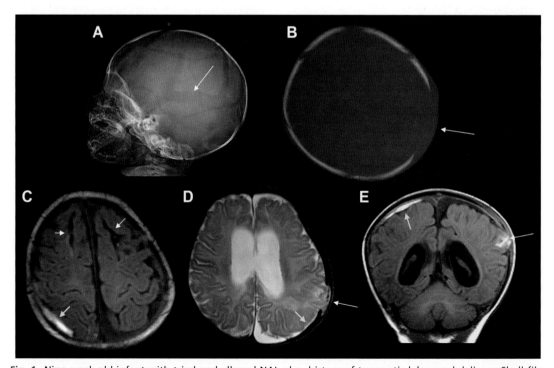

Fig. 1. Nine-week-old infant with triad and alleged NAI; also, history of traumatic labor and delivery. Skull film (*A*), CT (*B*) plus FLAIR (*C*), T2 (*D*), and T1 (*E*) MR imaging shows bilateral skull fractures with left growing fracture (*long white arrows*), chronic bifrontal cerebral white matter clefts (*short white arrows*) (*C*) plus acute, subacute, and chronic SDHs/rehemorrhages (*yellow arrows*).

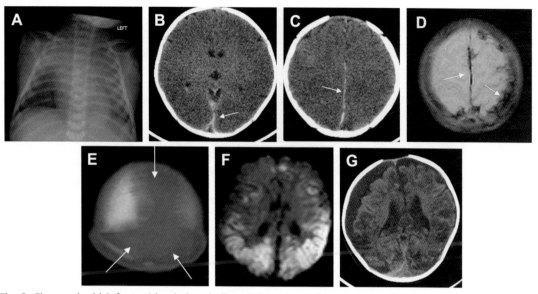

Fig. 2. Five-week-old infant with triad and alleged NAI; also, cold symptoms, vitamin D undersupplemented, acute choking episode during feeding, and status epilepticus. Chest film (A) shows bilateral lung opacities. CT (B, C) plus T2* MR imaging (D) shows bilateral cerebral edema with bilateral thin, acute-subacute hemorrhages (or thromboses) about the falx, tentorium, and convexities (arrows). Vertex CT (E) shows suture diastasis versus pseudodiastasis (arrows) (craniotabes?). DWI (F) shows global hypoxic-ischemic injury. Later CT (G) shows atrophy and chronic SDH.

undermines the SBS hypothesis by imposing a shaking-impact syndrome. Also, the inclusion criteria provided in many reports are criticized as arbitrary. Examples include suspected abuse, presumed abuse, likely abuse, and indeterminate.[21,22] Furthermore, the diagnostic criteria often seem to follow circular logic, such that the inclusion criteria (eg, the triad equals SBS/NAI) becomes the conclusion (ie, SBS/NAI equals the triad).

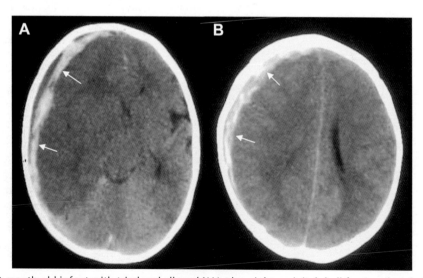

Fig. 3. Eight-month-old infant with triad and alleged NAI; also, right occipital skull fracture (age indeterminate; not shown) and 4- to 6-week-old wrist fracture. Hyperacute right SDH versus chronic SDH with rehemorrhage? CT (A, B) shows mixed high- plus low-density right extracerebral collection (arrows) with right cerebral edema, mass effect, and left shift. Question of subdural membrane on autopsy.

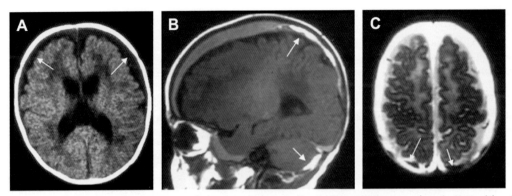

Fig. 4. Six-month-old infant with macrocephaly, the triad, and alleged NAI: BECC versus chronic SDH with rehe-morrhage versus acute SDHG plus SDH? CT (*A*) shows bilateral frontal isohypodense extracerebral collections (*arrows*) with minute high densities (not shown). T1 MR imaging (*B*) shows smaller extracerebral high intensities (*arrows*) superimposed on larger isohypointensities. T2 MR imaging (*C*) shows small extracerebral T2 hypointen-sities (*arrows*) superimposed on large isohyperintensities.

RULES OF EVIDENCE AND EXPERT TESTIMONY

Regarding rules of evidence within the justice system, there are legal standards for the admissi-bility of expert testimony.[7,8,11,23] The Frye stan-dard requires only that the testimony be generally accepted in the relevant scientific community. The Daubert standard requires assessment of the scientific reliability of the testi-mony. A criticism of the justice system is that the application of these standards varies with the juris-diction (eg, according to state versus federal law). Additional legal standards regarding proof are also applied in order for the trier of fact (eg, judge or jury) to make the determination of civil liability or criminal guilt. In a civil action (eg, medical malprac-tice lawsuit), money is primarily at risk for the

defendant health care provider, and proof of liability is based on a preponderance of the evidence (ie, at least 51% scientific or medical probability or certainty). In a criminal action, life or liberty is at stake for the defendant, including the permanent loss of child custody.[7,8,11,23,24] In such cases, the defendant has the constitutional protection of due process that requires a higher level of proof. This includes the principles of inno-cent until proved guilty beyond a reasonable doubt with the burden of proof on the prosecution and based on clear and convincing evidence. No percentage of level of certainty is provided, however, for these standards of proof in most jurisdictions. Furthermore, only a preponderance of the medical evidence (ie, minimum of 51% certainty) is required to support proof of guilt whether or not the medical expert testimony

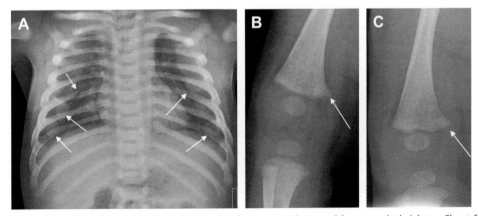

Fig. 5. Three-month-old infant with alleged NAI; also, history consistent with congenital rickets. Chest film (*A*) shows bilateral recent and old, healing rib fractures (pseudofractures? rachitic rosary? [*arrows*]). Knee films before (*B*) and after (*C*) vitamin D supplementation show healing classic metaphyseal lesions (*arrows*)?

complies with the Frye standard (ie, general acceptance requirement) or the Daubert standard (ie, scientific reliability requirement). Further criticism of the criminal justice process is that in NAI cases, medical experts have defined SBS/NAI as "the presence of injury (eg, the triad) without a sufficient historical explanation" and that this definition unduly shifts the burden to the defendant to establish innocence by proving the expert theory wrong.

THE MEDICAL PROSECUTION OF NAI AND ITS EBM CHALLENGES

Traditionally, the prosecution of NAI has been based on the presence of one or more aspects of the triad as supported by the premises that (1) shaking alone in an otherwise healthy child can cause SDH leading to death, (2) such injury can never occur on an accidental basis (eg, short-distance fall) because it requires a massive violent force equivalent to a motor vehicle accident or a fall from a multistory building, (3) such injury is immediately symptomatic and cannot be followed by a lucid interval, and (4) changing symptoms in a child with prior head injury indicates newly inflicted injury and not a spontaneous rebleed.[1–4,7,8,11] Using this reasoning, the last caretaker is automatically guilty of inflicted injury, especially if not witnessed by an independent observer. Also, it has been asserted that RHs of a particular pattern are diagnostic of SBS/NAI.

Reports from clinical, biomechanical, pathology, forensic, and legal disciplines, within and outside of the child maltreatment literature, have challenged the evidence base for NAI/SBS as the only cause for the triad.[5–12] Such reports indicate that the triad may also be seen with AI (including witnessed short-distance falls, lucid intervals, and rehemorrhage) (**Figs. 6** and **7**) as well as in medical conditions. These are the mimics of NAI and often present as acute life-threatening events (ALTEs).[25,26] The medical mimics include hypoxia-ischemia (eg, apnea, choking, or respiratory or cardiac arrest) (see **Figs. 2, 6,** and **7**), ischemic injury (eg, arterial versus venous occlusive disease) (**Fig. 8**), vascular anomalies (eg, arteriovenous malformation [AVM]) (**Fig. 9**), seizures (see **Fig. 2**), infectious or postinfectious conditions (**Fig. 10**), coagulopathies (**Fig. 11**), fluid-electrolyte derangement, and metabolic or connective tissue disorders, including vitamin deficiencies and depletions (eg, C, D, or K) (see **Figs. 1** and **5; Fig. 12**).[2,4]

Many ALTEs seem multifactorial and involve a combination, sequence, or cascade of predisposing and complicating events or conditions.[4,25] As an example, an infant may suffer a head impact,

or choking spell, followed by seizures or apnea, and then undergo a series of interventions, including prolonged or difficult resuscitation and problematic airway management with subsequent hypoxia-ischemia and coagulopathy (see **Figs. 2, 6, 7,** and **11**). Another example is a young infant with a predisposing condition, such as infectious illness, fluid-electrolyte imbalance, metabolic disorder, or a coagulopathy, who then suffers seizures, respiratory arrest, and resuscitation with hypoxia-ischemia (see **Figs. 10–12; Fig. 13**). In many cases of alleged SBS/NAI, it is often assumed that nonspecific premorbid symptoms (eg, irritability, lethargy, and poor feeding) in an otherwise healthy infant are indicators of ongoing abuse or that such symptoms become the inciting factor for the abuse. A thorough and complete medical investigation in such cases may reveal that the child is not otherwise healthy and is suffering from a medical condition that progresses to an ALTE.[2,4,25]

BIOMECHANICAL CHALLENGES

The mechanical basis for SBS as hypothesized by Guthkelch, Caffey, and other investigators,[27] was originally extrapolated from Ommaya,[28] who used an animal whiplash model to determine the angular acceleration threshold (ie, 40 g) for head injury (ie, concussion, SDH, and shear injury). It was assumed that manual shaking of an infant could generate these same forces and produce the triad. Duhaime and colleagues[29] measured the angular accelerations associated with adult manual shaking (ie, 11 g) and impact (ie, 52 g) in a 1-month-old infant anthropormorphic test device (ATD). Only accelerations associated with impact (4 to 5 times that associated with shakes) on an unpadded or padded surface exceeded the injury thresholds determined by Ommaya. In the same study, the Duhaime and colleagues reported a series of 13 fatal cases of NAI/SBS in which all had evidence of blunt head impact (more than half noted only at autopsy).[29] The investigators concluded that CNS injury in SBS/NAI in its most severe form is usually not caused by shaking alone. Their results contradicted many of the original reports that had relied on the whiplash mechanism as causative of the triad. They suggested the use of the new term, shaken-impact syndrome. More recently, Prange and colleagues,[30] using a 1.5 month-old ATD, showed that inflicted impacts against hard surfaces were more likely associated with brain injury than falls from less than 1.5 m or from vigorous shaking. With further improvements in ATDs, more recent experiments indicate that maximum head

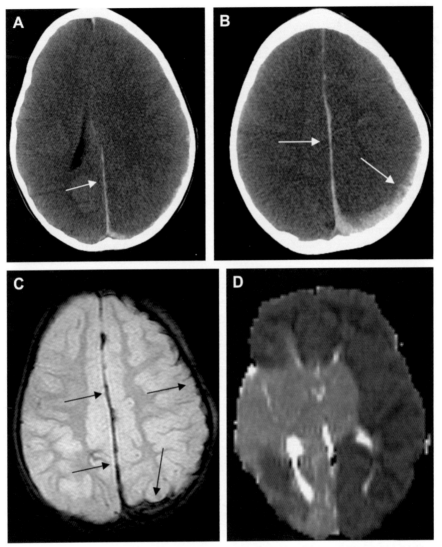

Fig. 6. Twenty-one–month–old toddler with triad and alleged NAI; also, history of prior head impact. Question prior injury with lucid interval versus hyperacute injury. CT (*A, B*) acute left convexity and interhemispheric SDH and SAH (*arrows*) with cerebral swelling, left more than right. T2* MR imaging (*C*) shows low intensity SDH (*arrows*) with T1/T2 isointensity (not shown). ADC map (*D*) shows asymmetric cerebral restricted diffusion (left > right). Autopsy confirms impact with acute SDH, SAH, and hypoxic-ischemic injury.

accelerations may exceed injury reference values at lower fall heights than previously determined (**Fig. 14**).[31] Critics of the Duhaime and Prange studies contend that there is no adequate human infant surrogate yet designed to properly test shaking versus impact.[32] Other reports also show that shaking alone cannot result in brain injury (ie, the triad) unless there is concomitant injury to the neck, cervical spinal column, or cervical spinal cord, because these are the weak links between the head and body of the infant.[33–35] Spinal cord injury without radiographic abnormality (SCIWORA), whether or not AI or

NAI, is an important example of primary neck and spinal cord injury with secondary brain injury (see **Fig. 7**).[35] For example, a falling infant experiences a head-first impact with subsequent neck hyperextension (or hyperflexion) from the force of the trailing body mass. There is resultant upper spinal cord injury without detectable spinal column injury on plain films or CT. Compromise of the respiratory center at the cervicomedullary junction results in hypoxic brain injury, including the thin SDH (see **Fig. 7**). CT often shows the brain injury, but only MR imaging may show the additional neck or spinal cord injury.

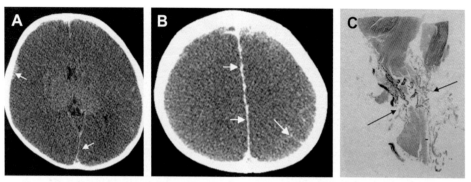

Fig. 7. Twenty-one—month—old with triad and alleged NAI; also, history of 4-ft fall. CT (A, B) with high-density SAH and thin SDH (*arrows*) plus cerebral edema. Sagittal plane photomicrograph (C) from autopsy shows upper cervical spinal cord disruption (*arrows*) resulting in global hypoxic-ischemic injury.

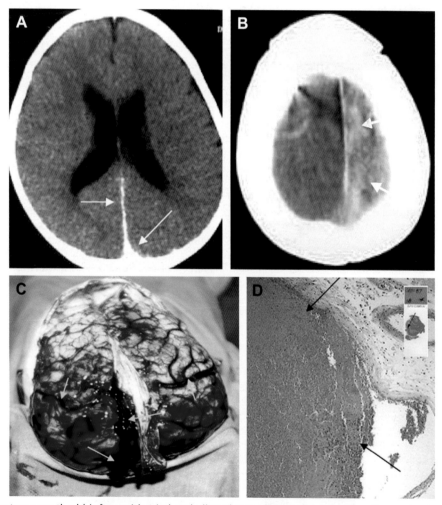

Fig. 8. Fourteen-month-old infant with triad and alleged NAI; also, recent infectious illness: dural and cortical venous sinus thrombosis with dural hemorrhage: CT (A, B) shows high densities along the falx and dural venous sinuses (*white arrows*). (C) Gross specimen—reflected superior sagittal sinus and cortical venous thromboses with distended veins (*yellow arrows*); (D) photomicrograph of cortical venous thrombus with inflammatory reaction (*black arrows*) plus SDH with neomembrane (7—14 days old; not shown). (*Pathology courtesy of J. Leestma, MD.*)

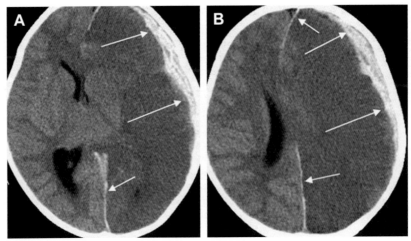

Fig. 9. Twenty-month-old infant with triad and alleged NAI. Left SDH with cerebral cortical and pial AVM at autopsy. CT (*A, B*) shows left mixed-density SDH and SAH (*long arrows*) plus interhemispheric hemorrhage (*short arrows*) with marked left cerebral swelling and shift.

The minimal force required to produce the triad has yet to be established. From the current biomechanical evidence base, however, it can be concluded that (1) shaking may not produce direct brain injury but may cause indirect brain injury if associated with neck and cervical spinal cord injury; (2) angular acceleration/deceleration injury forces clearly occur with impact trauma; (3) such injury on an accidental basis does not require a force that can only be associated with a motor vehicle accident or a multistory fall; (4) household (ie, short-distance) falls may produce direct or indirect brain injury; (5) in addition to fall height, impact surface and type of landing are important factors; and (6) head-first impacts in young infants not having developed a defensive reflex (eg,

extension of a limb to break the fall) are the most dangerous and may result in direct or indirect brain injury (eg, SCIWORA).

NEUROPATHOLOGY CHALLENGES

In their landmark neuropathology study of 53 victims of alleged SBS/NAI,[36,37] Geddes and colleagues showed in 37 infants (ages <9 months) that (1) 29 had evidence of impact with only one case of admitted shaking; (2) cerebral swelling was more often due to DAI of hypoxic-ischemic encephalopathy (HIE) rather than shear or traumatic axonal injury (TAI); (2) although fracture, thin SDH (eg, dural vascular plexus origin), and RH are commonly present, the usual cause of

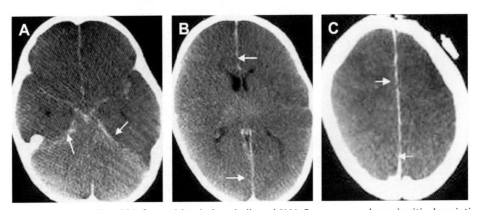

Fig. 10. Twenty-one–month–old infant with triad and alleged NAI. Pneumococcal meningitis, herniation, and hypoxic-ischemic injury confirmed at autopsy. CT (*A–C*) shows high-density thin SDH (*arrows*) plus cerebral edema.

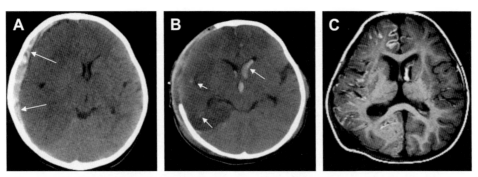

Fig. 11. Nine-month-old girl with triad and alleged NAI; also, recent fall and coagulopathy (later confirmed platelet disorder). Initial CT (*A*) shows mixed-density right SDH (*arrows*) with right cerebral edema. Postoperative CT 5 days later (*B*) shows other cerebral and intraventricular hemorrhages (*arrows*). T1 MR imaging (*C*) 11 days postoperatively shows evolving right cerebral high-intensity cortical injury and hemorrhages.

death was increased intracranial pressure from brain swelling associated with HIE (see **Fig. 2**); and (4) cervical epidural hemorrhage and focal axonal brainstem, cervical cord, and spinal nerve root injuries were characteristically seen in these infants (most with impact). Upper cervical cord/brainstem injury may result in apnea/respiratory arrest and be responsible for the HIE. In the 16 older victims (ages 13 months to 8 years), the pathology findings were primarily those of the battered child or adult trauma syndrome, including extracranial injuries (eg, abdominal), large SDH (ie, bridging vein rupture), and TAI. Additional neuropathology series by Geddes and colleagues[38] have shown that SDHs are also seen in nontraumatic fetal, neonatal, and infant brain injury cases and that such SDHs are actually of intradural vascular plexus origin rather than bridging cortical vein origin.

The common denominator in all these cases is likely a combination of vascular immaturity and fragility further compromised by HIE or infection, cerebral venous hypertension or congestion, arterial hypertension, and brain swelling (see **Fig. 2**). Although the unified hypothesis of Geddes and colleagues[13,14,39] has received criticism, their findings and conclusions have been validated by the research of Cohen and Scheimberg,[40] Croft and Reichard,[41] and others. In their postmortem series, Cohen and colleagues described 25 fetuses (26–41 weeks) and 30 neonates (1 hour–19 days) with HIE who also had macroscopic intradural hemorrhage (IDH), including frank parietal SDH in two-thirds. The IDH was most prominent along the posterior falcine and tentorial vascular plexuses (ie, interhemispheric fissure) (see **Fig. 2**). They concluded from their work, along with the findings of other cited

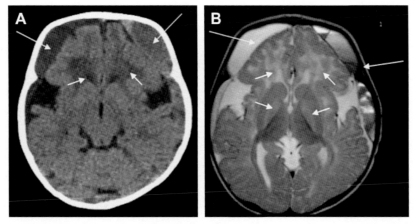

Fig. 12. Twelve-month-old infant with triad and alleged NAI. Glutaric acidopathy type 1. CT (*A*) and T2 MR imaging (*B*) shows bilateral SDH of varying age (*long arrows*), wide sylvian fissures plus basal ganglia, and cerebral white matter abnormalities (*short arrows*).

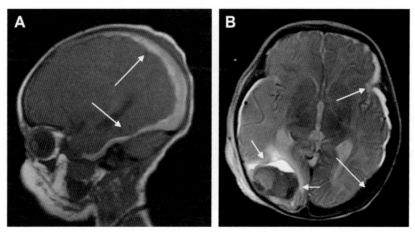

Fig. 13. Home-delivered newborn with seizures at 1 week of age; also, no vitamin K given at birth. T1 (*A*) and T2 (*B*) MR imaging shows acute-subacute left SDH (*long arrows*) plus right cerebral hemorrhage (*short arrows*); vitamin K deficiency confirmed and treated.

researchers, that IDH and SDH are commonly associated with HIE, particularly when associated with increases in central venous pressure. This also explains the frequency of RH associated with perinatal events.[42]

From the current forensic pathology evidence base, it may be concluded that (1) shaking may not cause direct brain injury but may cause indirect brain injury (ie, HIE) if associated with cervical spinal cord injury; (2) impact may produce direct

or indirect brain injury (eg, SCIWORA); (3) the pattern of brain edema with thin SDH (dural vascular plexus origin) may reflect HIE whether or not due to AI or NAI; and (4) the same pattern of injury may result from nontraumatic or medical causes (eg, HIE from any cause of ALTE). Furthermore, because the observed edema does not represent TAI (which results in immediate neurologic dysfunction), a lucid interval is possible, particularly in infants whose sutured skull and

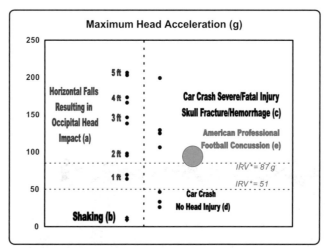

Fig. 14. Maximum head accelerations versus trauma mechanisms as correlated with injury thresholds. CRABI, child restraint air bag interaction; IRV, injury reference values. (*Data from* Van Ee C, PhD. Design research engineering. Available at: www.dreng.com. Accessed September 12, 2010; Leestma J. Forensic neuropathology. 2nd edition. Boca Raton [FL]: CRC Press; 2009; Mertz H. Anthropomorphic test devices. In: Melvin J, Nahum A, editors. Accidental injury: biomechanics and prevention. 2nd edition. New York: Springer; 2002. p. 84; Klinich JD, Hulbert G, Schneider LW. Estimating infant head injury criteria and impact response using crash reconstruction and finite element modeling. Society of Automotive Engineers Paper # 2002−22−0009, 2002; CRABI 12 [a, b]; CRABI 6 [c, d]; and [e] Pellman EJ, Viano DC, Tucker AM, et al. Concussion in professional football: reconstruction of game impacts and injuries. Neurosurgery 2003;53[4]:799−812.)

dural vascular plexus have the distensibility to tolerate early increases in intracranial pressure. Also, the lucid interval invalidates the premise that the last caretaker is always responsible in alleged NAI.

CLINICAL CHALLENGES

In the prosecution of NAI, it is often stipulated that short-distance falls cannot be associated with the triad, serious (eg, fatal) head injury, or a lucid interval. Traditionally, it has also been stipulated that nonintentional new bleeding in an existing SDH is always minor, that SDH does not occur in benign extracerebral collections (BECCs), and that symptomatic or fatal new bleeding in SDH requires newly inflicted trauma.[1–4,7,8,11] Several past and current reports refute the significance of low level falls in children, including in-hospital and outpatient clinic series.[43–51] There are other reports, however, including emergency medicine, trauma center, neurosurgical, and medical examiner series, that indicate a heightened need for concern regarding the potential for serious intracranial injury associated with minor or trivial trauma scenarios, particularly in infants.[52–74] This includes reports of skull fracture or acute SDH from accidental simple falls in infants, SDH in infants with predisposing wide extracerebral spaces (eg, BECCs of infancy, chronic subdural hygromas, arachnoid cyst, and so forth) (see **Fig. 4; Figs. 15** and **16**), and fatal pediatric head injuries due to witnessed, accidental short-distance falls, including those with a lucid interval, SDH, RH, and malignant cerebral edema (see **Fig. 6**). Also included are infants with chronic SDH from prior trauma (eg, at birth) who then develop rehemorrhage (see **Figs. 1, 4,** and **15**).

Short-Distance Falls, Lucid Intervals, and Malignant Edema

Hall and colleagues[44] reported that 41% of childhood deaths (mean age 2.4 years) from head injuries associated with AI were from low level falls (3 feet or less) while running or down stairs. Chadwick and colleagues[45] reported fatal falls of less than 4 feet in seven infants but considered the histories unreliable. Plunkett[56] reported witnessed fatal falls of 2 to 10 feet in 18 infants and children, including those with SDH, RH, and lucid intervals. Greenes and Schutzman[57] reported intracranial injuries, including SDH, in 18 asymptomatic infants with falls of 2 feet to 9 stairs. Christian and colleagues[63] reported three infants with unilateral RH and SDH/SAH due to witnessed accidental household trauma. Denton and Mileusnic[59] reported a witnessed, accidental 30-inch fall in a 9-month-old infant with a 3-day lucid interval before death. Murray and colleagues[60] reported more intracranial injuries in young children (49% <age 4 y; 21% <age 1 y) with reported low level falls (<15 ft), both AI and NAI. Kim and colleagues[61] reported a high incidence of intracranial injury in children (ages 3 mo to 15 y; 52% <age 2 y) accidentally falling from low heights (3 to 15 ft; 80% <6 ft; including 4 deaths). Because of the lucid intervals in some patients, including initially favorable Glasgow Coma Scale scores (GCS) with subsequent deterioration, Murray and colleagues[60] and others expressed concern regarding caretaker delays and medical transfer delays contributing to the morbidity and mortality in these patients.[53–56,58–61] Bruce and colleagues[54,55] reported one of the largest pediatric series of head trauma (63 patients, ages 6 months to 18 years), both AI and NAI, associated with malignant brain edema and SAH/SDH (see **Fig. 6**). In the higher GCS (>8) subgroup,

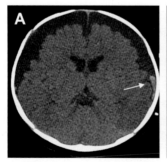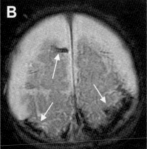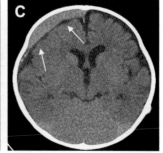

Fig. 15. Five-month-old infant with the triad and alleged NAI; also, macrocephaly from birth, recent seizure but no trauma. CT (*A*) and T2* MR imaging (*B*) shows large extracerebral collections with smaller recent hemorrhages (*arrows*). CT 3 months postdrainage (*C*) shows rehemorrhage (*arrows*). Diagnosis: BECC or chronic SDHG with rehemorrhage?

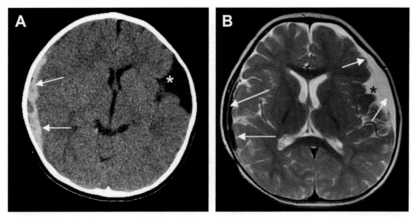

Fig. 16. Sixteen-month-old with triad (right RH) and alleged NAI; also, short-distance fall with right scalp impact. CT (*A*) shows left sylvian arachnoid cyst (*) and right hyperacute SDH (*arrows*). T2 MR imaging (*B*) 2 days later shows acute right SDH (*long arrows*) and smaller left sylvian arachnoid cyst (*) with subdural hygroma (*short arrows*).

there were 8 with a lucid interval and all 14 had complete recovery. In the lower GCS ($\leq$ 8) subgroup, there were 34 with immediate and continuous coma, 15 with a lucid interval, 6 deaths, and 11 with moderate to severe disability. More recently, Steinbok and colleagues[62] reported 5 children (4 <age 2 y; 3 falls) with witnessed AI, including SDH and cerebral edema detected by CT 1 to 5 hours post event. All experienced immediate coma with rapid progression to death (see **Fig. 6**).

Benign Extracerebral Collections

BECCs of infancy (also known as benign external hydrocephalus or benign extracerebral subarachnoid spaces) is a common and well-known condition characterized by diffuse enlargement of the subarachnoid spaces.[65–74] A transient disorder of cerebrospinal fluid (CSF) circulation, probably due to delayed development of the arachnoid granulations, is widely accepted as the cause and develops from birth. BECC is typically associated with macrocephaly but may also occur in infants with normal or small head circumferences, including premature infants. As with any cause of craniocerebral disproportion (eg, BECC, hydrocephalus, chronic SDH or hygroma, arachnoid cyst, or underdevelopment or atrophy), there is a susceptibility to SDH that may be spontaneous or associated with trivial trauma (see **Figs. 4** and **15**). A recent large series report and review by Hellbusch[73] emphasizes the importance of this predisposition and cites other confirmatory series and case reports (30 references). Papasian and Frim[68] designed a theoretic model that

predicts the predisposition of benign external hydrocephalus to SDH with minor head trauma. Piatt's[66] case report of BECC with SDH (27 references), including RH, along with McNeely and colleagues'[72] case series are further warnings that this combination is far from specific for SBS/NAI.

Birth Issues

In addition to the examples discussed previously (eg, short-distance falls and BECCs), another important but often overlooked factor is birth-related trauma.[1,4,75–89] This includes normal as well as complicated labor and delivery events (pitocin augmentation, prolonged labor, vaginal delivery, instrumented delivery, cesarean section, and so forth). It is well known that acute SDH often occurs even with the normal birth process and that this predisposes to chronic SDH, including in the presence of BECC (see **Figs. 1, 4,** and **15**). Intracranial hemorrhages, including SDH and RH, have been reported in several CT and MR imaging series of normal neonates including a frequency of 50% by Holden and colleagues,[81] 8% by Whitby and colleagues,[76] 26% by Looney and colleagues,[82] and 46% by Rooks and colleagues.[78] Chamnanvanakij and colleagues[75] reported 26 symptomatic term neonates with SDH over a 3-year period after uncomplicated deliveries. Long-term follow-up imaging has not been provided in many of these series, although Rooks and colleagues[78] reported one child in their series who developed SDH with rehemorrhage superimposed on BECC (**Fig. 17**).

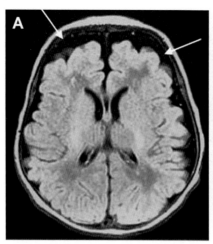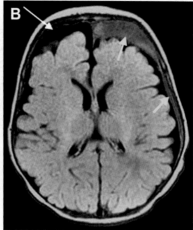

Fig. 17. BECC versus SDHG at birth (*A*) (*long arrows*) with SDH versus rehemorrhage 1 month later (*B*) (*yellow arrows*) on axial FLAIR MR images. (*Courtesy of* Veronica J. Rooks, MD, Tripler Army Medical Center, Honolulu, HI.)

Chronic SDH and Rehemorrhage

Chronic SDH is one of the most controversial topics in the NAI versus AI debate.[1–4,12,21,22,36–41] Unexplained SDH is often ascribed to NAI. By definition, a newly discovered chronic SDH started as an acute SDH that, for whatever reason, may have been subclinical. There is likely more than one mechanism for SDH that has prompted a revisiting of the concept of the subdural compartment.[12,40,41,90,91] Mack and colleagues[90] have provided an updated review on this important topic. In some cases of infant trauma, dissection at the relatively weak dura-arachnoid border zone (ie, dural border cell layer) may allow CSF to collect and enlarge over time as a dural interstitial (ie, intradural) hygroma. In other cases, there is bridging vein rupture within the dural interstitium that results in an acute subdural or intradural hematoma that extends along the dural border cell layer. Furthermore, traumatic disruption of the dural vascular plexus (ie, venous, capillary, or lymphatic), which is particularly prominent in young infants, may also produce an acute intradural hematoma. Some of these collections undergo resorption whereas others progress to become chronic SDH. Some progressive collections may represent mixed CSF-blood collections (see **Figs 1, 4,** and **15**).

The pathology and pathophysiology of neomembrane formation in chronic SDH, including rebleeding, is well established in adults and seems similar, if not identical, to that in infants.[83,92–112] Although acute SDH is most often due to impact or deformational trauma, whether or not AI or NAI, it must be differentiated from chronic SDH

with rehemorrhage. Progression of chronic SDH and rehemorrhage is likely related to capillary leakage and intrinsic thrombolysis.[92,93] Other factors include dural vascular plexus hemorrhage associated with increases in intracranial or central venous pressures (eg, birth trauma, congenital heart disease, venous thrombosis, or dysphagic choking) or with increased meningeal arterial pressure (eg, reperfusion after hypoxia-ischemia) with resultant acute hemorrhage (or rehemorrhage) in normal infants or superimposed on predisposing chronic BECC, hygromas, hematomas, or arachnoid cysts (see **Figs. 1, 2, 4,** and **15–17**).[12,38,40,65–74,90,91] The phenomenon of acute infantile SDH, whether or not AI or NAI, evolving to chronic SDH and rehemorrhage, including RH, is well documented in several neurosurgical series reports, including those by Aoki and colleagues,[97,98] Ikeda and colleagues,[99] Parent,[94] Howard and colleagues,[102] Hwang and Kim,[95] Vinchon,[103,104] and others.

Conclusions

From the clinical evidence base, in addition to the biomechanical and neuropathology evidence bases, it may be concluded that (1) significant head injury, including SDH and RH, may result from low fall levels; (2) such injury may be associated with a lucid interval; (3) in some, the injury may result in immediate deterioration with progression to death; (4) BECC predisposes to SDH; (5) SDH may date back to birth; and (6) rehemorrhage into an existing SDH occurs in childhood and may be serious.

RH CHALLENGES

Many guidelines for diagnosing NAI depend on the presence of RH, including those of a particular pattern (eg, retinal schisis, and perimacular folds) and based on the theory of vitreous traction due to inflicted acceleration/deceleration forces (eg, SBS).[1–4,113–132] The specificity of RH for NAI has been repeatedly challenged, however. Plunkett[56] reported RH in two-thirds of eye examinations in children with fatal AI. Goldsmith and Plunkett[132] reported a child with extensive bilateral RH in a videotaped fatal accidental short-distance fall. Lantz and colleagues[122] reported RH with perimacular folds in an infant crush injury. Gilles and colleagues[120] reported the appearance and progression of RH with increasing intracranial pressure after head injury in children. Obi and Watts[125] reported RH with schisis and folds in two children, one with AI and the other with NAI. Forbes and colleagues[126] reported RH with epidural hematoma in five infant AI cases. From a research perspective, Brown and colleagues[128] found no eye pathology in their fatal shaken animal observations. Binenbaum and colleagues[127] observed no eye abnormalities in piglets subjected to acceleration/deceleration levels greater than 20 times what Prange and colleagues[30] predicted possible in inflicted injury. Emerson and colleagues[129] found no support for the vitreous traction hypothesis as unique to NAI. The eye and optic nerve are an extension of, and therefore a window to, the CNS, including their shared vascularization, meningeal coverings, innervation, and CSF spaces. RH has been reported with a variety of conditions, including AI, resuscitation, increased intracranial pressure, increased venous pressure, subarachnoid hemorrhage, sepsis, coagulopathy, certain metabolic dis,orders, systemic hypertension, and other conditions.[121,123,131] The common pathophysiology seems to be increased intracranial pressure or increased intravascular pressure. Furthermore, many cases of RH (and SDH) are confounded by the sequence or cascade of multiple conditions (eg, the unified hypothesis of Geddes) that often has a synergistic influence on the type and extent of RH. For example, consider the common situation of a child who has had trauma (factual or assumed) followed by seizures, apnea, or respiratory arrest and resuscitation with resultant HIE or coagulopathy. In much of the traditional NAI/SBS literature, little if any consideration has been given to any predisposing or complicating factors, and often there is no indication of the timing of the eye examinations relative to the clinical course or the brain imaging.[113,114,119,130]

From the research and clinical evidence base, it may be concluded that (1) RH is not specific for NAI, (2) RH may occur in AI and medical conditions, and (3) predisposing factors and complicating cascade effects must be considered in the pathophysiology of RH.

MEDICAL CONDITIONS MIMICKING NAI

A significant part of the controversy is the medical conditions that may mimic the clinical presentations (ie, the triad) and imaging findings of NAI.[1,2,4,25,26,89,101] Furthermore, such conditions may predispose to or complicate AI or NAI, as part of a cascade that results in or exaggerates the triad. In some situations, it may be difficult or impossible to tell which of these elements are causative and which are the effects. These include HIE, seizures, dysphagic choking ALTE, cardiopulmonary resuscitation, infectious or post-infectious conditions (eg, sepsis, meningoencephalitis, or postvaccinial), vascular diseases, coagulopathies, venous thrombosis, metabolic disorders, neoplastic processes, certain therapies, extracorporeal membrane oxygenation, and other conditions.[4,25,89,101] Regarding pathogenesis of the triad (with or without other organ system involvement [eg, skeletal]) and whether or not due to NAI, AI, or medical etiologies, the pathophysiology seems to be a combination or sequence of factors, including increased intracranial pressure, increased venous pressure, systemic hypotension or hypertension, vascular fragility, hematologic derangement, and/or a collagenopathy imposed on the immature CNS, including the vulnerable dural vascular plexus as well as other organ systems.[4,12,25,38,90] Although the initial medical evaluation, including history, laboratory tests, and imaging studies, may suggest an alternative condition, the diagnosis may not be made because of a rush to judgment regarding NAI.[4–11] Such bias may have devastating effects on an injured child and family. It is important to be aware of these mimics, because a more extensive work-up may be needed beyond routine screening tests. Also, lack of confirmation of a specific condition does not automatically indicate the default diagnosis of NAI. In all cases, it is critical to review all past records dating back to the pregnancy and birth as well as the postnatal pediatric records, family history, more recent history preceding the acute presentation, details of the acute event itself, resuscitation, and the subsequent management, all of which may contribute to the clinical and imaging findings. An incomplete medical evaluation may result in unnecessary cost shifting to child protection and criminal justice systems and have further adverse effects regarding transplantation organ donation in brain death cases and custody/adoptive dispositions for the surviving child and siblings.

Sirotnak's[89] recent review, along with others', extensively catalogs the many conditions that may mimic NAI[4,25,101]:

Birth Trauma and Neonatal Conditions

Manifestations of birth trauma, including fracture, SDH, and RH, may persist beyond the neonatal period. Other examples are the sequelae of extracorporeal membrane oxygenation therapy, at-risk prematurity, and congenital heart disease. When evaluating a young infant with apparent NAI, it is important to consider that the clinical and imaging findings may actually stem from parturitional and neonatal issues.[75–112] These include hemorrhage or rehemorrhage into extracerebral collections existing from birth (see **Figs. 1, 4, 13**, and **15**). There may be associated skeletal findings of birth trauma (eg, new or healing clavicle, rib, or long bone fractures), particularly in the presence of a bone fragility disorder (see **Figs. 1, 2** and **5**).[133–137]

Developmental Anomalies and Congenital Conditions

Vascular malformations are rarely reported causes for the triad but may be underdiagnosed (see **Fig. 9**). BECCs and arachnoid cysts are also known to be associated with SDH and RH, spontaneously and with trauma (see **Figs. 4, 15–17**).[65–74]

Genetic and Metabolic Disorders

Several conditions in the genetic and metabolic disorders category may present with intracranial hemorrhage (eg, SDH) or RH. These include osteogenesis imperfecta, glutaric aciduria type I (see **Fig. 12**), Menkes' kinky hair disease, Ehlers-Danlos and Marfan syndromes, homocystinuria, and others.[4,89,101,138–142]

Hematologic Disease and Coagulopathy

Conditions in the hematologic disease and coagulopathy category predispose to intracranial hemorrhage and RH (see **Figs. 11** and **13**). The bleeding or clotting disorder may be primary or secondary. A more extensive work-up beyond the usual screening tests is needed, including a hematology consultation. Conditions in the category include the anemias, hemorrhagic disease of the newborn (vitamin K deficiency), the hemophilias, thrombophilias, disseminated intravascular coagulation and consumption coagulopathy, liver or kidney

disease, hemophagocytic lymphohistiocytosis, and anticoagulant therapy.[4,89,101,143–145] Venous thrombosis includes dural venous sinus thrombosis (DVST) and cerebral venous thrombosis (CVT). DVST or CVT may be associated with primary or secondary hematologic or coagulopathic states.[4,89,101,146–152] Risk factors include acute systemic illness, dehydration, fluid-electrolyte imbalance, sepsis, perinatal complications, chronic systemic disease, cardiac disease, connective tissue disorder, hematologic disorder, oncologic disease and therapy, head and neck infection, hypercoagulable, and trauma states. Infarction, SAH, SDH, or RH may be seen, especially in infants. High densities on CT may be present along the dural venous sinuses, tentorium, falx, or the cortical, subependymal, or medullary veins and be associated with SAH, SDH, or intracerebral hemorrhage (see **Fig. 8**). There may be focal infarctions, hemorrhagic or nonhemorrhagic, intraventricular hemorrhage, and massive, focal, or diffuse edema. Orbit, paranasal sinus, or otomastoid disease may be present. The thromboses and associated hemorrhages have variable MR imaging appearances depending on their age. CT venography (CTV) or magnetic resonance venography (MRV) may readily detect DVST but not CVT. The latter may be better detected as abnormal hypointensities on susceptibility-weighted T2* sequences but difficult to distinguish from hemorrhage (SDH or SAH), hemorrhagic infarction, contusion, or hemorrhagic shear injury.

Infectious and Postinfectious Conditions

Meningitis, encephalitis, or sepsis may involve the vasculature resulting in vasculitis, arterial or venous thrombosis, mycotic aneurysm, infarction, and hemorrhage.[4,89,101] SDH and RH may also be seen (see **Fig. 10**). Postinfectious illnesses may also be associated with these findings. Included in this category are the encephalopathies of infancy and childhood, hemorrhagic shock and encephalopathy syndrome, and postvaccinial encephalopathy.[4,89,101,153–158]

Toxins, Poisons, and Nutritional Deficiencies

The category of toxins poisons, and nutritional deficiencies includes lead poisoning, cocaine, anticoagulants, over-the-counter cold medications, prescription drugs, and vitamin deficiencies or depletions (eg, K, C, or D).[4,89,101,136,143,155–159] Preterm neonates, and other chronically ill infants, are particularly vulnerable to nutritional deficiencies and complications of prolonged immobilization that often primarily effect bone development. Furthermore, the national and international epidemic of vitamin D deficiency and insufficiency in pregnant mothers, their term fetuses, and their undersupplemented breastfed term neonates predisposes them to rickets (ie, congenital). Such infants, who have also been subjected to the trauma of birth, may have skeletal imaging findings (eg, multiple healing fractures or pseudofractures) that are misinterpreted as NAI, especially in the presence of the triad (see **Figs. 2 and 5**).[136,137]

Dysphagic Choking ALTE as a Mimic of NAI

Apnea is an important and common form of ALTE in infancy whose origin may be central, obstructive, or combined.[25] The obstructive and mixed forms may present with choking, gasping, coughing, or gagging due to mechanical obstruction. When paroxysmal or sustained, the result may be severe brain injury or death due to a combination of central venous hypertension and hypoxia-ischemia. It is this synergism that produces cerebral edema and dural vascular plexus hemorrhage with SDH, SAH, and RH (see **Fig. 2**; **Fig. 18**). Examples include dysphagic choking (eg, aspiration of a feed or gastroesophageal reflux), viral airway infection (eg, RSV), and pertussis, particularly when occurring in a predisposed child (eg, prematurity, Pierre Robin syndrome, or sudden infant death syndrome).[25,160–167]

IMAGING CHALLENGES AND THE IMPORTANCE OF A DIFFERENTIAL DIAGNOSIS
CT

Because of the evidence-based challenges to NAI, imaging protocols should be designed to evaluate not only NAI versus AI but also the medical mimics.

Noncontrast CT has been the primary modality for brain imaging because of its access, speed, and ability to show lesions (eg, hemorrhage and edema) requiring immediate neurosurgical or medical intervention.[4,77,83–99,102–112,168–181] Cervical spinal CT may also be needed. CT angiography (CTA) or CTV may be helpful to evaluate the cause of hemorrhage (eg, vascular malformation or aneurysm) or infarction (eg, dissection or venous thrombosis). A radiographic or scintigraphic skeletal survey should also be obtained according to established guidelines.[179,180]

MR Imaging

Brain and cervical spinal MR imaging should be done as soon as possible because of its sensitivity and specificity regarding pattern of injury and timing parameters.[4,104,181–190] Brain MR imaging should include T1, T2, T2*, fluid-attenuated inversion recovery (FLAIR), and diffusion-weighted imaging/apparent diffusion coefficient (DWI/ADC). Gadolinium-enhanced T1 images should probably be used along with MRA and MRV. T1 and T2 are necessary for estimating the timing of hemorrhage, thrombosis, and other collections using published criteria.[4,104,181] T2* techniques are most sensitive for detecting hemorrhage or thromboses but may not distinguish new (eg, deoxyhemoglobin) from old (eg, hemosiderin). DWI plus ADC can be quickly obtained to show hypoxia-ischemia or vascular occlusive ischemia.[4,154,189,190] Restricted or reduced diffusion, however, may be seen with other processes, including encephalitis, seizures, or metabolic disorders, and with suppurative collections and some tumors.[4,154,189,190] Gadolinium-enhanced sequences and MRS can be used to evaluate for these other processes. Additionally, MRA and

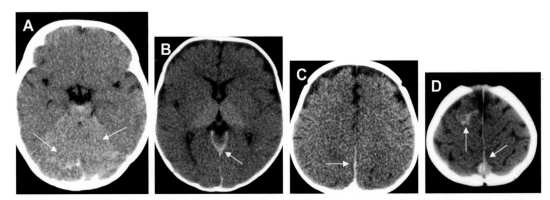

Fig. 18. Six-month-old infant with triad and alleged NAI; acute choking event while feeding. CT (*A–D*) shows bilateral cerebral edema with acute SAH and SDH (*arrows*), including along the falx, and tentorium. Autopsy confirmed the hemorrhages, a subdural membrane, and hypoxic-ischemic brain injury. (*Courtesy of* The Wisconsin Innocence Project.)

MRV are important to evaluate for arterial occlusive disease (eg, dissection) or venous thrombosis, although they cannot rule out small vessel disease. The STIR technique is particularly important for cervical spine imaging.

Scalp and Skull Abnormalities

Scalp injuries (eg, edema, hemorrhage, and laceration) are difficult to precisely time on imaging studies and depend on the nature and number of traumatic events or other factors (circulatory compromise, coagulopathy, medical interventions, and so forth).[1,4] Skull abnormalities may include fracture and suture splitting. Fracture may not be readily distinguished from sutures, synchondroses, their normal variants, or from wormian bones (eg, osteogenesis imperfecta) on CT or skull films. 3-D–CT surface reconstructions may be needed. In general, the morphology of a fracture cannot differentiate NAI from AI and must be correlated with the trauma scenario (eg, biomechanically) (see **Fig. 1**). Skull fractures are also difficult to time because of the lack of periosteal reaction.[1,4] Suture diastasis may be traumatic or a reflection of increased intracranial pressure but must be distinguished from pseudodiastasis due to a metabolic or dysplastic bone disorder (eg, congenital rickets) (see **Fig. 2**).[1,4,136,137] The growing fracture (eg, leptomeningeal cyst) is not specific for NAI and may follow any diastatic fracture in a young infant, including birth related (see **Fig. 1**).[1,2,4] Nondetection of scalp or skull abnormalities on imaging should not be interpreted as the absence of impact injury.

Intracranial Collections

It should not be assumed that such collections are always traumatic in origin. A differential diagnosis is always necessary and includes NAI, AI, coagulopathy (hemophilic and thrombophilic conditions), infectious and postinfectious conditions, metabolic disorders, and so forth.[2,4,22,89,90,101,106–110] It may not be possible to specify with any precision the components or age of an extracerebral collection because of meningeal disruptions (eg, acute or subacute subdural hygroma [SDHG] versus chronic SDH, or subarachnoid versus thin SDH).[1,4,103,104,173–176,181] Vezina[181] has recently summarized the literature regarding the complexity of timing of intracranial collections. Subarachnoid and subdural collections, hemorrhagic or nonhemorrhagic, may be localized or extensive and may occur about the convexities, interhemispheric (along the falx), and along the tentorium. With time and gravity, these collections may redistribute to other areas, including into or out of the spinal canal, and cause confusion.[4,177,181,191] For example, a convexity SDH may migrate to the peritentorial and posterior interhemispheric regions or into the intraspinal spaces. SDH migration may lead to a misinterpretation that there are hemorrhages of different timing. The distribution or migration of the sediment portion of a hemorrhage with blood levels (ie, hematocrit effect) may cause further confusion because density/intensity differences between the sediment and supernatant may be misinterpreted as hemorrhages (and trauma) of differing age and location.[4,104,178,181] Prominent subarachnoid CSF spaces are commonly present in infants (ie, BECCs). This entity predisposes infants to SDH, which may be spontaneous or associated with trauma of any type (eg, dysphagic choking ALTE) (see **Figs. 4, 15,** and **17**).[4,65–73] A hemorrhagic collection may continually change or evolve with regard to size, extent, location, and density/intensity characteristics. Rapid spontaneous resolution and redistribution of acute SDH over a few hours to 1 to 2 days has been reported.[4,177,191] A tear in the arachnoid may allow SDH washout into the subarachnoid space or CSF dilution of the subdural space.

For apparent CT high densities, it may be difficult to differentiate cerebral hemorrhage from subarachnoid hemorrhage or from venous thrombosis (see **Figs. 2, 3, 6–11, 15, 16,** and **18**).[4] According to the literature, hemorrhage or thromboses that are high density (ie, clotted) on CT (ie, acute to subacute) have a wide timing range of 0 to 3 hours up to 7 to 10 days.[4,104,178,181] Hemorrhage that is isohypodense on CT (ie, nonclotted) may be hyperacute (<3 h) or chronic (>10 d) (see **Figs. 3** and **11**). The low density may also represent pre-existing, wide, CSF-containing subarachnoid spaces (eg, BECC) or SDHG (ie, CSF-containing) that may be acute or chronic (see **Figs. 3, 12** and **15**).[4,103,104,175,181] Blood levels are unusual in the acute stage unless there is coagulopathy.[4,104,181,188] CT cannot distinguish acute hemorrhage from rehemorrhage on existing chronic collections (BECC or chronic SDHG) (see **Figs. 3** and **15**).[4,66,72,92–104,173,178,181] Traditionally, the interhemispheric SDH as well as mixed-density SDH were considered characteristic, if not pathognomonic, of SBS/NAI.[1,2,4,168,171–173] This has been proved unreliable. Interhemispheric SDH may be seen with AI or with nontraumatic conditions (eg, HIE, venous thrombosis, venous hypertension, or dysphagic choking ALTE) (see **Figs. 2, 6–10**).[178] Mixed-density SDH also occurs in AI as well as in other conditions (see **Figs. 3, 9,** and **11**).[178] Furthermore, SDH may occur in BECC spontaneously or result from minor trauma (ie, AI), and rehemorrhage within SDH may occur spontaneously or with minor AI (see **Figs. 1, 4, 15, and 17**).[4,12,38,40,72,90,104,178,181]

Only MR imaging may provide more precise information than CT regarding pattern of injury and timing, particularly with regard to (1) hemorrhage versus thromboses (**Table 1**) and (2) brain injury.[104,181–190] As a result, MR imaging has become the standard and should be done as soon as possible. Mixed-intensity collections, however, are problematic regarding timing.[181] Matching the MR imaging findings with the CT findings may help along with follow-up MR imaging. Blood levels may indicate subacute hemorrhage versus coagulopathy. The timing guidelines are better applied to the sediment than to the supernatant. With mixed-intensity collections, MR imaging cannot reliably differentiate BECC with acute SDH from acute SDHG/SDH, from hyperacute SDH, or from chronic SDH or chronic SDHG with rehemorrhage (see **Figs. 1, 4, and 13–17**).[4,104,181] T2* hypointensities are iron sensitive but may not differentiate hemorrhages from venous thromboses that are not detected by MRV (eg, cortical, medullary, or subependymal).

BRAIN INJURY

Edema or swelling in pediatric head trauma may represent primary injury or secondary injury and be acute-hyperacute (eg, minutes to a few hours) or delayed (eg, several hours to a few days), including association with short-distance falls and lucid intervals.[4,53–62] The edema or swelling may be further subtyped as traumatic, malignant, hypoxic-ischemic, or related to (or combined with) other factors. Traumatic edema is related to areas of primary brain trauma (ie, contusion or shear) or to traumatic vascular injury with infarction (eg, dissection, herniation, or spasm) (see **Figs. 3, 6, 9, and 11**). Traumatic edema is usually focal or multifocal, whether or not hemorrhagic. CT, however, may not distinguish focal or multifocal cerebral high densities as hemorrhagic contusion, hemorrhagic shear, or hemorrhagic infarction.[4] Focal or multifocal low density edema may also be seen with infarction (eg, arterial or venous occlusive), encephalitis, demyelination (eg, ADEM), or seizure edema.[4,89,146–154] Also, MR imaging often shows shear and contusional injury as focal/multifocal restricted diffusion, GRE hypo-intensities, and/or T2/FLAIR high intensities.[4] Focal/multifocal ischemic findings may also be due to traumatic arterial injury (eg, dissection) or venous injury (eg, tear or thrombosis), arterial spasm (as with any cause of hemorrhage), herniation, or edema with secondary perfusion deficit or seizures (eg, status epilepticus) (see **Figs. 2, 6, and 11**).[4,64,154,189,192] These may not be reliably differentiated, however, from focal/multifocal ischemic or hemorrhagic infarction from nontraumatic causation (eg, dissection, vasculitis, venous, or embolic) even without supportive MRA, CTA, MRV, or angiography. Also, similar cortical or subcortical intensity abnormalities (including restricted diffusion) may also be observed with

Table 1
MR imaging of intracranial hemorrhage and thrombosis[a]

Stage	Biochemical Form	Site	T1—MR Imaging	T2—MR Imaging
Hyperacute (+ edema) (<12 hours)	Fe II oxyHb	Intact RBCs	Iso-low I	High I
Acute (+ edema) (1–3 days)	Fe II deoxy Hb	Intact RBCs	Iso-low I	Low I
Early subacute (+ edema) (3–7 days)	Fe III metHb	Intact RBCs	High I	Low I
Late subacute (−edema) (1–2 weeks)	Fe III metHb	Lysed RBCs (extracellular)	High I	High I
Early chronic (−edema) (>2 weeks)	Fe III transferrin	Extracellular	High I	High I
Chronic (cavity)	Fe III ferritin and hemosiderin	Phagocytosis	Iso-low I	Low I

[a] Fe II, ferrous; Fe III, ferric; Hb, hemoglobin; I, signal intensity; Iso, isointense; RBCs, red blood cells; +, present; −, absent.
Data from Refs. [4,188,189]

encephalitis, seizures, and metabolic disorders. Therefore, a differential diagnosis is always required.[4,154,189,192]

Malignant brain edema, a term used for severe cerebral swelling after head trauma, may lead to rapid deterioration.[1,4,54,55,62] The edema is usually bilateral and may be related to cerebrovascular congestion (ie, hyperemia) as a vasoreactive rather than an autoregulatory phenomenon and associated with global ischemia. A unilateral form may also occur in association with an ipsilateral SDH that progresses to bilateral edema (see **Figs. 3** and **6**).[64] There may be rapid or delayed onset (ie, lucid interval). Predisposing factors are not well established but likely include a genetic basis. Hyperemic edema may appear early as accentuated gray-white matter differentiation on CT, then progresses to loss of differentiation.

Global hypoxia (eg, apnea or respiratory failure) or ischemia (eg, cardiovascular failure or hypoperfusion) is likely a major cause of or contributor to brain edema in a child with head trauma (eg, malignant edema).[4,38,40,54,55,62] HIE, depending on its severity and duration, may have a diffuse appearance acutely (ie, diffuse or vascular axonal injury) with decreased gray-white differentiation throughout the cerebrum on CT (eg, white cerebellum sign) and then evolve to a more specific pattern on CT or MR imaging (eg, border zone or watershed, basal ganglia/thalamic, cerebral white matter necrosis, reversal sign) (see **Figs. 2, 6, 7, 10,** and **18**).[4,189] It is typically bilateral but may not be symmetric. This more diffuse pattern may distinguish HIE from the multifocal pattern of primary traumatic injury, although they may coexist. Hypoxia-ischemic brain injury due to apnea/respiratory arrest may occur with head trauma or with neck/cervical spine/cord injuries (eg, SCIWORA) whether or not AI or NAI (see **Fig. 7**).[4,35,54,55,62] It may also occur with any nontraumatic cause (choking, paroxysmal coughing, aspiration, and so forth) (see **Figs. 2** and **18**).[4,25,160-166] In addition to the diffuse brain injury, there may be associated subarachnoid and SDH without mass effect (see **Figs. 2, 7, 10,** and **18**).[4,38,40,54,55,62] MR imaging shows hypoxic-ischemic injury, depending on timing, as diffuse-restricted diffusion on DWI/ADC plus matching T1/T2 abnormalities as the injury evolves (see **Figs. 2, 6** and **11**).[4,189] Other important contributors to edema or swelling include such complicating factors as seizures (eg, status epilepticus [see **Fig. 2**], fluid-electrolyte imbalance, other systemic or metabolic derangements (eg, hypoglycemia, hyperglycemia, hyperthermia), or hydrocephalus.[4] It is well known that many of these may also be associated with restricted diffusion along

with other nontraumatic processes (encephalitis, seizures, and metabolic disorders).[4,154,186,187,189] Again, a differential diagnosis is required.

SUMMARY

An extensive review of the literature to date fails to establish an evidence base for reliably distinguishing NAI from AI or from the medical mimics. The medical and imaging findings alone cannot diagnose intentional injury. Only a child protection investigation may provide the basis for inflicted injury in the context of supportive medical, imaging, or pathologic data. The duty of a radiologist is to give a detailed description of the imaging findings, provide a differential diagnosis, and communicate the concern for NAI, directly to the primary care team in a timely manner. Radiologists should be prepared to consult with child protection services; other medical and surgical consultants, including a pathologist or biomechanical specialist; law enforcement investigators; and attorneys for all parties as appropriate. Radiologists must also be aware of certain conditions that are known to have clinical and imaging features that may mimic abuse. These should be properly evaluated, and the possibility of combined or multifactorial mechanisms with synergistic effects should also be considered. Furthermore, a negative medical evaluation does not make NAI the default diagnosis. A timely and thorough multidisciplinary evaluation may be the difference between appropriate child protection versus an improper breakup of a family or a wrongful indictment and conviction.

REFERENCES

1. Kleinman P. Diagnostic imaging of child abuse. New York: Mosby Year Book; 1998.
2. Frasier L. Abusive head trauma in infants and children. St Louis (MO): GW Medical Publishing; 2006.
3. Kellogg N. Committee on child abuse and neglect. Evaluation of suspected child physical abuse. Pediatrics 2007;119:1232–41.
4. Barnes P, Krasnokutsky M. Imaging of the CNS in Suspected or Alleged NAI. Top Magn Reson Imaging 2007;18:53–74.
5. Donohoe M. Evidence-based medicine and shaken baby syndrome part I: literature review, 1966–1998. Am J Forensic Med Pathol 2003;24: 239–42.
6. Leestma J. Case analysis of brain injured admittedly shaken infants, 54 cases 1969–2001. Am J Forensic Med Pathol 2005;26:199–212.

7. Lyons G. Shaken baby syndrome: a questionable scientific syndrome and a dangerous legal concept. Utah Law Rev 2003;1109:1–22.

8. Gena M. Shaken baby syndrome: medical uncertainly casts doubt on convictions. Wis L Rev 2007;701:1–26.

9. Goudge Hon ST. Report of the inquiry into pediatric forensic pathology in Ontario. Ontario Ministry of the Attorney General. Queen's Printer for Ontario September 30, 2008. Available at: www.goudgeinquiry.ca. Accessed September 12, 2010.

10. Mackey M. After the court of appeal: R v Harris and others [2005] EWCA crim 1980. Arch Dis Child 2006;91:873–5.

11. Tuerkheimer D. The next innocence project: shaken baby syndrome and the criminal courts. Wash U L Rev 2009;87(1):1–58.

12. Squier W. Shaken baby syndrome: the quest for evidence. Dev Med Child Neurol 2008;50:10–4.

13. David TJ. Non-accidental head injury—the evidence. Pediatr Radiol 2008;38(Suppl 3):S370–7.

14. Jaspan T. Current controversies in the interpretation of non-accidental head injury. Pediatr Radiol 2008;38(Suppl 3):S378–87.

15. Guyatt, Haynes RB, Jaeschke RZ, et al. Users' guides to the medical literature. XXV. Evidence-based medicine. JAMA 2000;284:1290–6.

16. Collins J. Evidence-based medicine. J Am Coll Radiol 2007;4(8):551–4.

17. Blackmore C, Medina LS. Evidence-based radiology and the ACR appropriateness criteria. J Am Coll Radiol 2006;3(7):505–9.

18. Crosskerry P. The importance of cognitive errors in diagnosis and strategies to minimize them. Acad Med 2003;78:775–80.

19. Newman, DH. Physician says medical ideology "gets in the way" of evidence-based medicine. New York Times 4-2-2009; AMA News 4-3-09 [online].

20. Groopman J, Hartzband P. Why 'quality care' is dangerous. Wall St J. Available at: WSJ.com. Accessed April 8, 2009.

21. Feldman K, Bethel R, Shugerman P, et al. The cause of infant and toddler subdural hemorrhage: a prospective study. Pediatrics 2001;108:636–46.

22. Hobbs C, Childs A, Wynne J, et al. Subdural haematoma and effusion in infancy: an epidemiological study. Arch Dis Child 2005;90:952–5.

23. Keierleber J, Bohan T. Ten years after Daubert: the status of the states. J Forensic Sci 2005;50:1–10.

24. Udashen G, Sperling C. Texas v. Hurtado (Daubert), 2006.

25. DeWolfe CC. Apparent life-threatening event: a review. Pediatr Clin North Am 2005;52:1127–46.

26. Bonkowsky J, Guenther E, Filoux F, et al. Death, child abuse, and adverse neurological outcome of infants after an apparent life-threatening event. Pediatrics 2008;122:125–31.

27. Uscinski R. Shaken baby syndrome: fundamental questions. Br J Neurosurg 2002;16:217–9.

28. Ommaya A. Whiplash injury and brain damage. JAMA 1968;204:75–9.

29. Duhaime A, Gennerelli T, Thibault L, et al. The shaken baby syndrome. A clinical, pathological, and biomechanical study. J Neurosurg 1987;66:409–15.

30. Prange M, Coats B, Duhaime A, et al. Anthropomorhic simulations of falls, shakes, and inflicted impacts in infants. J Neurosurg 2003;99:143–50.

31. Leestma J, editor. Forensic neuropathology. 2nd edition. Boca Raton (FL): CRC Press; 2009. p. 603.

32. Pierce MC, Bertocci G. Injury biomechanics and child abuse. Annu Rev Biomed Eng 2008;10:85–106.

33. Ommaya A, Goldsmith W, Thibault L. Biomechanics and neuropathology of adult and paediatric head injury. Br J Neurosurg 2002;16:220–42.

34. Bandak FA. Shaken baby syndrome: a biomechanics analysis of injury mechanisms. Forensic Sci Int 2005;151:71–9.

35. Barnes P, Krasnokutsky M, Monson K, et al. Traumatic spinal cord injury: accidental vs. nonaccidental injury. Semin Pediatr Neurol 2008;15:178–84.

36. Geddes J, Hackshaw A, Vowles G, et al. Neuropathology of inflicted head injury in children. I. Pattern of brain injury. Brain 2001;124:1290–8.

37. Geddes J, Vowles G, Hackshaw A, et al. Neuropathology of inflicted head injury in children. II. Microscopic brain injury in infants. Brain 2001;124:1299–306.

38. Geddes J, Tasker R, Hackshaw A, et al. Dural haemorrhage in noñ-traumatic infant deaths: does it explain the bleeding in 'shaken baby syndrome'? Neuropathol Appl Neurobiol 2003;29:14–22.

39. Byard R, Blumbergs P, Rutty G, et al. Lack of evidence for a causal relationship between hypoxic-ischemic encephalopathy and subdural hemorrhage in fetal life, infancy, and early childhood. Pediatr Dev Pathol 2007;10:348–50.

40. Cohen M, Scheimberg I. Evidence of occurrence of intradural and subdural hemorrhage in the perinatal and neonatal period in the context of hypoxic ischemic encephalopathy. Pediatr Dev Pathol 2009;12:169–76.

41. Croft P, Reichard R. Microscopic examination of grossly unremarkable pediatric dura mater. Am J Forensic Med Pathol 2009;30:10–3.

42. Emerson M, Pieramici D, Stoessel K, et al. Incidence and rate of disappearance of retinal hemorrhage in newborns. Ophthalmology 2001;108:36–9.

43. Chadwick D, Bertocci G, Castillo E, et al. Annual risk of death resulting from short falls among children. Pediatrics 2008;121:1213—24.

44. Hall J, Reyes H, Horvat M, et al. The mortality of childhood falls. J Trauma 1989;29:1273—5.

45. Chadwick D, Chin S, Salerno C, et al. Deaths from falls in children: how far is fatal. J Trauma 1991;31:1335.

46. Helfer R, Slovis T, Black M. Injuries resulting when small children fall out of bed. Pediatrics 1977;60:533—5.

47. Reiber G. Fatal falls in childhood. Am J Forensic Med Pathol 1993;14:201—7.

48. Williams R. Injuries in infants and small children resulting from witnessed and corroborated free falls. J Trauma 1991;31:1350—2.

49. Lyons T, Oates R. Falling out of bed: a relatively benign occurrence. Pediatrics 1993;92:125—7.

50. Oehmichen M, Meissner C, Saternus K. Fall or shaken: traumatic brain injury in children caused by falls or abuse at home—a review on biomechanics and diagnosis. Neuropediatrics 2005;36:240—5.

51. Duhaime A, Alario A, Lewander W, et al. Head injury in very young children: mechanisms, injury types, and ophthalmologic findings in 100 hospitalized patients younger than 2 years of age. Pediatrics 1992;90:179—85.

52. Schutzman SA, Barnes PD, Duhaime A-C, et al. Evaluation and management of children younger than two years old with apparently minor head trauma: proposed guidelines. Pediatrics 2001;107:983—93.

53. Stein S, Spettell C. Delayed and progressive brain injury in children and adolescents with head trauma. Pediatr Neurosurg 1995;23:299—304.

54. Bruce D. Delayed deterioration of consciousness after trivial head injury in childhood. Br Med J (Clin Res Ed) 1984;289:715—6.

55. Bruce D, Alavi A, Bilaniuk L, et al. Diffuse cerebral swelling following head injuries in children: the syndrome of malignant brain edema. J Neurosurg 1981;54:170—8.

56. Plunkett J. Fatal pediatric head injuries caused by short-distance falls. Am J Forensic Med Pathol 2001;22:1—12.

57. Greenes D, Schutzman S. Occult intracranial trauma in infants. Ann Emerg Med 1998;32:680—6.

58. Arbogast K, Margulis S, Christian C. Initial neurologic presentation in young children sustaining inflicted and unintentional fatal head injuries. Pediatrics 2005;116:180—4.

59. Denton S, Mileusnic D. Delayed sudden death in an infant following an accidental fall. Am J Forensic Med Pathol 2003;24:371—6.

60. Murray J, Chen D, Velmahos G, et al. Pediatric falls: is height a predictor of injury and outcome? Am Surg 2000;66:863—5.

61. Kim K, Wang M, Griffith P, et al. Analysis of pediatric head injury falls. Neurosurg Focus 2000;8:1—9.

62. Steinbok P, Singhal A, Poskitt K, et al. Early hypodensity on CT scan of the brain in accidental pediatric head injury. Neurosurgery 2007;60:689—95.

63. Christian CW, Taylor AA, Hertle RW, et al. Retinal hemorrhages caused by accidental household trauma. J Pediatr 1999;135:125—7.

64. Durham SR, Duhaime A- C. Maturation-dependent response of the immature brain to experimental subdural hematoma. J Neurotrauma 2007;24:5—14.

65. Azais M, Echenne B. Idiopathic pericerebral effusions of infancy (external hydrocephalus). Annales Pediatr (Paris) 1992;39:550—8.

66. Piatt J. A pitfall in the diagnosis of child abuse: external hydrocephalus, subdural hematoma, and retinal hemorrhages. Neurosurg Focus 1999;7(4):1—8.

67. Pittman T. Significance of subdural hematoma in a child with external hydrocephalus. Pediatr Neurosurg 2003;39:57—9.

68. Papasian N, Frim D. A theoretical model of benign external hydrocephalus that predicts a predisposition towards extra-axial hemorrhage after minor head trauma. Pediatr Neurosurg 2000;33:188—93.

69. Hangique S, Das R, Barua N, et al. External hydrocephalus in children. Ind J Radiol Imag 2002;12:197—200.

70. Mori K, Sakamoto T, Mishimura K, et al. Subarachnoid fluid collection in infants complicated by subdural hematoma. Childs Nerv Syst 1993;9:282—4.

71. Ravid S, Maytal J. External hydrocephalus: a probable cause for subdural hematoma of infancy. Pediatr Neurol 2003;28:139—41.

72. McNeely PD, Atkinson JD, Saigal G, et al. Subdural hematomas in infants with benign enlargement of the subarachnoid spaces are not pathognomonic for child abuse. Am J Neuroradiol 2006;27:1725—8.

73. Hellbusch L. Benign extracerebral fluid collections in infancy: clinical presentation and long-term follow-up. J Neurosurg 2007;107:119—25.

74. Mori K, Yamamoto T, Horinaka N, et al. Arachnoid cyst is a risk factor for chronic subdural hematoma in juveniles. J Neurotrauma 2002;19:1017—27.

75. Chamnanvanakij S, Rollins N, Perlman J. Subdural hematoma in term infants. Pediatr Neurol 2002;26:301—4.

76. Whitby E, Griffiths P, Rutter S, et al. Frequency and natural history of subdural hemorrhages in babies and relation to obstetric factors. Lancet 2004;363:846—51.

77. Hayashi T, Hashimoto T, Fukuda S, et al. Neonatal subdural hematoma secondary to birth injury. Childs Nerv Syst 1987;3:23–9.

78. Rooks V, Eaton J, Ruess L, et al. Prevalence and evolution of intracranial hemorrhage in asymptomatic term infants. AJNR Am J Neuroradiol 2008; 29:1082–9.

79. Volpe JJ. Neurology of the newborn. 4th edition. Philadelphia: WB Saunders; 2000.

80. Ney J, Joseph K, Mitchell M. Late subdural hygromas from birth trauma. Neurology 2005;65:517.

81. Holden K, et al. Cranial MRI of normal term neonates: a pilot study. J Child Neurol 1999;14: 708–10.

82. Looney C, Smith J, Merck L, et al. Intracranial hemorrhage in asymptomatic neonates: prevalence on MRI and relationship to obstetric and neonatal risk factors. Radiology 2007;242: 535–41.

83. Powers C, Fuchs H, George T. Chronic subdural hematoma of the neonate. Pediatr Neurosurg 2007;43:25–8.

84. Ross M, Fresquez M, El-Hacklad M. Impact of FDA advisory on reported vacuum-assisted delivery and morbidity. J Matern Fetal Med 2000;9:321–6.

85. Towner D, Castro M, Eby-Wilkens E, et al. Effect of mode of delivery in nulliparous women on neonatal intracranial injury. N Engl J Med 1999;341: 1709–14.

86. Polina J, Dias M, Kachurek D, et al. Cranial birth injuries in term newborn infants. Pediatr Neurosurg 2001;35:113–9

87. Alexander J, Leveno K, Hauth J, et al. Fetal injury associated with cesarean delivery. Obstet Gynecol 2006;108:885–90.

88. Doumouchtsis S, Arulkumaran S. Head trauma after instrumental births. Clin Perinatol 2008;35: 69–83.

89. Sirotnak A. Medical disorders that mimic abusive head trauma. In: Frasier L, editor. Abusive head trauma in infants and children. St Louis (MO): GW Medical Publishing; 2006. p. 191–226.

90. Mack J, Squier W, Eastman J. Anatomy and development of the meninges: implications for subdural collections and cerebrospinal fluid circulation. Pediatr Radiol 2009;39:200–10.

91. Haines D, Harkey H, Al-Mefty O. The subdural space: a new look at an outdated concept. Neurosurgery 1993;32:111–20.

92. Kawakami Y, Chikama M, Tamiya T, et al. Coagulation and fibrinolysis in chronic subdural hematoma. Neurosurgery 1998;25:25–9.

93. Murakami H, Hirose Y, Sagoh M, et al. Why do chronic subdura hematomas continue to grow slowly and not coagulate? J Neurosurg 2002;96: 877–84.

94. Parent AD. Pediatric chronic subdural hematoma. A retrospective comparative analysis. Pediatr Neurosurg 1992;18:266–71.

95. Hwang S, Kim S. Infantile head injury, with special reference to the development of chronic subdural hematoma. Child's Nerv Syst 2000;16:590–4.

96. Fung E, Sung RY, Nelson EA, et al. Unexplained subdural hematoma in young children: is it always child abuse. Pediatr Int 2002;44:37–42.

97. Aoki N, Masuzawa H. Infantile acute subdural hematoma. J Neurosurg 1984;61:273–80.

98. Aoki N. Chronic subdural hematoma in infancy. J Neurosurg 1990;73:201–5.

99. Ikeda A, Sato O, Tsugane R, et al. Infantile acute subdural hematoma. Child's Nerv Syst 1987;3:19–22.

100. Dyer O. Brain haemorrhage in babies may not indicate violent abuse. BMJ 2003;326:616.

101. Hymel K, Jenny C, Block R. Intracranial hemorrhage and rebleeding in suspected victims of abusive head trauma: addressing the forensic controversies. Child Maltreat 2002;7:329–48.

102. Howard M, Bell B, Uttley D. The pathophysiology of infant subdural haematomas. Br J Neurosurg 1993; 7:355–65.

103. Vinchon M, Noizet O, Defoort-Dhellemmes S, et al. Infantile subdural hematomas due to traffic accidents. Pediatr Neurosurg 2002;37: 245–53.

104. Vinchon M, Noule N, Tchofo P, et al. Imaging of head injuries in infants: temporal correlates and forensic implications for the diagnosis of child abuse. J Neurosurg 2004;101:44–52.

105. Maxeiner H. Demonstration and interpretation of bridging vein ruptures in cases of infantile subdural bleeding. J Forensic Sci 2001;46:85–93.

106. Minns R. Subdural haemorrhages, haematomas, and effusions of infancy. Arch Dis Child 2005;90: 883–4.

107. Hobbs C, Childs A, Wynne J, et al. Subdural haematoma and effusion in infancy. Arch Dis Child 2005;90:952–5.

108. Datta S, Stoodley N, Jayawant S, et al. Neuroradiological aspects of subdural haemorrhages. Arch Dis Child 2005;90:947–51.

109. Kemp A. Investigating subdural haemorrhage in infants. Arch Dis Child 2002;86:98–102.

110. Jayawant S, Rawlinson A, Gibbon F, et al. Subdural haemorrhages in infants: population based study. BMJ 1998;317:1558–61.

111. Jayawant S, Parr J. Outcome following subdural haemorrhages in infancy. Arch Dis Child 2007;92: 343–7.

112. Trenchs V, Curcoy A, Navarro R, et al. Subdural haematomas and physical abuse in the first two years of life. Pediatr Neurosurg 2007;43: 352–7.

113. Galaznik J. Eye findings and allegations of shaking and non-accidental injury: post-publication peer review (8 August 2007). Pediatrics 2007;19: 1232–41.

114. Galaznik J. Shaken baby syndrome: letter to the editor. Dev Med Child Neurol 2008;50:317–9.

115. Levin A, Wygnanski-Jaffe T, Shafiq A, et al. Post-mortem orbital findings in shaken baby syndrome. Am J Ophthalmol 2006;142:233–40.

116. Morad Y, Kim Y, Armstrong D, et al. Correlation between retinal abnormalities and intracranial abnormalities in the shaken baby syndrome. Am J Ophthalmol 2002;134:354–9.

117. Kirshner R, Stein R. The mistaken diagnosis of child abuse. A form of medical abuse? Am J Dis Child 1985;139:873–5.

118. Tongue A. The ophthalmologists role in diagnosing child abuse. Ophthalmology 1991;98:1009–10.

119. Gardner H. Correlation between retinal abnormalities and intracranial abnormalities in the shaken baby syndrome. Am J Ophthalmol 2003;135: 745–6.

120. Gilles E, McGregor M, Levy-Clarke G. Retinal hemorrhage asymmetry in inflicted head injury: a clue to pathogenesis? J Pediatr 2003;143:494–9.

121. Gilliland M, Luthert P. Why do histology on retinal hemorrhages in suspected nonaccidental injury. Histopathology 2003;43:592–602.

122. Lantz P, Sinal S, Staton C, et al. Perimacular retinal folds from childhood head trauma: evidence-based case report. BMJ 2004;328: 754–6.

123. Aryan H, Ghosheh F, Jandial R, et al. Retinal hemorrhage and pediatric brain injury: etiology and review of the literature. J Clin Neurosci 2005; 12:624–31.

124. Lueder GT, Turner JW, Paschall R. Perimacular retinal folds simulating nonaccidental injury in an infant. Arch Ophthalmol 2006;124:1782–3.

125. Obi E, Watts P. Are there any pathognomonic signs in shaken baby syndrome. J AAPOS 2007;11: 99–100.

126. Forbes B, Cox M, Christian C. Retinal hemorrhages in patients with epidural hematomas. J AAPOS 2008;12:177–80.

127. Binenaum G, Forbes B, Raghupathi R, et al. An animal model to study retinal hemorrhages in nonimpact brain injury. J AAPOS 2007;11:84–5.

128. Brown S, Levin A, Ramsey D, et al. Natural animal shaking: a model for inflicted neurotrauma in children? J AAPOS 2007;11:85–6.

129. Emerson MV, Jakobs E, Green WR. Ocular autopsy and histopathologic features of child abuse. Ophthalmology 2007;114:1384–94.

130. Gardner H. Retinal folds. Arch Ophthalmol 2007; 125:1142.

131. Lantz PE. Postmortem detection and evaluation of retinal hemorrhages. Abstract, presented at the AAFS Annual meeting. Seattle, Washington, February, 2006. Am Acad Forens Sci 2006.

132. Goldsmith W, Plunkett J. Biomechanical analysis of the causes of traumatic brain injury in infants and children. Am J Forensic Med Pathol 2004;25: 89–100.

133. Jenny C. Committee on Child Abuse and Neglect. Evaluating infants and young children with multiple fractures. Pediatrics 2006;118:1299–303.

134. Bishop N, et al. Unexplained fractures in infancy: looking for fragile bones. Arch Dis Child 2007;92: 251–6.

135. Kleinman P. Problems in the diagnosis of metaphyseal fractures. Pediatr Radiol 2008;38(Suppl 3): S388–94.

136. Keller K, Barnes P. Rickets vs. abuse: a national and international epidemic. Pediatr Radiol 2008; 38:1210–6.

137. Keller KA, Barnes PD. Rickets vs. abuse – the evidence: reply to editorial commentaries. Pediatr Radiol 2009;39:1130.

138. Ganesh A, Jenny C, Geyer J, et al. Retinal hemorrhages in type I osteogenesis imperfecta after minor trauma. Ophthalmology 2004;111:1428–31.

139. Groninger A, Schaper J, Messing-Juenger M, et al. Subdural hematoma as clinical presentation of osteogenesis imperfecta. Pediatr Neurol 2005;32: 140–2.

140. Strauss K, Puffenberger E, Robinson D, et al. Type I glutaric aciduria, part 1: natural history of 77 patients. Semin Med Genet 2003;121C:38–52.

141. Nassogne MC, Sharrad M, Hertz-Pannier L, et al. Massive subdural haematomas in Menkes disease mimicking shaken baby syndrome. Childs Nerv Syst 2002;18:729–31.

142. Ernst L, Sondheimer N, Deardorff M, et al. The value of the metabolic autopsy in the pediatric hospital setting. J Pediatr 2006;148:779–83.

143. Brousseau T, Kissoon N, McIntosh B. Vitamin K deficiency mimicking child abuse. J Emerg Med 2005;29:283–8.

144. Rooms L, Fitzgerald N, McClain KL. Hemophagocytic lymphohistiocytosis masquerading as child abuse. Pediatrics 2003;111:636–40.

145. Liesner R, Hann I, Khair K. Non-accidental injury and the haematologist: the causes and investigation of easy bruising. Blood Coagul Fibrinolysis 2004;15(Suppl 1):S41–8.

146. Roach E, Golomb M, Adams R, et al. Management of stroke in infants and children. Stroke 2008;39: 2644–91.

147. Carvalho KS, Bodensteiner JB, Connolly PJ, et al. Cerebral venous thrombosis in children. J Child Neurol 2001;16:574–85.

148. Fitzgerald KC, Williams LS, Garg BP, et al. Cerebral sinovenous thrombosis in the neonate. Arch Neurol 2006;63:405–9.

149. DeVeber G, Andrew M, Group CPISS. Cerebral sinovenous thrombosis in children. N Engl J Med 2001;345:417–23.

150. Barnes C, deVeber G. Prothrombotic abnormalities in childhood ischaemic stroke. Thromb Res 2006; 118:67–74.

151. Sebire G, Tabarki B, Saunders D, et al. Cerebral venous sinus thrombosis in children: risk factors, presentation, diagnosis, and outcome. Brain 2005;128:477–89.

152. Krasnokutsky M, Barnes P. Cerebral venous thrombosis: a mimic of nonaccidental injury. Scientific Paper Session. Miami (FL): Society for Pediatric Radiology; 2007.

153. Menge T, Hemmer B, Nessler S, et al. Acute disseminated encephalomyelitis. An update. Arch Neurol 2005;62:1673–80.

154. Moritani T, Smoker W, Sato Y, et al. Diffusion-weighted imaging of acute excitotoxic brain injury. AJNR Am J Neuroradiol 2005;26:216–28.

155. Yazbak F. Multiple vaccinations and the shaken baby syndrome. National Vaccine Information Center. The Vaccine Adverse Event Reporting System (VAERS) of the Center for Disease Control and Prevention (CDC) and the Food and Drug Administration (FDA). Available at: www.nvic.org/doctors_corner/ed_yazbak_shaken-baby_syndrome.htm. Accessed September 12, 2010.

156. Innis M. Vaccines, apparent life-threatening events, Barlow's disease, and questions about Shaken baby syndrome. J Am Phys Surg 2006; 11:17–9.

157. Clemetson CA. Is it "shaken baby," or Barlow's disease variant? J Am Phys Surg 2004;9:78–80.

158. Clemetson CA. Caffey revisited: a commentary on the origin of "shaken baby syndrome". J Am Phys Surg 2006;11:20–1.

159. Marinetti L, Lehman L, Casto B, et al. Over-the-counter cold medications—postmortem findings in infants and the relationship to cause of death. J Anal Toxicol 2005;29:738–43.

160. Geddes J, Talbert D. Paroxysmal coughing, subdural, and retinal bleeding: a computer modeling approach. Neuropathol Appl Neurobiol 2006;32:625–34.

161. Talbert D. The sutured skull and intracranial bleeding in infants. Med Hypotheses 2006;66:691–4.

162. American Academy of Pediatrics red book online. Pertussis. 2003:472. Available at: http://www.aapredbook.aappublications.org/cgi/content/full/2003/1/3.9. Accessed September 12, 2010.

163. Surridge J, Segedin E, Grant C. Pertussis requiring intensive care. Arch Dis Child 2007;92:970–5.

164. CDC National Immunization Program. General pertussis information. 2000:2. Available at: http://www.cdc.gov/doc.do/id/0900f3ec80228696. Accessed September 12, 2010.

165. Page M, Jeffery H. The role of gastro-oesophageal reflux in the aetiology of SIDS. Early Hum Dev 2000;59:127–49.

166. Mohan P. Aspiration in infants and children. Pediatr Rev 2002;23:330–1.

167. Barnes P, Galaznik J, Krasnokutsky M, et al. CT in infant dysphagic choking acute life threatening event (ALTE – a mimic of child abuse). Scientific Session. Scottsdale (AZ): Society for Pediatric Radiology; 2008.

168. Zimmerman RA, Bilaniuk LT, Bruce D, et al. Interhemispheric acute subdural hematoma. A computed tomographic manifestation of child abuse by shaking. Neuroradiology 1979;16:39–40.

169. Cohen RA, Kaufman RA, Myers PA, et al. Cranial computed tomography in the abused child with head injury. AJNR Am J Neuroradiol 1985;6:883–8.

170. Bird CR, McMahan JR, Gilles RH, et al. Strangulation in child abuse: CT diagnosis. Radiology 1987;163:373–5.

171. Hymal KP, Rumack CM, Hay TC, et al. Comparison of intracranial CT findings in pediatric abusive and accidental head trauma. Pediatr Radiol 1997;27:743–7.

172. Ewings-Cobbs L, Prasad M, Kramer L, et al. Acute neuroradiologic findings in young children with inflicted or noninflicted traumatic brain injury. Childs Nerv Syst 2000;16:25–33.

173. Barnes PD, Robson CD. CT findings in hyperacute nonaccidental brain injury. Pediatr Radiol 2000;30:74–81.

174. Wells R, Vetter C, Laud P. Intracranial hemorrhage in children younger than 3 years. Arch Pediatr Adolesc Med 2002;156:252–7.

175. Wells R, Sty J. Traumatic low attenuation subdural fluid collections in children younger than 3 years. Arch Pediatr Adolesc Med 2003;157:1005–10.

176. Stoodley N. Neuroimaging in non-accidental head injury: if, when, why and how. Clin Radiol 2005;60:22–30.

177. Duhaime AC, Christian C, Armonda R, et al. Disappearing subdural hematomas in children. Pediatr Neurosurg 1996;25(3):116–22.

178. Tung GA, Kumar M, Richardson RC, et al. Comparison of accidental and nonaccidental traumatic head injury in children on noncontrast computed tomography. Pediatrics 2006;118(2):626–33.

179. Slovis TL, Smith WL, Strain JD, et al. Expert panel on pediatric imaging. Suspected physical abuse–child. Reston (VA): American College of Radiology (ACR); 2005 [online].

180. Di Pietro MA, Brody AS, Cassady CI, et al for Section on Radiology; American Academy of Pediatrics. Diagnostic imaging of child abuse. Pediatrics 2009;123:1430–5.

181. Vezina G. Assessment of the nature and age of subdural collections in nonaccidental head injury with CT and MRI. Pediatr Radiol 2009;39:586–90.

182. Ewing-Cobbs L, Kramer L, Prasad M, et al. Neuroimaging, physical, and developmental findings after inflicted and non-inflicted traumatic brain injury in young children. Pediatrics 1998;102:300–7.

183. Rooks VJ, Sisler C, Burton B. Cervical spine injury in child abuse: report of two cases. Pediatr Radiol 1998;28:193–5.

184. Chabrol B, Decarie JC, Fortin G. The role of cranial MRI in identifying patients suffering from child abuse and presenting with unexplained neurological findings. Child abuse Negl 1999;23:217–28.

185. Barlow KM, Gibson RJ, PcPhillips M, et al. Magnetic resonance imaging in acute nonaccidental head injury. Acta Pediatr 1999;88:734–40.

186. Suh D, Davis P, Hopkins K, et al. Non-accidental pediatric head injury: diffusion-weighted imaging findings. Neurosurgery 2001;49:309–20.

187. Ichord R, Naim M, Pollack A, et al. Hypoxic-ischemic injury complicates inflicted and accidental traumatic brain injury in young children: the role of diffusion-weighted imaging. J Neurotrauma 2007;24:106–18.

188. Zuerrer M, Martin E, Boltshauser E. MRI of intracranial hemorrhage in neonates and infants at 2.35 Tesla. Neuroradiology 1991;33:223–9.

189. Barkovich A. Pediatric neuroimaging. Philadelphia: Lippincott-Raven; 2005. p. 190–290.

190. Barnes P. Pediatric brain imaging. In: Blickman J, Parker B, Barnes P, editors. Pediatric radiology: the requisites. 3rd edition. Philadelphia: Elsevier; 2009. p. 221–7.

191. Zouros A, Bhargava R, Hoskinson M, et al. Further characterization of traumatic collections of infancy. J Neurosurg 2004;100:512–8.

192. Fullerton HJ, Johnston SC, Smith WS. Arterial dissection and stroke in children. Neurology 2001;57:1155–60.

Index

Note: Page numbers of article titles are in **boldface** type.

Radiol Clin N Am 49 (2011) 231–236
doi:10.1016/S0033-8389(10)00230-7
0033-8389/11/$ – see front matter © 2011 Elsevier Inc. All rights reserved.